CANARY

In a (POST)

COVID WORLD

MONEY, FEAR AND POWER

VOL 2

A COLLECTION OF ESSAYS FROM
37 CONTEMPORARY THOUGHT LEADERS

Edited by C.H. Klotz

Canary House Publishing

Three dollars from each "Canary in a Covid World" book sold will be donated to three important organizations: React19, to support vaccine-injured individuals and their advocacy efforts; Children's Health Defense (CHD); and Informed Consent Action Network (ICAN). Both CHD and ICAN are actively engaged in litigation against government and institutional censorship, overreach, propaganda, and corruption.

Please support our mission by rating and reviewing this book on Amazon. Your reviews will help more people discover the book and uncover the truth behind COVID. Stay connected:

- *Follow us on Substack: https://canaryinacovidworld.substack.com*
- *Follow us on X (formerly Twitter): Canary_Covid"*

AMAZON #1 BEST SELLER

CANARY
In a
COVID WORLD

HOW PROPAGANDA WORKS AND CENSORSHIP
CHANGED OUR (MY) WORLD

VOL. 1

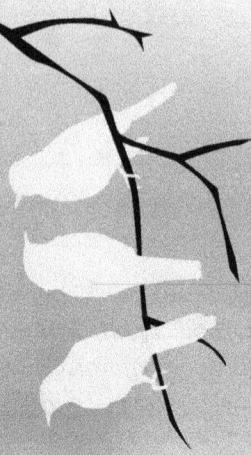

A collection of essays from
34 contemporary thought leaders.

CANARY IN A COVID WORLD   VOL. 1

Canaries:

Colin McAdam - Novelist

Brianne Dressen - Vaccine Injured co-founder of React 19

Dr. George Fareed - Family Physician who treated over 20,000 Covid patients.

Sir Christopher Chope - Ten term British MP from Christchurch.

Dr. Pierre Kory - Co-founder of the FLCCC, ICU Specialist

Elizabeth Woodworth - Medical Librarian

Dr. Michael Nevradakis - Journalist

Edward Dowd - Wall Street Analyst and best selling author

Dr. Jessica Rose - Researcher

Dr. Joseph Fraiman - Physician & Researcher

Trish Wood - Journalist - former CBC Fifth Estate Anchor & Podcaster

Dr. Ryan Cole - Pathologist

Dr. Aseem Malhotra - British Cardiologist

Senator Ron Johnson - Three term American Senator from Wisconsin.

Dr. Peter McCullough - Internist & Cardiologist

Dr. Norman Fenton - Professor Emeritus of Risk, Queen Mary University of London

Rodney Palmer - Retired CBC / CTV Journalist

Dr. Paul Marik - Co-founder of FLCCC & Critical Care Specialist

Dr. Jay Bhattacharya - Professor of Medicine, Health Research Policy, Stanford University.

Dr. Joseph Ladapo - Florida Surgeon General

Drs. Robert & Jill Malone - Scientist, Physician and Inventor of the base mRNA vaccination technology

Lord Sumption - Retired Senior UK Supreme Court Judge

Professor Bruce Pardy - Professor of Law, Queen's University.

Drs. James & Maggie Thorp - Obstetrician and Gynecologist

Dr. Naomi Wolf - Author of 7 nonfiction best sellers

Steve Kirsch - Journalist & technology entrepreneur

John Leake - Historian and best selling author

Dr Mary O'Connor - Family Physician

Dr. Harvey Risch - Professor Emeritus of Epidemiology, Yale

Dr. Sam Dubé - Mathematician, Physician, Broadcaster

Margaret Anna Alice - Writer and Blogger

Dr. Michael Rectenwald - Professor & Author

Dr. Peter & Ginger Breggin - Psychiatrist

Professor Denis Rancourt - Scientist

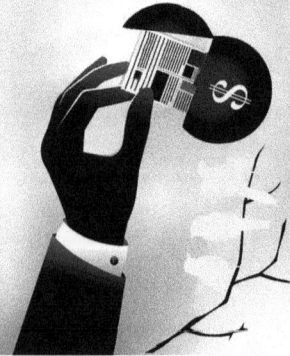

CANARY HOUSE PUBLISHING
EDITED BY C.H. KLOTZ

A heartfelt thank you to these 34 Canaries who generously contributed their insights and expertise to this second volume of Canary in a Covid World. Their invaluable perspectives have illuminated the truth behind the censorship and propaganda that shaped the COVID narrative, ensuring that future generations learn from these pivotal experiences.

Dr. Julie Ponesse - Public intellectual, former Ethics Professor, author of *My Choice* and *Our Last Innocent Moment.*

Dr. Joel Wallskog- Co-founder of React19 and an Orthopaedic Surgeon.

Scott W Atlas MD - Robert Wesson Senior Fellow Health Policy at the Hoover Institution of Stanford University. Former Professor and Chief of Neuroradiology at Stanford University Medical Center for 14 years and in academic medicine for 25 years.

Dr. Byram Bridle - Tenured professor of Immunology and Virology and a cancer therapeutics expert at the University of Guelph, Ontario, Canada.

Dr. Ramesh Thakur - Former United Nations Assistant Secretary-General, and a Brownstone Institute Senior Scholar. Emeritus Professor in the Crawford School of Public Policy, The Australian National University.

Dr. Charles Hoffe - South African trained general practitioner and emergency room doctor, practising in Lytton, British Columbia, Canada.

Professor Mattias Desmet - Professor of Clinical Psychology at Ghent University (Belgium) and author of *The Phycology of Totalitarianism.*

Robert F. Kennedy Jr. - Environmentalist, attorney and former US Presidential candidate.

Andrew Bridgen - Four term British Member of Parliament.

Seamus Bruner - Vice President and Executive Director, Research at Peter Schweizer's Government Accountability Institute (GAI) and the author of three bestselling books.

Dr. Michael Neveradakis - Journalist and senior reporter for The Defender and CHD TV host.

Meredith Miller - Holistic coach, author and speaker.

Regina Watteel - PhD Statistics and author of Fisman's Fraud.

Dr. Peter McCullough - Practising Internist and Cardiologist and co-author of "The Courage to Face Covid-19"

Dr. Angus Dalgleish - Professor of Oncology at St George's, University of London.

Dr. Dubé - Mathematician, physician, strength coach and broadcaster.

Dr. James Thorp - Board-certified in obstetrics and gynaecology (OB/GYN) as well as a specialist in maternal-fetal medicine.

Dr. Roger Hodkinson - Royal College certified general pathologist (FRCPC). Former fellow of the College of American Pathologists (FCAP) for forty years and a Fellow of the Royal College of Physicians and Surgeons of Canada.

Professor James Allan - Garrick Professor of Law at the University of Queensland, Australia.

Dr. Mike Yeadon - Former Vice President & Chief Scientific Officer of Allergy & Respiratory at Pfizer Global R&D.

Dr. David Bell - A former medical officer and scientist at the World Health Organization (WHO). A clinical and public health physician with a PhD in population health and background in internal medicine, modelling and epidemiology of infectious disease.

Jeffrey Tucker - Founder, author, and president at Brownstone Institute; Senior Economics columnist for Epoch Times.

Dr. Meryl Nass MD Internal medicine physician and activist with expertise in hydroxychloroquine, anthrax and bioterrorism; her interest is in prevention, investigation, amelioration, and safe and effective medical response.

Margaret Anna Alice - Writer who blogs about propaganda, mass control, psychology, politics and health with a focus on Covid.

Tamara Lich - Activist and organiser of the Canadian Freedom Convoy.

Paul Thacker - Investigative journalist and founder of The DisInformation Chronicle, a newsletter that reports on corruption in science and medicine.

Dr. Mary Talley Bowden - Dr. Mary Talley Bowden is an otolaryngologist and sleep medicine specialist in Houston, Texas who treated over 6,000 COVID patients during the pandemic.

Catherine Austin Fitts - American investment banker, former Assistant Secretary of Housing/Federal Housing Commissioner in the first Bush Administration and founder of the Solari Report.

Dr. Peter Parry - Associate professor of psychiatry affiliated with University of Queensland, Australia.

Professor Ian Brighthope - Australian Physician and Agricultural Scientist. Director of Nutritional and Environmental Medicine at the National Institute of Integrative Medicine in Melbourne, Australia.

Dr. Kat Lindley - Board-certified family physician. President and co-founder of the Global Health Project.

Shawn Buckley - Constitutional Lawyer and founding member of the National Citizens Inquiry in Canada.

Ivor Cummins - Irish chronic disease researcher, public speaker and host of the Fat Emperor podcaster.

Joshua Walkos - Independent journalist and researcher.

CJ Hopkins - Award-winning playwright, novelist, and political satirist.

Robin Monotti - London based Italian architect, designer, architectural, urban, film & cultural theorist and commentator.

Jason Christoff - Researcher in behaviour modification & psychological manipulation.

Contents

Introduction

In this second Canary book, *Canary in a (Post) Covid World; Money, Fear and Power,* our contributors tell the story in great detail how the COVID-19 pandemic was used to change our world. It is a rich, varied and disturbing story, told by many of the world's bravest and most qualified voices, of how health care, information and financial systems have been compromised in the name of profit and control.

While the first volume, *Canary in a Covid World; How Propaganda and Censorship Changed Our (My) World,* looked closely at the pandemic and how we were all fed a diet of propaganda, while the media prevented the dissemination of truth and diverse perspectives on so many topics, this follow-up takes us deeper into the motives and machinery of governments, banks, pharmaceutical giants, tech corporations and global institutions.

This time, we hear from 37 more Canaries: doctors and scientists, lawyers and politicians, academics and journalists, financial experts, creatives, a satirist, an architect, and an ethicist. What unites them is their courage to stand up and say one powerful word: **No** — no to mandates, lockdowns and censorship; no to experimental vaccines, school closures, digital IDs and central bank digital currencies; no to fear and to the silence and self-censorship it breeds.

These contributors have paid a high price for their convictions. They have seen their licenses threatened or revoked; reputations besmirched. Others have been jailed or seen families fractured under the weight of pressure and division. Yet they persist because they understand that *No* is the last line of defense against tyranny and the erosion of our most basic freedoms: to speak, to move, to question, and to choose what happens to our bodies and our property.

At the heart of this crisis lie three forces: **money, fear, and power**. Fear of COVID-19 was manufactured and amplified through relentless propaganda and the suppression of dissent. Powerful interests, especially within the pharmaceutical industry, seized that fear to drive profit and governments used it to extend control.

The vaccine rollout was never solely about public health, it was about money and control. Tragically, this has led to the destruction of millions of lives: through vaccine mandates and their devastating side effects and through the immense economic and societal collapse brought by lockdowns and social isolation. These measures reordered so much of what we once believed to be true and good in society. Meanwhile, the harms were buried under the hollow slogan "safe and effective" — a phrase we now know concealed more than it revealed. The politicization of medicine has devastated lives and shattered trust.

Meanwhile, power continues to consolidate into the hands of unelected institutions like the WHO and the UN, which now seek to dictate national health policy through binding treaties. The digitization of health and financial systems threatens to transform rights into privileges, conditional and revocable, controlled by centralized authorities far removed from the people.

This book like the volume before it is a call for truth, unity and remembrance. It is an act of defiance and hope: a gathering of voices that, though diverse, harmonize in their pursuit of freedom and truth. As we wrote in the first volume, *"The endeavour of this book is to bring thoughtful voices together to sing as one choir. The diversity of these voices that harmonize may allow others to hear the music."* May you hear that music now through the courage, clarity, and conviction of these 37 Canaries and the 34 before them in Volume 1. They refused to stay silent and in doing so, they became beacons for us all. Their courage reminds us that freedom of speech is the foundation for a free society. By speaking truth even in the face of overwhelming opposition, they have revealed to us the bigger picture and they continue to show us the way forward.

CHAPTER 1

Our Last Innocent Moment

Dr. Julie Ponesse

Public Intellectual, Former Ethics Professor

Dr. Ponesse has a PhD in Ethics and Ancient Philosophy from Western University, a Masters in Philosophy with Collaborative Specialization in Bioethics from the University of Toronto, and a Diploma in Ethics from the Kennedy Institute of Ethics at Georgetown University. She was a 2023 Brownstone Institute Fellow, and has authored two books, My Choice (2021) and Our Last Innocent Moment (2024). In the fall of 2021, her credentials were put to the test when she challenged her university's COVID-19 mandate. In true "when one door closes" fashion, she was launched into a new world where she has been able to reach more people than she ever did in the classroom. She has been fortunate to interview with some of our foremost public voices including Bret Weinstein, Jordan Peterson, Zuby, and Mathias Desmet. She has spoken at numerous events, including the Freedom Convoy in Ottawa, and even returned to Western, the university that terminated her, to speak at a student-organized rally in 2022. Dr. Ponesse continues to write and is now developing a suite of online ethics courses to help us navigate these surreal times. Access to these courses can be found at www.julieponesse.com.

Do you remember where you were when it happened? Who you were with?

That moment when you first felt the ground shift beneath you.

When your friends seemed a little less familiar, family a little more distant.

When your trust in our highest institutions — government, medicine, law, journalism —started to unravel.

The last time your naive optimism allowed you to believe that the world is, generally, as it seems.

Our last innocent moment.

* * *

If you are reading this, then there is a good chance you have your own last moment of innocence, even if the details of it are a little hazy. Sometime in 2020, there was a fundamental shift in how many of us view the world. The delicate network of core beliefs about what makes it possible to navigate life with some measure of stability and reliability — that medicine is a patient-focused institution, that journalists pursue truth, that the courts track justice, that our friends would behave in certain predictable ways — started to unravel.

There was a paradigm shift in how we live and relate to each other. A shift in attitude. A shift in trust. A shift away from a world we can never revisit ...

Now, an almost unfathomable four years after the World Health Organization declared COVID-19 a global pandemic, our once seemingly stable world is unrecognizable. Medicine and science have proven themselves to be closed systems, echo chambers in which even the most minute deviation from their orthodoxies cannot survive. Journalism is now a powerful narrative spin machine. Our courts offer show trials that employ predetermined conclusions as matters of professional practice, and even our most promising politicians seem to undergo a mystical transformation to silence and conformity once admitted to office.

We have, in general, become untethered from a world that seemed to be spinning with a certain cadence, from the relationships that framed our days and our futures, and maybe even from who we were as individuals. We have set ourselves adrift from life framed by core Western liberal values — liberty, equality, and autonomy, most fundamentally — and we find ourselves broken and unrecognizable without them. And, most treacherously, we seem to be tinkering with the fundamental principles of civility: toleration, patience, respect, and kindness.

Even now, each day brings yet another set of unfathomable revelations. We learned that calls for emergency medical services decreased in 2020 and then spiked in 2022, contradicting the narrative that COVID-19 killed unprecedented numbers of people and that the COVID-19 shots are perfectly "safe and effective." We learned that the Chief Justice of the Supreme Court co-chaired a committee on COVID-19 with the federal Minister of Justice since 2020. And Sheila Lewis, the transplant patient removed from a transplant list because of her vaccination status, died on the day the Liberal government posted on Twitter "Every Canadian deserves access to the health care they need, when they need it." Every Canadian?

Our world has become a house of mirrors, a patchwork of shattered layers of institutions and narratives and individuals that have shown themselves to be illogical and capricious, and yet somehow capable of invading the most intimate corners of our lives. We face a health care crisis, an economic crisis, a housing crisis, a food crisis, and a land crisis. Our children are losing their childhoods and, with it, their innocence. Families are imploding. The world is burning, literally and metaphorically.

We find ourselves in a hellish reality that the Freedom Convoy made poignant to us. Canada no longer feels like home. It is no longer a safe haven. Parents are struggling to feed their families, to educate their children, to navigate a crumbling health care system. Neighbours feel like strangers. Friend groups are torn apart. Our flag waves weakly and "Best country in the World" is now an empty phrase.

And, on top of all of this, we face a deep constitutional crisis, not in the technical sense — though I think our Canadian constitution has proven itself to be useful only to the degree that it is in capable hands — but a crisis of who we are as a people, what we are made of, what constitutes us in a very literal sense.

Looking back, there were no clear signs, no cautionary tales, no warnings from friends that could have prepared us for what was to come. There have always been corporations that couldn't be trusted, collective missteps, and historical atrocities, but we were making progress, weren't we? Hadn't we learned from the past? Weren't we becoming a little more enlightened? A little more tolerant and patient? Weren't our institutions, for the most part, getting us somewhere, or a sign that we had gotten somewhere?

Before 2020, our relationships were framed by probabilities, by predictions about what and who we could rely on in times of crisis, who would protect us and what sacrifices people would make when 'push came to shove.'

Well, we were shoved. And shoved hard. Those probabilities played themselves out. COVID-19 pulled back the curtain revealing dark corners of our world, our relationships and ourselves. It revealed who the "Little Hitlers" are and the ordinary people who became extraordinary heroes. And it revealed in each of us both our tipping points and the wells of strength that we had, unknowingly, started filling long before.

COVID-19 was a "black swan" event, what I think of as a "Babel moment" that shifted us from our last moment of innocence to something darker but at the same time more raw and more real. It held our feet to the fire, forcing us to confront the messy realities of our world. COVID had a way of hitting particular buttons like no religious or political issue I have known, and the ideological divide it created attained an almost spiritual status. I know couples who weathered the trials of infidelity and bankruptcy and child loss but who separated over COVID-19.

Our world has been turned upside down and we are the unwitting bobble-heads reverberating from every unanticipated new jostle.

IN PLAIN SIGHT

There is no doubt that the government response to COVID-19 is the largest public health disaster in modern history.

But what most interests and worries me is not that the authorities demanded our compliance, not that the media failed to ask the right questions, but that we submitted so freely, that we were so easily seduced by the assurance of safety over freedom, and the invitation to applaud shame and hatred of the non-compliant. What shocks me still is that so few fought back.

And so the question that keeps me up at night is, how did we get to this place? Why didn't we know?

I think part of the answer, the part that is hard to process, is that we did know. Or at least the information that would have allowed us to know was hiding in plain sight.

In 2009, Pfizer (the company we are told exists to "change patients' lives" and "make the world a healthier place") received a record-setting $2.3 billion fine for illegally marketing its painkiller Bextra and for paying kickbacks to compliant doctors. At the time, associate U.S. attorney general Tom Perrelli said the case was a victory for the public over "those who seek to earn a profit through fraud."

Well, yesterday's victory is today's conspiracy theory. And, unfortunately, Pfizer's misstep is not a moral anomaly in the pharmaceutical industry.

Those familiar with the history of psychopharmacology will know of the drug industry's profile of collusion and regulatory capture: the Thalidomide disaster of the 1950s and 1960s, the Opioid epidemic of the 1980s, Anthony Fauci's mismanagement of the AIDS epidemic, the SSRI crisis of the 1990s, and that just scratches the surface. The fact that drug companies are not moral saints should never have surprised us.

So why didn't that knowledge get the traction it deserved? How did we get to the point where our blind adherence to "follow the science" ideology led us to be more unscientific than arguably at any other moment in history?

HOW MUCH FREEDOM IS YOUR SAFETY WORTH?

If you heard one of my speeches over the last couple of years, you might be familiar with the parable of the camel.

On a cold night in the desert, a man is sleeping in his tent, having tied his camel outside. As the night grows colder, the camel asks his master if he can put his head in the tent for warmth. "By all means," says the man, and the camel stretches his head into the tent. A little while later, the camel asks if he may also bring his neck and front legs inside. Again, the master agrees.

Finally, the camel, who is now half in, half out, says "I'm letting cold air in. May I not come inside?" With pity, the master welcomes him into the warm tent. But once inside, the camel says. "I think that there is not room for both of us here. It will be best for you to stand outside, as you are the smaller." And with that the man is forced outside of his tent.

Let me put my head in, then my neck and front legs, then my whole self. Then, please step outside. Wear the arm-band, show your papers, pack a suitcase, move to the ghetto, pack another suitcase, get on the train. "Arbeit Macht Frei" until you find yourself in a lineup for the gas chamber.

How does this happen?

The camel's lesson is that you can get people to do just about anything if you break the unreasonable down into a series of smaller, seemingly reasonable 'asks.' It is the humble petition of the camel—just to put his head in the tent—that is so modest, so pitiful, that it seems unreasonable to refuse.

Isn't this what we've seen over the last two years?

It's been a master class in how to influence a person's behaviour one step at a time by encroaching a tiny bit, pausing, then starting from this new place and encroaching again, all the while unwittingly transferring what matters to us most to whoever is coercing us.

This idea that our liberties are something authorities can wantonly suspend is reflected in the eery reasoning of British epidemiologist Neil Ferguson, who said this about what inspired his recommendation of the lockdowns:

"I think people's sense of what is possible in terms of control changed quite dramatically between January and March... We couldn't get away with it in Europe, we thought.... And then Italy did it. And we realized we could."

We got to this point because we consented to tiny encroachments that we never should have consented to, not because of the size but the nature of the ask. When we were first asked to lock down but had questions, we should have refused. When doctors were first asked to deny available therapeutics for COVID, they should have refused. Today's physicians who are ordered to follow the CPSO's guideline to prescribe psycho-pharmaceuticals and psychotherapy for vaccine-hesitant patients should object.

We got to this point not because we consider autonomy to be a reasonable sacrifice for the public good (although there are surely some of us who do). We got to this point because we are suffering from "moral blindness," a term ethicists apply to those who would otherwise act ethically but because of temporary pressures (like a coercive medical body or a myopic obsession to "do our part") are therefore temporarily unable to see the harms we do.

How can little things like autonomy and consent possibly stack up against saving the human race? How could freedom possibly win out over purity, safety, and perfection?

THE FEAR FACTOR

One of the great lessons of the last four years is just how powerfully we are all affected by fear, how it can alter our capacities for critical thinking and emotional regulation, shifting us to abandon existing beliefs and commitments, and become irrationally pessimistic.

We saw how fear makes us particularly susceptible to the media's negative framing that focuses on case and death numbers and not on the fact that, for most, COVID causes only mild symptoms. We saw how fear reframes how we relate to one another, making us more suspicious, more ethnocentric, more intolerant, more hostile toward out-groups, and more susceptible to a saviour stepping in (think of Canada's Transport Minister frequently claiming that everything the government has done over last two years is to "keep you safe").

We are also starting to understand how our manipulated fears caused the mass hysteria to set in, and how our moral panic was generated in the first place. Parents are still paranoid that their children are at great risk from COVID even though in Canada not one child has died from COVID without a comorbidity.

Our fear didn't develop naturally. The nudging didn't emerge *ex nihilo* in 2020. Our blindness, our reflex to persecute those who threatened our ideas of purity, is the culmination of a long-term cultural revolution and devolution of all the institutions we trust so deeply: government, law, media, medical colleges and professional bodies, academia, and private sector industries. It would take a book to explore all the ways our institutions have undergone a synchronised implosion over the last several decades. Maybe I'll write that book one day.

But for now, I think of how prescient were the words of Antonio Gramsci who said that to achieve a wholesale shift in thinking, we must "capture the culture." Couple this with Rudi Dutschke's exhortation to take a "long march through the institutions" and you have the perfect recipe for the cultural revolution that brought us to this point.

Each of the core institutions that we have been trained to trust was transformed by a paradigm shift in values, a shift towards the "politics of intent" which assumes that, if your intentions are noble and your compassion boundless, you are virtuous, even if your actions ultimately lead to disaster on a colossal scale. Those who refuse to surrender moral turf to the so-called 'progressives' are shamed or cancelled into oblivion so that the Utopian world of absolute purity can be realized.

This is the social operating system that has proven its ability to reshape society without limitation, that led to my termination, that tells Kelly-Sue Oberle "correlation isn't causation," that upheld the suspension of Dr. Crystal Luchkiw for giving a COVID vaccine exemption to a high-risk patient, that led you to read the words on this page now. And the fallout from this progressive shift is the moral blindness that plagues us now, the hijacked moral consciences, the belief that our compliance is harmless or even impeccably virtuous.

SCIENTISM IN THE AGE OF COVID

It is said that ours is an age of entitlement, or at least that millennials — the "Me, Me, Me," generation — have an attitude of entitlement. Our culture caters and markets so fully to every whim that a desire for making our own choices is the last thing you might expect us to give up on. So why did we give up on it?

I believe that the decline of informed consent has coincided not just with the specific events related to COVID-19, but more generally with the ascent of a particular scientific ideology called "scientism."

It's important to be clear that scientism is not science. In fact, it has very little to do with science itself. It is an ideology, a way of viewing the world that reduces all complexities, and all knowledge, to a single explanatory approach. At its most benign, scientism offers a complete view of the human condition, appealing to science to explain who we are, why we do what we do, and why life is meaningful. It is a meta-scientific view about what science is capable of and how it should be viewed relative to other areas of inquiry including history, philosophy, religion, and literature. Scientism has become so ubiquitous that it now influences every sphere of life from politics to economic policy to spirituality. And, like every dominating ideology that has imposed itself on the world, scientism has its own shamans and wizards.

The practical upshot of this is that, because scientism uses science to resolve conflicts outside its proper domain, conversations about whether it is right to disinvite an unvaccinated sibling from Thanksgiving dinner, for example, frequently devolve into the rhetorical "What, don't you believe in science?" The question assumes that science, by itself, can answer all relevant questions, including those about etiquette, civility, and morality. Hurt feelings, broken relationships, and moral missteps are all justified by appealing to the fact that the shunned individual excused herself from moral consideration by not following "the science."

One particularly devastating feature of scientism is that it obliterates debate and discussion, ironically hallmarks of the scientific method. Think of the frequent invocation of "#Trustthescience" or even just "#Science" in social media communications, used not as a prelude to argument and the presentation of scientific evidence but as a stand-in for them, rendering alternative viewpoints impotent and heretical.

Political scientist Jason Blakely identifies the locus of this feature of scientism as the "overextension of scientific authority." As Blakely wrote in his cover story for Harper's Magazine in August 2023, "scientific expertise has encroached on domains in which its methods are unsuited to addressing, let alone resolving, the issue at hand." The fact that a microbiologist understands the elements of DNA is, today, unquestionably used to grant that person supreme authority in matters of morality and public policy.

YOUR CHOICE

"Your." "Choice."

Who could have guessed prior to 2020 just how controversial these two little words would become. Simple on their own but, put together, they create an affirmation of yourself, your worth and your abilities, and a declaration of your right to be the author of your own life. They give you the confidence to reflect, consider, question, and resist, and in so doing, make yourself and your place in the world.

To choose is not just to randomly opt for one option over another. It is not an act of indulgence nor is it selfish. It defines who and what we are, as individuals and as a people. In one act of choice, we bring to fruition a lifetime of self-development. In one act of choice, we become human.

As it is, our scientism has put us into a moral deficit that is destroying our own moral capacities and the moral bonds between us.

Though we think being scientific means leaving the insights of the humanities and social sciences behind, we forget that not even two hundred years after the Scientific Revolution came the Enlightenment, the 17th century intellectual movement that asserted the natural and inalienable rights to life, liberty, and property, and especially personal autonomy and the capacity for choice. The capacity for choice was seen by Enlightenment thinkers not just to serve individual interests but to be able to produce societies that are more equitable and just, and unbeholden to the unchecked powers of misguided and corrupt leaders.

Unfortunately, the lessons of the Enlightenment didn't stick.

We find ourselves now in desperate need of a 21st century Enlightenment, a renaissance of informed consent and personal choice. Such a renaissance will mean the coexistence of choices that are different from one another, and therefore messy and varied. But, in being so, they will also be perfectly imperfect. They will be, as Friedrich Nietzsche wrote, "human, all too human."

IN PLAIN SIGHT

One of the things we have learned over the last four years is just how much regulatory capture factored into the COVID response, how economics turned vaccine technology into an industrial profit machine. One crucial piece of evidence for this came from the Pfizer report, released last year by the FDA as part of a U.S. court order, containing what Naomi Wolf calls "evidence of the greatest crime against humanity in the history of our species."

The report shows massive incongruity between how the vaccines were marketed to the public and what Pfizer knew about them prior to their release to market. It shows:

- Pfizer knew their gene-based injections had negative efficacy as early as November 2020 (with the third most common side effect of the vaccine being COVID, itself)
- shortly after the vaccines came to market, Pfizer hired 2,400 full-time employees to process the adverse event reports (a stunning fact given the culture of silence that prevented so many adverse events even from being reported to, or processed by, physicians)
- that the vaccines cause myocarditis within a week after injection
- the shot's lipid nanoparticles do not remain at the injection site but are quickly bio-distributed throughout the body to the brain, liver, spleen, and ovaries where they may remain permanently
- an asymmetry between the adverse events that were disclosed to the public (chills, fatigue, swelling at injection site) and those contained in the documents (haemorrhages, blood clots, neurological disorders, Bell's Palsy, Guillain-Barré syndrome)
- there were 61 deaths from stroke, half of which took place within 48 hours of injection

These are the things Pfizer knew. These are the things Pfizer did not reveal to the public. These are the things that made us the turkeys and Pfizer, the butcher.

It has been said that there is no historical parallel to the COVID vaccines: a vigorously marketed experimental product on a global scale, which garnered almost perfect support from policymakers. The scale of money involved is almost beyond comprehension. Pfizer's 2023 "Annual Review" states: "2022 was a year in which we set all-time highs in several financial categories." That year, Pfizer's revenue was a record-setting $100.3 billion, 38% coming from the Pfizer-BioNTech vaccine.

While it's no secret that pharmaceutical companies spend large portions of their budgets on marketing, it's hard to think of pharmaceutical products being marketed like cars or lipstick. But they are. Perhaps even more so. In 2022, Pfizer spent $2.8 billion on marketing, a mere 2% of the revenue they earned from the Pfizer-BioNTech vaccine. But just how pharmaceutical products are marketed is a complex business.

One thing we find in the Pfizer report is a long list of donations to organizations that encouraged vaccine use, and/or directly addressed vaccine hesitancy. Pfizer couldn't produce ads endorsing mandates — that would have been too obvious — but they could fund various lobbying groups, healthcare colleges, media, and even medical journals that promote vaccine use, address vaccine hesitancy, and support mandates.

WHY SO NAIVE?

One lesson black swan events teach is just how fragile are our systems of thought. Being innocent of the contents of the Pfizer report and of the history of pharmaceutical collusion, more generally, makes the harms of the COVID response not just extreme but tragic, because they were foreseeable and, therefore, preventable. The truth is that, whether we saw, or didn't see, relevant information is what helped to create the COVID harms. We were complicit. And there are two common, and quite reasonable, ways of thinking that made us prone to being caught off guard in the ways that we were.

One is the idea that the past is a reliable predictor of the future. One of the most powerful pieces of propaganda in the COVID response was "All vaccines on the market are safe, therefore the COVID vaccine is safe too." We are vulnerable to this error in thinking because of our belief that the future will roughly resemble the past. And for many things in life, this is a reasonable way of forming beliefs. But it isn't an infallible one. As the philosopher Bertrand Russell pointed out in 1948, with respect to certain phenomena — markets and stock prices, for example — a pattern in the past is no guarantee of that pattern holding true in the future. The observance of a single black swan negated the long-held presumption that all swans we will see will be white. A set of conclusions can easily be undone once any of its fundamental premises is proven false. Our belief that something being on the market, or being endorsed by an institution (or even the totality of institutions), makes it safe, unfortunately is not a reliable indication that it is so.

The second common way of thinking that allows us to be caught off guard is that we are vulnerable to "salience bias," which predisposes us to misjudging the importance or likelihood of events by giving excessive weight to information that is more obvious. Commercial air travel is statistically 1,000 times safer than driving a car. But most people are more afraid of flying as plane crashes are, in some sense at least, more dramatic and more salient. The problem with salience bias is that it distorts our perception, memory, problem-solving abilities, and ultimately, our decision-making.

When it came to COVID decision-making, salience bias came into play as we began to give disproportionate attention to information about infections and deaths, which were widely publicized, versus information about vaccine side effects and the negative impacts of COVID restrictions, which were not. Our collective disregard for the less salient information became so perilous that, in May 2020, a group of over 600 physicians sent a letter to President Trump pointing out that "the downstream health effects...are being massively underestimated and under-reported." The authors called the lockdowns a "mass casualty incident" with "exponentially growing negative health consequences." The negative effects of the COVID response, the authors claimed, were being massively under-estimated and under-reported.

In reality, suicide hotline calls and liquor sales both increased by 600% and 150,000 Americans per month experienced missed cancer diagnoses. "This is an order of magnitude error," the authors wrote. The letter was signed by over 500 physicians including Richard Amerling, Marilyn Singleton, and Amit Gupta. But this letter, like all other attempts to point out the harmful consequences of the response, went largely ignored.

Our lives are made up of moments, some more memorable than others, some with more impact than others. Sometime in 2020, we had what I have come to think of as our last innocent moment. Our last moment of being unaware of what was to come and how we would hurt each other. Our last moment of understanding what really drives us and what we had done, or allowed to happen, that got us to this place. Our last moment of knowing how everything to come would put us on a new course.

Whatever happened over the last few years, we have been fundamentally changed by it. There's no reclaiming the innocence we lost. Life is more serious now. Our obligations are more weighty, or just more apparent. There are certain truths we came to see that can never be unseen. And everything is so much more complicated than we thought.

One thing COVID showed is that how well a society endures a crisis or rebounds from one says a lot about how strong it was when it entered the crisis. And how we endured COVID is more telling than it might be comfortable to admit.

"Let them die."

The fact that these words were strewn not in orange spray paint on the dirty walls of an overpass but in bold, carefully chosen font on the front page of our country's largest newspaper and the fact that they received so little criticism — when that kind of bigotry moves out of the shadows and into the public square — means that it's not about the hated, themselves. It's about those who do the hating. It's about the state of our nation and the cultural forces that festered long and strong enough to gain the momentum they needed to parade, unapologetically, in public spaces. It's a sign of a deep social pathology. It's a symptom of our self-destruction. And it's an explanation for why the most educated and elevated among us responded to these words with savagery rather than civility.

And this is also why, of the many horrible things COVID did to us, it trained us to focus on numbers (though not, in my view, very accurately). But numbers are just symbols, ways we organize a chaotic environment. They represent things about our lives but they are not life itself. An adverse event number is a woman suffering so many strokes that she fears she will wake up and not know who she is, a teenager who takes her life during a third lockdown, a longed-for baby who is "born sleeping." The COVID narrative wants to teach us that we are insignificant, that our voices are silenceable, and that our individual lives are made meaningful only by sacrificing ourselves at the altar of scientism and perfectionism. This is the reality to which our complicity, and our moral blindness, has brought us.

FORESIGHT IS 20/20

My thoughts kept returning to the comment "Hindsight is 20/20," as though our COVID mistakes were justified because we simply didn't know better. But we didn't need hindsight; we had foresight. We had all the pieces of the puzzle going into 2020 — about the history of pharmaceutical collusion with government, about how the vaccine industry became captured by politico-economic forces, about how scientism and perfectionism were filtering into our highest institutions, and about how complacency has taken hold in our culture and in our souls.

Everything that should have shown the COVID response to be a massive failure — the Pfizer report, the National Citizens Inquiry (2023) and Public Order Emergency Commission (2022), the breakthrough cases, the displacement of informed consent with Behavioural Insights strategies — failed. Everything that should have quelled our fears — the reality of IFRs, the availability of effective early treatments — only stoked them. The questions that should have been asked every day by every person weren't asked. Why were pregnant women so willing to experiment on their unborn children? Why did the vaccinated who contracted COVID insist that "it could have been so much worse?" Why did we turn so hostile and hateful? Why didn't basic critical thinking help us? Why did the lesson of failed hubris die in Corinth or on the plains of Shinar or in a German courtroom in 1946? Why do we need to keep learning these lessons time and time again?

So many times over the last four years I heard people say, "I can't wait until the mandates lift," as though that would restore the freedom we lost. But that's not a remedy for the fear that put us here. It's not a therapeutic for the normalization of cancellation and hatred. And it's not a remedy for the complacency that allowed our situation to become rabid and entrenched. None of those things got fixed when the mandates started to lift. None of them have disappeared since. And we shouldn't have expected them to do so.

What the mandates did brilliantly was to create a first-round elimination test, weeding out of our professions and highest institutions the conscientious objectors, the whistleblowers, the critically thoughtful, and the most fearless. By eliminating those who were right to resist, we have homogenized the workforce and, with it, the ways policies will be determined and enforced, how we will receive medical care, how we will be represented in court, and how our children will be educated. How much less likely will it be now for judges, doctors, educators, and politicians to resist when those who proved most able to do so have been eliminated?

Those who challenged the narrative will never be at the top of the fields they once loved; there will be no questioners who make partner, no dissenters who become Chief of Staff, no courageous academics made Full Professor. These are honours reserved now only for the most compliant among us. The mandates, and our submission to them, created a globally compliant workforce waiting patiently, and compliantly, for the next push on our liberty, a push that will only need to be minimal at best.

Sometimes I allow myself to make a wishlist for the future. If I could change the world with a snap of my fingers, what would I wish for?

Some things are pretty clear. We need technology to follow our values rather than create values for us. We need our scientists to cling fearlessly to independence, curiosity, and uncertainty. We need our physicians to rise above their culture of compliance and, as cliché as it sounds, protect their patients whatever the costs to their reputation or bank account. We need journalists to report facts, and not feed the narrative spin machine. We need our courts to abandon judicial notice. And, we need individualism to triumph over collectivism, humility over hubris, and as controversial as it may be to say, nationalism over globalism.

Over the last four years, we've seen humanity move quickly and disloyally from one heroic figure to another: Tam and Fauci to Gates, and then Zuckerberg and, even in the freedom camp, from Elon Musk who will 'save the world' by purchasing Twitter, to Danielle Smith or Robert Kennedy, Jr. or some other Olympian political figure who will "bring fire to the people." Without a moral compass to tether our lives, we've become conditioned to outsource our thinking to the current saviour of the moment. But the truth is, there is no politician who will save us, no billionaire who will cure what's really broken in us.

If we are waiting to be rescued, or for those who wronged us to make amends, I fear we will be waiting a very long time. We can wish for grand sweeps of political and cultural change. But, at the end of the day, the only thing we can control are the shifts in ourselves. We need to think better, remember better, vote better. We need to resist when it would be easier to give in, to charge ahead when it means leaving the warm embrace of the crowd. We need to learn how to stand up and say "no," to hold tightly to the mast even as the torrent blows around us.

Yes, we must regain control of our captured institutions but, first and foremost, we must regain control of ourselves.

So where do we start? First, we need to confront the true costs of our compliance. So many kind and thoughtful people I know even to this day defend their compliance. "The grocery store wouldn't let me in without a mask, so I had to wear one," a young mother of five recently told me. "If I don't comply, I won't be able to help anyone," nurses have said. But this is all 'little picture' stuff. I know how scary it is to stick out one's oar into a tumultuous sea. I can see how it might even feel right in the moment and how good it feels to make a noble concession for the sake of possibly doing something bigger and better.

But, as Hannah Arendt showed us, just 'following orders' will always incur a debt that will be difficult to pay. And getting the engines of autonomy going again, overcoming moral inertia, is a lot harder once its gears have ground to a halt.

Is it enough to resist tyranny in your heart and hope that by doing so you've somehow sidestepped the next atrocity?

Is it enough to talk about loyalty and then shun your noncompliant friend from the coffee circle?

Will courage and integrity suddenly appear the next time your liberty is 'pinched?'

I think it's unlikely. The COVID narrative, and our compliance with it, has created a powerful cultural force that will now be even more difficult to resist.

As a citizen, a student of history and a mother, all of this terrifies me. I'm terrified that the politico-economic forces that wrote the chapters of the COVID crisis will now move into even more intimate zones of our lives and that, next time, it will not be so easy to resist. I'm terrified that those who managed to say "no" the first time around won't have the strength to manage the next crisis as well. I'm terrified that the lessons of history that should have prevented all of this will be permanently shut up in the tombs of our memory. I'm terrified by what we've done, and by what this has shown us to be capable of.

But I am also reminded of the Ancient Greek idea that courage isn't the absence of fear; it's finding a way to move through the fear so as not to become paralyzed by it. It's finding a way to let our fears shape us into people who are stronger than we would have been without them. From difficult times come courageous people, it is often said. And quite rightly.

CHAPTER 2

Stories of Vaccine Injury: React19's Mission to Support the Injured and Push for Recognition

By: Dr. Joel Wallskog

Orthopedic Surgeon and Co-Founder of React19

Joel earned his medical degree from the University of Wisconsin and completed an orthopedic surgery residency at the Medical College of Wisconsin. He completed specialty fellowship training at Case Western Reserve University. He subsequently built a large successful orthopedic practice, focusing on joint replacement. He was also a clinical faculty member of the Medical College of WI throughout most of his career. After his one Moderna injection on 12/30/2020, his health acutely deteriorated. He soon had to retire because of his medical disability secondary to his adverse event from his COVID-19 shot. Since November of 2021, Joel has been the co-founder of React19.

In December 2020, I, like many others, received my first dose of the Moderna COVID-19 vaccine. I followed the CDC's guidelines, waiting three months after my antibody diagnosis before getting vaccinated. I never imagined that this decision would drastically alter my life. Approximately one week after the shot, I began experiencing numbness, weakness, and balance issues. What followed was a diagnosis of transverse myelitis—a condition that has left me unable to return to my work as an orthopedic surgeon or enjoy the outdoor activities I once loved.

My story isn't unique. Across the country, tens of thousands of individuals have experienced life-altering adverse reactions following COVID-19 vaccination. Yet, their stories, like mine, have often been dismissed, downplayed, or outright censored. That's why I co-founded React19—an organization committed to supporting those who have suffered similar injuries and advocating for the recognition and care they deserve.

React19 is a community built on real people and their experiences. On our website, you'll find over 1,460 personal stories from people all over the country who have been impacted by COVID-19 vaccines. These stories are just from those who have found us, but we represent over 36,000 injured people in the United States and have 20 global partnerships with groups advocating for the vaccine injured. Similar groups like ours exist across the country and the world. The extent of these injuries is truly massive, and yet they remain largely unacknowledged.

Every story of vaccine injury is deeply personal and tells a story of loss—loss of health, livelihood, and in some cases, loved ones. People who once led active, vibrant lives are now struggling with debilitating conditions that range from chronic fatigue and joint pain to neurological disorders and cardiovascular issues. These stories reflect the human side of a broader crisis, where individuals trusted the system, did what they believed was right, and were left suffering without answers or meaningful support. Now, most of them are abandoned. Abandoned by their government, their health care providers, their employers, their friends, and often their families.

Take the story of **Heiko Sepp**, a highly accomplished extreme triathlete from Norway. Known for competing in some of the world's most grueling endurance sports, Sepp's life changed after his second COVID-19 vaccine dose in 2021. He developed severe heart inflammation and was later diagnosed with an autoimmune disease, which led to debilitating chest pain, extreme fatigue, and muscle inflammation. Once at the peak of physical fitness, Sepp found himself struggling to regain his former health and athletic abilities. He documented his experience in the film *My Biggest Battle*, using his platform to raise awareness about vaccine injuries and advocate for greater recognition and support for those similarly affected.

Or consider **Brianne Dressen**, a preschool teacher and co-founder of React19, who participated in the AstraZeneca COVID-19 vaccine trial. Shortly after receiving the vaccine in November 2020, she experienced severe neurological symptoms, including paresthesia, motor dysfunction, and blurred vision. These symptoms confined her to her bedroom for months, isolating her from her family and rendering her unable to perform even basic daily tasks. Despite being a participant in a clinical trial, Brianne struggled to receive acknowledgment or adequate treatment, as her symptoms were consistently downplayed by medical professionals. She was completely ignored and abandoned by AstraZeneca.

Professional mountain biker **Kyle Warner** also found his life transformed after receiving his second dose of the Pfizer COVID-19 vaccine in June 2021. Once a professional elite athlete; three-time North American Enduro Tour Mountain Bike Champion, Warner began experiencing heart palpitations, dizziness, and extreme fatigue that left him bedridden for months. Eventually diagnosed with pericarditis and Postural Orthostatic Tachycardia Syndrome (POTS), Warner's athletic career was derailed, and he found himself battling not just his health issues but the medical community's reluctance to link his symptoms to the vaccine. Through React19, Warner found the support and validation he needed to begin his journey toward recovery, but his story—like so many others—highlights the struggles vaccine-injured individuals face when seeking care and recognition.

Eric Clapton, legendary guitarist, also experienced severe side effects after receiving the AstraZeneca vaccine. Already dealing with peripheral neuropathy, Clapton suffered extreme numbness and burning in his hands and feet—symptoms he described as "disastrous." Fearing that he might never play guitar again, Clapton criticized the lack of transparency surrounding the vaccine's risks, especially for individuals with pre-existing conditions. His experience resonated with many who felt they had been misled about vaccine safety.

Jessica Sutta, a former member of the Pussycat Dolls, developed vaccine-induced lupus after receiving her second Moderna vaccine dose. She suffered extreme joint pain and muscle spasms, which left her unable to walk or care for her child. Sutta has since become a vocal advocate for raising awareness about vaccine injuries and has connected with support groups like React19, underscoring the need for greater recognition of long-term complications.

Then there is the tragic story of **Ernest Ramirez**, who lost his 16-year-old son, Ernesto Ramirez Jr., just days after receiving the Pfizer vaccine. Ernesto collapsed while running with friends and was later pronounced dead from myocarditis, a recognized side effect of the vaccine in young males. Ernest has been vocal in sharing his son's story, advocating for greater awareness of vaccine risks, especially in children. However, his efforts have been met with resistance and censorship on social media platforms, where posts about vaccine injuries are often labeled as misinformation.

Each of these individuals faced unique physical challenges post-vaccination, but their stories share common themes: initial difficulty in receiving proper diagnosis, the shock of seeing their lives and careers disrupted, and a sense of abandonment by collective society that assured vaccine safety. Their public accounts contribute to the growing vaccine hesitancy, calling for greater transparency, more nuanced medical advice, and acknowledgment of the risks involved, particularly for those with underlying conditions or sensitivities.

Social media platforms like Facebook, YouTube, and Twitter have been actively removing or suppressing vaccine injury content, labeling it as misinformation. Entire support groups for vaccine-injured individuals were shut down, and people trying to share their personal experiences were given account strikes or permanently banned. Algorithms suppressed any news or posts about vaccine injuries, keeping them out of the public view. Even today, algorithms continue to block or bury posts that criticize the vaccines or raise concerns about vaccine injuries, even if such statements relay factual scientific information. This has created an environment where vaccine-injured individuals are not only ignored by the medical community but also silenced on public platforms, unable to share their stories or seek support.

React19 was born out of this vacuum—an organization founded by the injured, for the injured. "There's no one coming to help us," one of our members shared. "There's no one coming to save us, so we needed to do it ourselves." React19 began as a small community of individuals who found each other through their shared experiences, and it has since grown into a global movement. Our mission is simple: to offer financial, physical, and emotional support to those suffering from long-term vaccine injuries and to raise awareness about the scale of this issue. We also demand adequate medical care and seek fair and just compensation for our injuries.

Beyond sharing stories, React19 is about action. Through initiatives like the CARE fund, we provide direct financial assistance to vaccine-injured individuals struggling to cover their medical expenses. For many, the financial burden of treatment is overwhelming. They've lost their ability to work and are faced with mounting medical bills that insurance won't cover. The CARE fund provides grants of up to $10,000 to help cover these expenses, offering a lifeline to those who otherwise might not be able to afford the care they need. To date, the CARE fund has awarded $880,000 to those harmed, double what the US government has awarded. We are doing what our government should be doing.

Consider the story of one mother who shared how the CARE fund made a world of difference for her daughter: "Without the CARE fund, my daughter would still be in a wheelchair. I wouldn't have been able to pay for the treatments she needed." Stories like this underscore the importance of financial support in helping vaccine-injured individuals regain some semblance of their former lives.

We also recognize that financial support alone is not enough. The lack of research into vaccine injuries has left many without answers or effective treatments. To address this, React19 is pushing for more research into vaccine-related injuries, including studies like the biomarker study, which aims to identify biological markers in vaccine-injured individuals. This research is critical in developing better treatment protocols and understanding the underlying causes of these injuries. Through collaborations with research institutions and medical professionals, we hope to bring much-needed clarity to the medical community and pave the way for more effective interventions.

At React19, we're focused on shedding light on the full extent of vaccine-related injuries. The Vaccine Adverse Event Reporting System (VAERS), established in 1990 to track potential vaccine-related injuries, has seen an unprecedented rise in reports since the introduction of COVID-19 vaccines. As of the latest data, over 2.6 million reports of adverse events have been filed in relation to COVID-19 vaccines, including 37,910 deaths. It's important to note that VAERS is a passive reporting system—meaning not all injuries are reported. In fact, studies suggest that VAERS historically captures only about 1% of actual vaccine injuries, making the true scale far greater than the reported figures.

The Joseph Fraiman et al. study, published in August 2022, analyzed the Phase 3 Pfizer and Moderna clinical trial data and revealed that 1 in 800 people experienced serious adverse events following COVID-19 vaccination. The CDC was forced to release this trial data by court order after attempting to hide it for 75 years. These findings highlight the importance of transparency and accountability, as millions of people have been harmed.

At React19, we know that this isn't about being anti-vaccine. It's about being pro-transparency and accountability. We are advocating for a compensation fund, funded by the billions of dollars in profits made by companies like Pfizer and Moderna, to support those who have been injured. The Countermeasures Injury Compensation Program is a failure, with a 98% denial rate. It's time to acknowledge that while vaccines have helped many, they've also harmed a significant number of people—and those people deserve recognition, care and compensation.

This fight for transparency extends beyond the United States. Around the world, similar groups like React19 have emerged as people from all walks of life grapple with the aftermath of their vaccine injuries. The global nature of this issue demands a concerted effort to raise awareness, push for better research, and advocate for policy changes that prioritize the health and well-being of those affected. Vaccine injuries know no borders, and the scale of this crisis is far larger than what most people realize. The stories on our website represent just a fraction of the true number of people impacted by vaccine injuries worldwide.

The work we are doing at React19 is just the beginning. We have a long way to go in terms of educating the public, advocating for policy changes, and ensuring that the vaccine-injured are no longer marginalized and dismissed. But we are determined to continue this fight because, as one of our members said, "People's lives are counting on this work."

If you'd like to learn more or support our mission, I invite you to visit our website, where you can read the personal stories of vaccine-injured individuals. These are real people, whose lives have been turned upside down by the very thing they believed would protect them. Their stories are a testament to the resilience of the human spirit and the urgent need for recognition and care.

Finally, every purchase of *Canary In a Covid World* (both volumes) contributes $1 to the CARE fund, helping those injured by the vaccines get the care they need. We are grateful to the editors, and to all the Canaries who have bravely shared their stories. Together, we can make a real difference.

CHAPTER 3

Civil Discourse and the Free Exchange of Ideas

Scott W. Atlas, MD

Robert Wesson Senior Fellow Health Policy at the
Hoover Institution of Stanford University.

Scott W. Atlas, MD is the Robert Wesson Senior Fellow in health policy at the Hoover Institution of Stanford University. He investigates the impact of government and the private sector on access, quality, and pricing in health care, trends in health care innovation, and key economic and civil liberties issues related to health policies. He is a frequent policy advisor to policymakers in the United States and other countries. He has served as senior advisor for health policy to several candidates for President, members of the US Congress, and health agencies. From August through November, 2020, he served as Special Advisor to the President and a member of the White House Coronavirus Task Force.

In June 2023, I was invited by the New College of Florida to give their commencement speech. That's a small school in Sarasota, where Governor DeSantis is trying to make a change, getting back to what's called "classical liberalism" instead of what might be called "wokism" as the thrust of the university. You can imagine the reception I was given.

What excited me most about speaking there was New College's stated commitment "to free speech and civil discourse" because in my opinion that is the most urgently needed change in the country today. Both civil discourse and the free exchange of ideas must be restored. We have lost our basic humanity to our fellow Americans.

The college campus is supposed to be America's center for the free exchange of ideas, essential to finding truth fundamental to all free societies. College is here, I told them, to challenge young people it's not to protect them from ideas that they may not like. It is crucial for students to hear ideas from many sources, especially ideas they don't agree with. That is the key part of learning how to think critically. It is literally impossible to learn critical thinking without hearing different views, and critical thinking is the most important lesson to learn in college.

In most ways, life after college is one with far more freedom than that environment, and there is no country with greater freedom, with more choices, than this country. But with that freedom comes responsibility, and our country needs help from our younger generation.

I was asked to help our country during the biggest health care crisis in a century. As a health policy scholar for more than 15 years and a medical scientist and physician for more than 30 years, I was called up by the White House in July of 2020. I was asked "would you come to speak to the President?" and of course I said yes. I remembered at the time the words of my friend and Hoover colleague General Jim Mattis, on the day he was headed to Washington to be President Trump's Secretary of Defense. He said to me "Scott, the President of the United States asked me to serve, and the answer is yes Sir, period."

After a day of meetings in the White House, I was asked by Jared Kushner to help advise President Trump. I replied "okay, but I just want to tell you what you're going to get here." I said "I'm not going to sign on to any group statement that somebody else wants me to if I don't agree with it. I'm not going to agree with something that someone else says just because I'm told to agree, and I'm not going to change my mind if I don't agree. I don't care who tells me to change my mind." And Jared said to me "that's exactly why we want you." I said, "I'm really happy to hear that" and then he warned "but I'm concerned they're going to try to destroy you once it's public." I was shocked – first, because I didn't think he would actually care if they destroyed me, but second, because that didn't sound so great to me. I wasn't a political person. I had no intention of being a political person. So I said "how about if I go back to California? I'm going to try from there," and he said "okay let's do that."

Within a few days it was obvious it was not going to work. This was in late July 2020, the country was panicking, the decisions were being made, the President was being fed wrong, harmful policies pushed by career bureaucrats who lacked both knowledge and critical thinking. So I went back.

My concern, my work, my entire motivation in the White House was focused on one thing - to stop people from dying from the pandemic and its management, both the harms of the virus and the impact on the public health of the policies.

That is the importance of having people who are health policy experts. That's my field; much broader scope of expertise than that of any virologist or epidemiologist and certainly more than any career government bureaucrat.

On reflection about that experience, it is a great blessing to have been given the opportunity. It's a rare opportunity to help your country in a time of crisis. Most people never get that chance, to try to do so much good for so many.

I always like to say to young people, and there are a few in this audience who might find themselves in this situation and some undoubtedly will, that no matter how difficult it may seem to speak the truth - even against a tidal wave of hostility, character assassination in national and international media, death threats requiring 24/7 police security surrounding my home and in my driveway for weeks, backstabbing from my own employer - it was never even a remote consideration to stop speaking up.

Why not? Because people were dying, and I know right from wrong.

They were dying from the Birx-Fauci lockdowns that were contrary to the data, to fundamental biology, and to simple logic. That had to be called out. I knew the data; I had to try to change that.

Second, it became apparent, although I wasn't aware of this when I first started, that so many people needed to hear those facts spoken logically and clearly. I received hundreds of emails per day, thousands from everyday working people, seniors, doctors and scientists, teachers, priests praying for me, fathers and mothers whose husbands and daughters had committed suicide from the isolation and the lockdowns, who begged me in their emails to keep speaking because they were afraid, because they were afraid to speak up and I would never let them down.

The press never understood that motivation - my responsibility to others completely dwarfed the media's slurs and criticisms and the politicized attacks from Stanford University, my own employer.

And third, I had the backing of the strongest, most ethical person I have ever known - my wife.

Let's briefly consider some facts.

We must acknowledge of course the pandemic was a great tragedy, there is no doubt about that. But it also exposed profound issues in the United States that threaten the very principles of freedom that we Americans take for granted. Under two administrations, Trump and Biden, the United States management of the pandemic was a failure in COVID deaths per million, among the worst compared to our peer nations - a straight line of increase if you look at a graph from March 1st, 2020 through April 2022, two full years, no change in the rate of deaths per day even after vaccine on December 16 2020. Any Judgement of the U.S. response lies at the hands of doctors Deborah Birx, Anthony Fauci, the CDC, and the university "experts" who convinced officials to implement their lockdown strategy, and on our elected leaders who abrogated the responsibility to lead and instead hid behind those incompetent people.

The lockdowners got what they wanted. Their policies were implemented throughout most of this country in almost all states. Their policies failed - they failed to stop the death, they failed to stop the infection from spreading, but in addition they inflicted massive health damages, death and destruction, particularly, heinously, on low-income families and our children. This was the biggest, the most tragic, the most unethical breakdown of public health leadership in modern history.

America's media is slowly acknowledging facts that refute the original reasons behind lockdowns and school closures. It shouldn't be partisan, because both the Trump and Biden administrations rejected the standard pandemic science outlined in Henderson's 2006 classic review 15 years earlier, that clearly stated two things: lockdowns were not effective, and lockdowns were extremely harmful. Both these administrations rejected the alternative - targeted protection, the safer, scientifically valid, and standard pandemic management that was first advised in national media in March of 2020 by three people separately and independently: John Ioannidis, David Katz, and myself, independently and then repeatedly for months. The recommendation of targeted protection – which means increasing the protection of known high-risk population and ending the destructive isolation and lockdowns destroying low-risk people and children – was then echoed seven months later in October 2020 by a document, the Great Barrington Declaration, reiterating that 1) we should increase protection of the elderly and the higher risk people, because the lockdowns were not protecting them, and 2) reopen schools and businesses to stop destroying children and the poor.

And to clarify, the relevant data was not "learned" in late 2020, or 2021, or 2022. *It was all known in spring of 2020*, from data all over the world. Unfortunately, my advice was rejected with rare exceptions, like a state you hear about in the news, Florida. People in Florida were the lucky ones. They had open schools, no lockdowns since late summer 2020, and they have been living normally. Florida avoided the lockdown harms, and yes, even with its elderly high-risk population, after two full years had better age-adjusted COVID deaths than 60 percent of the states; Florida had lower excess death increase, that is death beyond what you would have without a pandemic, than my own much younger state of California. That's fact. Americans need to learn to disregard fabrications of untruthful media and politicians.

Why did Americans accept these draconian, unprecedented, and illogical lockdowns? This is the question.

First, two lies were told to convince the public, both of which frightened them. Number one: if you're against lockdowns, you're choosing the economy over lives. That was contrary to decades of economic literature showing severe economic downturns literally kill people. It was always lives versus lives. Number two: if you're against lockdowns you're for "letting it rip" - the so-called "herd immunity strategy". This was an outright lie - no one ever suggested doing that; that was never even mentioned in any White House meeting I ever attended; I never advised it to President Trump; I never even heard it discussed. And that is not the same thing as targeted protection.

What really are those lies used to convince the public? They are called propaganda - that's evil propaganda, distributed through a dishonest media reminiscent of lies that were told during the most heinous regimes in modern history to demonize opposing groups as dangerous to others.

We must live in a society where facts matter. This is the data:

- Bjornskov, March 2021: "more severe lockdown policies have not been associated with lower mortality." The lockdowns did not reduce the deaths;

- Bendavid, Stanford January 2021: "we do not find significant benefits on case growth." That means the lockdowns did not prevent the spread of the infection;

- Agarwal, Rand Institute and USC June 2021: "the lockdown policies in 43 countries and across the United States individual states led to *more* excess deaths; the deaths were coming down and then the lockdowns were instituted, and more people died."

- Herby, Johns Hopkins January 2022: Covid mortality was reduced by only 0.2 percent and "should be rejected as a pandemic policy."

- Kerpen, Moore, and Mulligan, University of Chicago February 2023: "Florida and South Dakota, states that opened early, were among the states with the best performance on death, education and employment; the worst performing states were those with the most stringent lockdowns - Illinois 46th, California 47th, New Mexico 48th, New York 49th, Washington DC 50th, and New Jersey 51st."

The lockdowners got their policies implemented. Their policies failed. That's fact. That's the data. That's not arguable. And to say otherwise is like saying the Earth is flat.

But those same people - the lockdowners - now run from accountability, and even worse, using logic that sounds like Kafka or Alice in Wonderland's Mad Hatter - and in fact sounds like the circular arguments and nonsensical discussions in the Task Force to me - lockdowners blame those who disagreed with the lockdowns and mandates for the failure of the lockdowns and mandates that were implemented!

Truth may be prevailing, but being proven right is not the point. We have witnessed something more fundamental than pandemic mismanagement. We have witnessed a shocking ethical breakdown in this country a failure of leadership, one that has created a crisis of trust in public health and institutions we need as a democratic and diverse society.,

Human rights were violated in the United States. guarantees of the most fundamental freedoms upon which this country was founded - speech, religion assembly - were suddenly reversed by lockdowners under the guise of "the science" or "safety." Any free society, especially this one founded on guaranteed liberty from government power in its Constitution and Bill of Rights, must be managed in concert with its system of laws even during health emergencies. And in this nation with its Declaration of Independence explicitly defining freedoms of individuals as, "endowed by their creator with certain unalienable rights," it is a stunning violation that Liberty fell so quickly and thoroughly by government decree and that the people allowed it.

And we must all recognize something else, the other reality unacknowledged by those in power: when Freedom disappears, it mostly harms minorities and the poor, not the affluent, not those in power.

And now we are faced with a tremendous challenge as a nation - how to restore that trust and the values required of an ethical society.

Do we truly have a problem with ethical leadership in this country?

Let's consider America's school lockdown policies. Almost all of Western Europe recognized the data in 2020 proving the minuscule risk to healthy children for serious illness. They opened their schools even during otherwise stringent lockdowns in 2020-21. America's Governors mostly closed in-person schools for that school year, as advised by our largest teachers unions and supported, whether you like to hear it or not, by most teachers - who by that behavior have wholly disqualified themselves from being entrusted to teach our children.

What happened during America's school closures?

- hundreds of thousands of child abuse cases went unreported since schools are the number one agency where child abuse is noticed

- severe child abuse exploded;

- mental health disorders - severe anxiety and depression in teenagers and college age kids skyrocketed;

- self-harm by teenagers - putting out cigarettes on their skin slashing their wrists - doubled to triple compared to the previous year;

- overdoses and substance use disorders in teenagers increased by 40 to 120 percent;

- massive learning losses directly from the shutdowns: the largest score drops in math since the first assessments more than 30 years ago and as highlighted by Unicef's 2022 update these harms and learning losses "disproportionately affected students from disadvantaged backgrounds and are concentrated among poor students."

The Birx-Fauci lockdowns were a luxury of the rich. They spared the affluent; they shifted the burden of this illness and this response to the working clas, to minorities, and to the poor. I thought we were a society that cared about the poor and low-income families? One that prioritizes our children?

Let's compare America's COVID vaccine policies in children to our peer nations:

- the UK September 21 "the margin of benefit is too small to support universal vaccination of otherwise healthy teenagers."

- Finland June 2021 "people under 16 who are not in a high-risk group will not be vaccinated in Finland."

- Norway 2020 and again in 2022 "for children who are offered the vaccine, vaccination is voluntary."

- Denmark 2022 "it will no longer be possible for children and young people under 18 to get the vaccine."

- the U.S.? October 26 2021 "we're never going to learn about how safe the vaccine is unless we start giving it, that's just the way it goes." That was Eric Rubin, MD, Editor-in-Chief, New England Journal of Medicine and advisor to the FDA committee on pediatric vaccines.

Nelson Mandela said, "There can be no keener revelation of a society's soul than the way in which it treats its children."

Across the U.S., almost all colleges and universities required testing, vaccination, and boosters in healthy asymptomatic young people, and some still did even in 2023. Yet back in October 2020 before any vaccine, when the virus was in its most lethal form, the CDC had posted on its website for schools "it is unethical and illegal to test someone who doesn't want to be tested." That CDC posting has been removed. It cannot be found.

Meanwhile, many of our so-called elite medical centers – Duke, Johns Hopkins, Stanford where I work, engage in a clinical trial sponsored by money from Pfizer, the vaccine maker, injecting healthy infants and toddlers with their experimental drug for a disease they have no significant risk to contract serious illness or die from. Is that now America's standard for medical ethics?

And even if it were true that the vaccines prevent the spread of the infection - which it does not by all of the world's data - what kind of society uses its children as human shields for adults?

I am a father. I am a shield for my children. They are not to be used as shields for me.

Beyond the death and destruction, beyond the exploding psychological harms, the self-harms, the suicides, the anxiety, the depression, the explosion in hospitalizing kids under 16 for eating disorders - all from the isolation, not the virus - we have set up a public health disaster in our younger kids. During the lockdown, more than half of college-aged kids had an unwanted weight gain that averaged 28 pounds. That's an obesity epidemic. And we have taught very young children, toddlers, that they are a disease vector, that they are a danger to everyone and everyone is a danger to them.

Where I live in Palo Alto you see people walking their toddlers with masks on, even today. Kids, babies in their strollers, with masks on in Palo Alto California.

Mackie said, "Of all the offspring of time, error is the most ancient, and is so old and familiar an acquaintance that truth, when discovered, comes upon most of us like an intruder and meets the intruder's welcome."

What was the response to hearing truth, especially on our university campuses, the centers for the free exchange of ideas? The response was censorship, intimidation, character assassination, and censure. And let's understand clearly - when you censor science and health policy, it's not simply an abstract evil, a less-than-ideal environment for diverse views or creative thinking. People die. And people died from the censorship of correct science policy.

I fear for our students and our country. Without permitting, without indeed encouraging open debate, we might never solve any future crisis. But it's not only the matter of academic freedom that needs comment. Many faculty members of our acclaimed universities are now dangerously intolerant of opinions contrary to their favoured narrative, and some employ toxic smears and organized rebukes against those of us who disagreed with what was implemented and who dared to help the country - our country, their country - under a president they happened to despise, apparently the ultimate transgression.

But defamatory attacks, character assassination - this is not acceptable in a civilized society, let alone in our great universities. Worse than a violation of ethical behaviour among colleagues, it does not meet any standard of simple human decency. If influential university board members, if illustrious graduates, if academic leaders fail to step up and renounce that shameful conduct, many experts, many more with a reputation to lose will be unwilling to serve their country in contentious times. As parents, as citizens, as educators, that would be the worst possible legacy to leave to our children, the next generation of stewards of this country.

Some call for simply forgiving and forgetting the unconscionable decisions to close schools and Implement these reckless lockdowns. No - that must not be allowed. Why? Because truth matters in an ethical society. The public needs to know the truth, especially after all they've been through. Because we must succeed in the next pandemic, the next inevitable crisis. And not if we want to restore trust. That requires us to start demanding the admission of failure and a public apology by lockdown advocates - to add accountability so they never impose these policies again.

Now I'm not naïve enough to think that they will give that apology - they will not apologize, they will never apologize. In fact, I was quoted in an Israeli interview two years ago that they will never admit that COVID is finished, and I'm not sure that they will ever admit that in parts of this country.

Aristotle argued that the distinct function of a human being is reasoning, or thinking critically; that what he called "the life worth living," is one in which we reason well. He explained that freedom is the necessary predicate to reason and to choose a virtuous life. During the 2020 pandemic, America fell short as a virtuous society by all definitions, whether secular or religious. And that failure is now on display throughout our society. It's beyond the pandemic - the pandemic exposed these issues, it did not create them.

So what can we do now?

First, each one of us has the burden of becoming critical thinkers, to make the best decisions for ourselves and our families. The era of accepting what so-called experts say simply based on their titles alone must be over. Learn the facts, use critical thinking, and then form the opinion - that's the order, not the reverse.

Second, we have a disastrous void in courage in American society today. Of the four cardinal virtues, courage is the predicate for all the others. As C.S Lewis said, "courage is not simply one of the virtues but the form of every virtue at the testing point."

If our democracy with its defining freedoms is to survive, we need good people, individuals with integrity, and there are many, to rise up. What does "rise up" mean? "Rise up" means speak up - as we are allowed, as we are expected to do in a free society, or we have no chance.

And third, we have a shocking deficit of moral, virtuous leadership in America. Amidst America's recovery from this debacle, our country urgently needs unity and strength, yet Americans have become more divided. Instead of unifying our citizens, our elected leaders including several presidents have been divisive, oblivious to their larger responsibility after they are elected to represent all Americans, even those who did not vote for them.

We need our younger generation to reinstate the moral backbone, the ethical compass, and the basic civility that is disappearing from this country. We cannot have a civil society if it is filled with people, led by people, who refuse to allow discussion of views contrary to their own. We desperately need leadership that unites, not divides; leaders with a moral compass who know right from wrong, who believe in strong family values; leaders who are not afraid to defend our precious freedoms, America's hard-earned freedoms that uniquely provide opportunities sought by millions the world over. We need leaders with Integrity, or this country as an ethical society, as a virtuous society, as a free and diverse society, is in serious trouble.

Finally, we must teach our children to have courage and to never forget what GK Chesterton said: "Right is right, even if nobody does it. Wrong is wrong, even if everybody is wrong about it."

CHAPTER 4

Public Health Officials
Broke Public Trust
Through Deception

Dr. Byram W. Bridle

Tenured Associate Professor of Immunology and Virology,
and a cancer therapeutics expert

Dr. Byram Bridle, PhD, is a distinguished Canadian Associate Professor of Viral Immunology at the University of Guelph in Ontario, Canada. As a member of the Canadian COVID Care Alliance (CCCA), he is known for his commitment to evidence-based science and his advocacy for informed consent and accurate risk-benefit assessments of novel medical interventions. Dr. Bridle has dedicated his career to studying immune responses to viruses, with a specialization in the development, optimization, and safety testing of vaccines for infectious diseases and cancers.

In his role as an educator, Dr. Bridle teaches immunology, virology, and cancer biology to students at undergraduate, graduate, and post-graduate levels and has received multiple prestigious awards in recognition of his contributions to both research and teaching. An accomplished researcher, he has an extensive publication record in peer-reviewed scientific literature and is frequently cited as a top-tier reviewer for Canada's national medical research granting agency.

Dr. Bridle's groundbreaking work includes being one of the first to raise concerns regarding the systemic distribution and potential harm of modified RNAs encapsulated in lipid nanoparticles. His dedication to the precautionary principle and transparent scientific discourse has made him a leading voice for rigorous safety standards in emerging medical technologies.

An Early Lie from Public Health Officials

When the COVID-19 pandemic was declared I was recognized as a Canadian expert in vaccinology. When the 'warp speed' development of vaccines against severe acute respiratory syndrome-coronavirus-2 (SARS-CoV-2) was underway I was sought after by many legacy media outlets to answer their questions. From the beginning I expressed concerns, noting that the dramatically truncated timeline opened the potential for corners to be cut, not to mention preventing accrual of long-term safety data. During this time, I also spoke openly about draconian policies promoting isolated quarantine of healthy children that had been introduced in some school districts. These were leading to abuse of kids by subjecting them to what was akin to long-term solitary confinement in the absence of reasonable scientific justifications. It quickly became clear to me that many public health policies were not actually 'following the science'. But at least dissenting opinions could be voiced in those early days.

For me, this all changed on May 27, 2021. On that day I gave an interview on a radio show as I had done so many times before[1]. The host asked me if I thought there might be a potential link between the modified RNA (modRNA) COVID-19 shots and cases of heart inflammation, also known as myocarditis, that were being observed in young males in Israel. I did think there was a potential association.

When a correlation is observed between a medical intervention and a serious side-effect a good scientist assesses whether there are biological mechanisms to potentially establish a cause-and-effect relationship. In that radio interview I presented just two out of a myriad of mechanisms that might explain a possible link between modRNA shots and damage to the heart. These two ideas provided a plausible connection between an injection into the shoulder leading to inflammation of the heart. I noted studies looking at how SARS-CoV-2 could cause severe disease had identified the spike protein from the virus as being responsible for a substantial amount of harm to the body; and the modRNA shots were designed to get cells in the body to manufacture the spike protein. But what could connect the potentially harmful spike protein with the heart? This is when I publicized my knowledge of a biodistribution study that was buried on the website of Japan's health regulatory agency[2]; a

[1] https://archive.org/details/new-peer-reviewed-study-on-covid-19-vaccines-suggests-why-heart-inflammation-bl (accessed November 5, 2024)

[2] https://uoguelphca-my.sharepoint.com/:b:/g/personal/bbridle_uoguelph_ca/EaWa5UjoAmZF m6TU06lgjY0B7CjuYj18Eq5ZApP90YYQ9Q?e=yT4al3

document that was brought to my attention by Dr. Peter Doshi from the University of Maryland. This document showed the lipid nanoparticles (LNPs) designed to carry the modRNA encoding the spike protein could migrate throughout the body via the blood. This identified a reasonable mechanism whereby the toxic spike protein and/or other toxic components of the shots could gain access to the heart.

Within twenty-four hours of this interview a highly organized global campaign was launched to destroy my career. Among many things, this included the creation of a defamatory website using my domain name that continues to be used to criminally impersonate me. And global networks of well-funded self-proclaimed 'misinformation experts' have been incessantly harming my professional reputation. I experienced a loss of academic freedom and had censorship imposed at my university, and legacy media ostracized me. I ended up being one of three experts invited to express concerns about censorship of scientists and physicians at a parliamentary press conference hosted by Member of Parliament, Derek Sloan[3]. Ironically, this was the first-ever parliamentary press conference in Canada's history to be censored. The chronic destruction of my career continues despite my concerns about COVID-19 shots having been repeatedly and definitively proven correct by an ever-growing avalanche of primary scientific data. Why?

I have often described what occurred in the days following my interview on May 27, 2021, as being like a nuclear bomb going off in my world. I suspect one reason for this was because I drew the attention of the public to an egregious lie that they had been told by public health 'experts' in which many people had placed their trust.

When the modRNA shots were being brought to market many people were worried about the possibility of this novel genetic technology causing

---

[3] https://www.cpac.ca/covid-19-canada-responds/episode/mp-derek-sloan-raises-concerns-over-censorship-of-doctors-and-scientists?id=cd50ce93-5138-4489-a88f-bb8065b7aa32 (accessed November 5, 2024)

their DNA to be altered. In response, public health and government officials assured everyone that the modRNA shots function like traditional vaccine technologies. They went on to explicitly state what they meant by this, which was that the shots would largely remain in the shoulder muscle where they were injected, with some portion going to the draining lymph nodes where an immune response would be initiated.

As an expert vaccinologist I was surprised by this messaging because I knew the modRNA shots relied upon small bubbles of fat, called LNPs, as a delivery mechanism. The LNPs were originally developed to deliver drugs and gene therapies throughout the body, to target diseases like brain cancers, Parkinson's disease, and many others. In other words, historical scientific data showed the LNPs got widely distributed throughout the body. However, I also knew there were proprietary aspects to the modRNA shots that had not been disclosed. So, I naturally assumed that one of these proprietary secrets had involved altering the LNP technology to prevent these little bubbles of fat from getting widely distributed in the body.

When I reviewed the biodistribution study provided by Pfizer to the Japanese government I was shocked by how it contradicted public messaging. It showed the LNPs behaved as they had consistently in the past; they went far and wide throughout the body. I realized the public had been lied to about the technology. This concept of systemic biodistribution was debated for a long time. But eventually it was confirmed when the United States Food and Drug Administration (FDA) was ordered by a court order to release documents that Pfizer had submitted to them and that they were trying to hide for 75 years. Among these was a version of Pfizer's biodistribution study that was even more egregious than the one provided to the Japanese government[4]. The US version included a previously unseen failed study in which rats died from the systemically distributed LNPs. It also demonstrated that Pfizer had cherry-picked the 'best' data for their

[4] https://uoguelphca-my.sharepoint.com/:b:/g/personal/bbridle_uoguelph_ca/EefRuVxKMHh Bjc52D7DgwMgBCLc6InFMy1AThT9wRAaSrA?e=7Rlmow

Japanese version and that Pfizer had covered up the fact that LNPs were accumulating exponentially in the tissues of females. Pfizer had pooled data from males and females to hide this from the Japanese government...

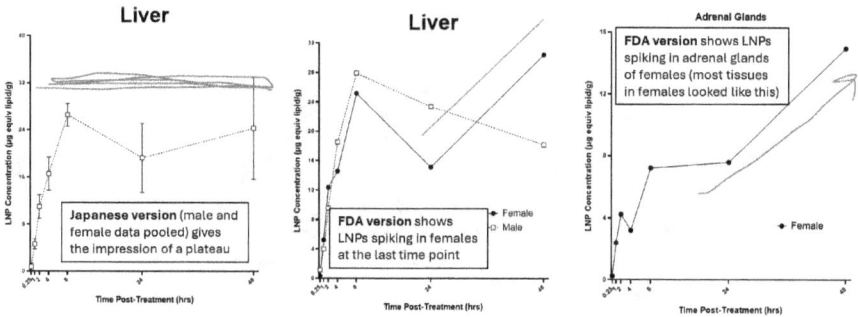

I also discovered that the FDA's version of the study hid damning evidence and then lied about it. As an example, the FDA's biodistribution study had highly redacted data like that shown below on the left. But the image of the mice in the bottom left corner was part of a larger set of pictures that can be seen in the Japanese figure on the right...

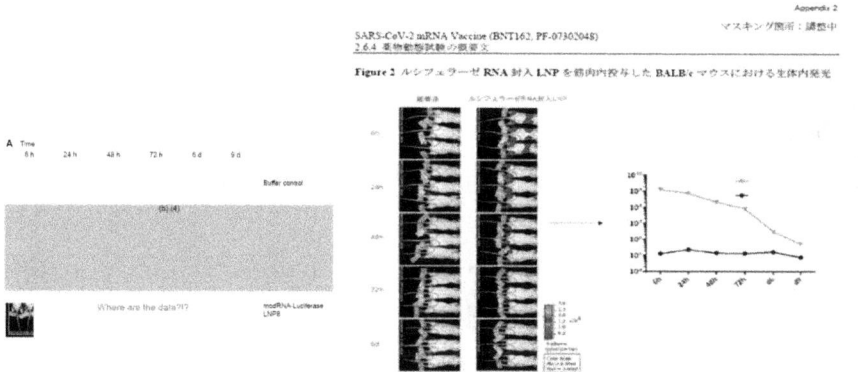

...here are the two relevant images placed side-by-side:

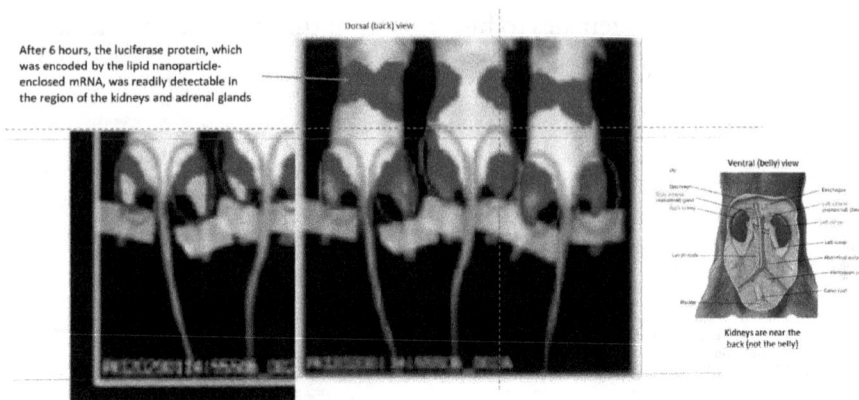

After 6 hours, the luciferase protein, which was encoded by the lipid nanoparticle-enclosed mRNA, was readily detectable in the region of the kidneys and adrenal glands

Dorsal (back) view

Ventral (belly) view

Kidneys are near the back (not the belly)

...the image in the FDA's document was cropped to give the impression that the signal for accumulation of LNPs (the bluish circles) was restricted to the injection site, which, in this case, was the hind leg muscles of mice. However, the unredacted image in the Japanese study showed an obvious accumulation of LNPs in the region of the kidneys and adrenal glands. The FDA's document declared there was no signal in this region, which represents an egregious lie from a health regulator the public is told it can trust.

At the present time, the problem I highlighted back in May of 2021 is well accepted in the scientific literature and has even been assigned the term 'spikeopathy'[5].

So, along with the abusive treatment I received from a massive number of 'experts' from around the world for revealing the truth about the systemic biodistribution of LNPs, I had to contend with the fact that I could no longer trust public health organizations.

[5] Parry PI, Lefringhausen A, Turni C, Neil CJ, Cosford R, Hudson NJ, Gillespie J. 'Spikeopathy': COVID-19 Spike Protein Is Pathogenic, from Both Virus and Vaccine mRNA. Biomedicines. 2023 Aug 17;11(8):2287. doi: 10.3390/biomedicines11082287. PMID: 37626783; PMCID: PMC10452662.

It only takes one lie to be deemed a liar. It then takes a long time of consistent truth-telling to attempt to earn trust back. So, once the 'it remains at the injection site' lie was unveiled did public health officials endeavour to regain the trust of the public? The answer is a definitive no. Gaslighting of truth-tellers and ongoing deception prevail to this day in last-ditch efforts by public health officials to avoid receiving the 'liar, liar, pants on fire' label from the public. I will provide two recent examples from Canada's public health system to demonstrate how deception remains an ongoing issue.

Manipulating Data to Make COVID-19 Shots Appear Safer Destroyed Informed Consent

When it comes to evaluating the safety of a vaccine, isolated numbers taken from passive adverse event monitoring systems that rely on voluntary reporting are difficult to interpret because they lack an appropriate context. These systems substantially underestimate the true number of adverse events following immunization (AEFIs). One way to circumvent this problem would be to conduct a head-to-head comparison with the safety of a well-established vaccine for which there is relatively high uptake, using the same safety database. This would control for a myriad of otherwise confounding variables.

The flu vaccine would be an ideal comparator because there are robust, long-term data sets available for this, and many people have decades of familiarity with both the vaccine and the disease it targets. This means people have a lot of experience conducting their own risk-benefit assessments in the context of influenza. Further, the peer-reviewed scientific literature is clear that for people outside of the high-risk demographics, which are primarily the frail elderly and those with multiple chronic illnesses, COVID-19 was of similar risk as the flu; and less of a risk for children[67]. So, letting people know how the safety of COVID-19 shots compared to flu vaccines would have been extremely helpful for people to make informed decisions. However, such data were never compiled, at least, as I found out, not for public viewing.

Lee Turner is a lawyer in British Columbia, Canada, that obtained a 1,315-page report through an 'Access To Information and Privacy' (ATIP) request and shared it with me[8]. The report documents information shared among staff at the Centre for Disease Control in British Columbia, Canada (BC-CDC), and Dr. Bonnie Henry, the Chief Medical Officer of Health for the province. These leaders in public health did, in fact, pull data about AEFIs from the same safety database for both COVID-19 shots and flu vaccines. One could not ask for a better-controlled public health data set. These officials used these comparative data for months to help them place the information about COVID-19 shots into a readily understandable context for themselves. But the moment they released information to the public, the comparative data were stripped away, effectively removing any contextual meaning. Worse, the report demonstrated nefarious manipulation of the data to artificially and dramatically reduce the number of AEFIs that were shown to the public. Let me show you exactly what happened.

---

[6] Levin AT, Hanage WP, Owusu-Boaitey N, Cochran KB, Walsh SP, Meyerowitz-Katz G. Assessing the age specificity of infection fatality rates for COVID-19: systematic review, meta-analysis, and public policy implications. Eur J Epidemiol. 2020 Dec;35(12):1123-1138. doi: 10.1007/s10654-020-00698-1. Epub 2020 Dec 8. PMID: 33289900; PMCID: PMC7721859.

[7] https://www.canada.ca/en/public-health/services/vaccination-children/covid-19.html?utm_campaign=hc-sc-covidvaccine-22-23&utm_medium=sem&utm_source=ggl&utm_content=ad-text-en&utm_term=kids%20vaccine&adv=2223-249950&id_campaign=16905919192&id_source=137027578313&id_content=593179147886&gclid=CjwKCAjwzY2bBhB6EiwAPpUpZpLVhlcD-hWO2Sx5Fga9KqJ0dbQmnbK2lI7NqrKSsJHMk1dqnAu8ghoC06AQAvD_BwE&gclsrc=aw.ds. (accessed November 5, 2024)

[8] https://uoguelphca-my.sharepoint.com/:b:/g/personal/bbridle_uoguelph_ca/ERgEga093s5GjmyshonCnbcB93ZQULyWPjQB7em-_Wpq0A?e=Eamfxu

The report showed that for months leading up to public dissemination of safety data, health officials in British Columbia accumulated information about AEFIs for COVID-19 vaccines and placed them into the context of flu vaccines. Here are the data from their final weekly update meeting just prior to when they went public with it...

BC Centre for Disease Control
Provincial Health Services Authority

BC COVID-19 AEFI Summary Report - March 25, 2021

British Columbia received its first shipment of COVID-19 vaccines during the week of December 13, 2020, and by March 22, 2021 there have been a total of 619,895 distributed doses. As of March 25, 2021, there have been 523 reports of an adverse event following immunization (AEFI) associated with COVID-19 vaccines, for a rate of 84.4 reports per 100,000 distributed doses (Table 1, Table 2). Of the reports to date, 144 (27.5%) met one or more of the criteria to be considered serious (refer to relevant footnote in Table 1 for serious AEFI definition). Some AEFI reports may include more than one adverse event. To date, there have been 714 adverse events reported, giving a ratio of 1.4 events per COVID-19 AEFI report.

No serious safety concerns were identified in the clinical trials for the Pfizer or Moderna mRNA COVID-19 vaccines.[1,2] Lymphadenopathy was observed in 1% of vaccine recipients and more frequently than in placebo recipients. Bell's Palsy was identified rarely but more often in vaccine than placebo recipients, but there was no clear basis upon which to conclude a causal association. Delayed local reactions with onset seven days after vaccination were reported in the Moderna trial data.[2] Anaphylaxis has been identified in postmarketing surveillance, occurring at a rate of 1.11 events per 100,000 doses administered of the Pfizer mRNA vaccine[3] and 0.25 events per 100,000 doses administered for the Moderna mRNA vaccine.[4]

Table 1: Summary of reported AEFI following a COVID-19 vaccine, BC, Dec 20, 2020 to Mar 25, 2021 (N=523)

	1st 4 Weeks				To Present Date			Comparison to Historic Flu AEFI				Comparison to H1N1 Flu AEFI			
	2021-09	2021-10	2021-11	2021-12	Cumulative COVID19 Count	Cumulative COVID19 Rate (per 100,000)[a]	Proportion of COVID19 Reports N	Historic Flu Rate (per 100,000)[b,c]	RR vs Historic Flu	Proportion of Historic Flu Reports %[b]	PRR vs Historic Flu	H1N1 Flu Rate (per 100,000)[d,e]	RR vs H1N1 Flu	Proportion of H1N1 Flu Reports[d]	PRR vs H1N1 Flu
AEFI Reports															
Total AEFI	63	36	21	6	523	84.37	100.0	6.50	13.0	100.0	1.0	33.38	2.6	100.0	1.0
Serious AEFI	21	13	13	2	144	23.23	27.5	1.48	15.7	22.5	1.1	7.23	3.2	22.5	1.2
Events															
Anaphylaxis	15	11	12	0	94	15.16	18.0	0.47	32.3	7.1	2.5	2.70	5.6	8.3	2.2
Anaphylaxis Brighton level 1/2/3[f]	6	6	5	0	53	8.55	10.1	0.19	45.0	2.6	3.6	NA	—	NA	—
Other allergic	25	10	11	2	209	33.72	40.0	2.09	16.1	32.1	1.2	5.70	5.9	17.6	2.6
Bell's Palsy	1	0	0	0	4	0.65	0.8	0.02	32.5	0.3	2.7	0.06	10.5	0.2	4.0
GBS	0	0	0	0	0	0.00	0.0	0.01	—	0.1	—	0.12	—	0.4	—
Encephalitis	0	0	0	0	0	0.00	0.0	0.02	—	0.3	—	0.00	—	0.0	—
Transverse myelitis	0	0	0	0	1	0.16	0.2	0.00	—	0.0	—	0.00	—	0.0	—

...this shows data about AEFIs that accumulated from December 20, 2020, until March 25, 2021. The first two rows represent the total number of AEFIs and serious AEFIs. I highlighted these in yellow. I have also highlighted an important column for comparative purposes. The numbers in this column show the relative risk of the COVID-19 shots compared to historic flu vaccines. Note that there was a 15.7-fold higher incidence of serious AEFIs on a per-dose basis than what historically occurred for flu shots. This massive difference in the safety profile of the two sets of vaccines is of substantial concern when one understands that the risk associated with the two diseases is approximately equal for most people. And it gets worse when considers that most people only require a single dose of the flu shot, but many received at least two and often three doses of COVID-19 shots per year. Would it be important to let people know that the COVID-19 shots were potentially sixteen times more dangerous per dose than the traditional flu vaccines? I think so. Such disclosure certainly would have made it impossible to justify mandating COVID-19 shots.

Although the data set was small, there were 13.6-fold more hospitalizations and a 24-fold higher rate of deaths following administration of COVID-19 shots as compared to the flu shots. This should not have been trivialized. Instead, it should have triggered intensive active safety monitoring, if not a halt in the shots; neither of which were done. Here are the data that were held behind closed doors at the BC-CDC...

	2021-08	2021-09	2021-10	2021-11	Cumulative COVID19 Count	COVID19 Rate (per 100,000)*	Proportion of COVID19 Reports %	Historic Flu Rate (per 100,000)*	RR vs Historic Flu	Proportion of Historic Flu Reports*	PRR vs Historic Flu	H1N1 Flu Rate (per 100,000)*	RR vs H1N1 Flu	Proportion of H1N1 Flu Reports*	PRR vs H1N1 Flu
Transverse myelitis	0	0	0	0	1	0.16	0.2	0.00	–	0.0	–	0.00	–	0.0	–
Seizure	0	1	0	0	1	0.16	0.2	0.27	0.6	4.1	0.0	1.53	0.1	4.7	0.0
Anaesthesia/ paraesthesia	4	7	1	0	40	6.45	7.8	NA	–	NA	–	NA	–	NA	–
Thrombocytopenia	0	0	1	2	3	0.48	0.6	0.02	24.0	0.3	2.0	0.05	–	1.0	–
Cellulitis	1	0	0	0	25	4.03	4.8	0.27	14.9	4.1	1.2	0.31	13.0	3.5	1.5
Adenopathy/ lymphadenitis	1	1	0	0	19	3.07	3.6	0.07	43.3	1.0	3.6	0.43	7.1	1.2	1.3
Recommendations															
No further immunizations	1	2	0	0	34	5.48	6.5	0.25	21.9	3.9	1.7	0.67	8.2	2.1	3.1
Outcomes															
Hospitalization	1	2	1	2	16	2.58	3.1	0.19	16.8	2.6	1.1	1.00	6.8	4.3	0.5
Permanent disability	0	0	0	0	0	0.00	0.0	0.00	–	0.0	–	0.00	–	0.0	–
Death	0	1	0	0	3	0.48	0.6	0.02	24.0	0.3	2.0	0.16	2.7	0.4	1.0
Health Authority															
HA	18	10	11	1	136	131.45	26.0	10.10	13.0	24.4	1.1	66.52	2.0	34.5	0.8

And of substantial concern, the data that BC-CDC and Dr. Bonnie Henry were looking at showed that side-effects from COVID-19 shots were being reported at eight-fold higher frequency for women...

	Last 4 Weeks				To Present Date			Comparison to Historic Flu AEFI				Comparison to H1N1 Flu AEFI			
	2021-08	2021-09	2021-10	2021-11	Cumulative COVID19 Count	Cumulative COVID19 Rate (per 100,000)*	Proportion of COVID19 Reports %	Historic Flu Rate (per 100,000)*	RR vs Historic Flu	Proportion of Historic Flu Reports*	PRR vs Historic Flu	H1N1 Flu Rate (per 100,000)*	RR vs H1N1 Flu	Proportion of H1N1 Flu Reports*	PRR vs H1N1 Flu
HA	18	10	11	1	136	131.45	26.0	10.10	13.0	24.4	1.1	66.52	2.0	34.5	0.8
FHA	17	16	16	2	148	71.39	28.3	4.34	16.4	22.0	1.3	20.31	3.5	19.1	1.5
VCHA	11	1	3	0	84	55.91	16.1	2.25	26.3	10.4	1.5	10.19	5.9	9.7	1.7
VIHA	14	3	6	2	102	99.42	19.5	9.33	10.4	25.8	0.8	38.58	2.6	22.6	0.9
NHA	1	5	2	1	55	90.24	10.1	26.36	3.0	17.4	0.6	116.81	0.7	15.3	0.6
Age Group															
<18	0	0	0	0	0	0.00	0.0	3.03	–	45.1	–	21.73	–	35.0	–
18-64	63	71	29	3	442	13.49	84.5	1.35	9.7	46.1	1.8	10.42	1.3	58.5	1.4
65+	1	5	12	3	81	8.22	15.5	0.93	8.7	8.8	1.8	5.24	1.6	6.4	2.4
Gender															
Female	43	23	29	4	466	17.95	89.1	2.32	7.7	60.4	1.5	16.63	1.1	68.3	1.3
Male	20	3	6	2	57	2.24	10.9	1.56	1.4	39.5	0.3	7.36	0.3	20.1	0.4

...women should have been told the shots might be more dangerous for them, especially since this concern matched the extremely disconcerting biodistribution profile of LNPs in females that was previously discussed.

A short time later a highly manipulated version of this data set was released. It was stripped of all comparisons to the flu shot, and the number of serious AEFIs were substantially reduced. First, here is the communication following the internal review of the March 25, 2021, AEFIs dataset...

From:	Noftall, Kyle [BCCDC]
To:	Amos, Heather [BCCDC]; Naus, Monika [BCCDC]
Subject:	April 8 Public COVID19 AEFI report
Date:	Thursday, April 08, 2021 10:34:29 AM
Attachments:	COVID19_AEFI_Weekly_Report_2021-04-08.docx
	COVID19_AEFI_Weekly_Report_2021-04-08.pdf

Hi Heather,

Attached is the final version of this week's (and first!) public COVID-19 AEFI report. I've included a Word and PDF, but only the PDF would be posted to the website. You were still deciding where on the website it would make sense to include this report, as the COVID-19 Data section was being reworked.

Monika was going to send you some key messages related to the report as well.

Thanks,

Kyle

Kyle Noftall, MPH

Communicable Disease Epidemiologist

Communicable Diseases and Immunization Service (CDIS)

And here is a portion of what was released publicly. I am showing just two pages to highlight major concerns. This is from page 1 of the public release...

British Columbia Report

Adverse Events Following Immunization with COVID-19 Vaccines

December 13, 2020 to April 03, 2021

This report summarizes the reports of COVID-19 vaccine adverse events following immunization (AEFI) reported to the BC Centre for Disease Control up to and including April 03, 2021. Please refer to the BCCDC website for reporting guidelines.[1] Events can be reported even when there is no certainty of a causal association. Please refer to the Data Notes section at the end of this report for additional information on the source data.

Summary

No safety signals have been identified in the reports received in BC to date. These results are in keeping with observed events elsewhere in Canada and available reports from other jurisdictions, as well as the demonstrated safety of the vaccines in clinical trials prior to authorization for use.[2-4] BC is reporting higher rates of anaphylaxis than many other Canadian jurisdictions, but about half of these had lower level of diagnostic certainty and may reflect events such as anxiety or pre-syncopal (fainting) events, which are nevertheless managed and reported as anaphylaxis out of an abundance of caution. Serious events have not been reported at rates higher than expected compared to background rates.

...bold claims were made that, "No safety signals have been identified in the reports received in BC to date" and "Serious events have not been reported at rates higher than expected compared to background rates". Yet I just showed you the internal data that they looked at one week prior, which demonstrated that reports of serious adverse events were accruing at a 16-fold higher rate per dose for COVID-19 shots when compared to the historical gold standard flu shots.

And BC-CDC also released this table to the public, which covered data from December 13, 2020, to April 3, 2021; so, it included one week of additional data compared to the internal data set reviewed above...

Table 1: Description of adverse event reports following receipt of a COVID-19 vaccine, BC, Dec.13, 2020 - Apr.03, 2021 **(N=593)**

		COVID-19 Vaccine		
	All COVID-19 Vaccines	COVISHIELD	Moderna mRNA	Pfizer mRNA
Total reports	**593** 523	10	239	344
Non-serious reports	567	9	230	328
Serious reports	26 144 !!!	1	9	16
Proportion serious	4.4% 27.5% !!!	10%	3.8%	4.7%
Dose 1 reports	507 ↑	10	213	284
Dose 2 reports	86 As of Mar. 25	0	26	60
Total doses administered	857,644	34,058	144,338	679,248
Dose 1 administered	770,236	34,058	127,228	608,950
Dose 2 administered	87,408	0	17,110	70,298
Total reporting rate	69.1	29.4	165.6	50.6
Serious rate	3.0	2.9	6.2	2.4
Dose 1 rate	65.8	29.4	167.4	46.6
Dose 2 rate	98.4	--	152.0	85.4

Note: Rates calculated per 100,000 doses administered

...note that all comparisons to the flu shots were removed so the public could not place the numbers into an appropriate context. Worse, data were manipulated to substantially reduce the real number of serious

AEFIs. Key numbers in this first public release of data are highlighted in yellow. In red text I added the numbers from the internal report from one week prior, which you can review in the previously presented table.

One week prior to this public data release there were 523 total AEFIs. On April 3, 2021, there were 593 total AEFIs. So, with 70 new AEFIs added to the data set one must question how the total number of serious side-effects plummeted from 144 in the internal data set on March 25th to a mere 26 in the public data on April 3rd. At least 118 serious AEFIs were unaccounted for (possibly more, depending on the nature of the 70 newly reported AEFIs). This manipulation of numbers allowed public health officials to claim that only 4.4% of the total AEFIs were serious despite them knowing that 27.5% of the total AEFIs had been deemed serious the week before. Even if all 70 new reports represented non-serious side-effects, the lowest this could have dropped to was 24.3%. So, how was this disappearing act accomplished?

The answer was discovered by Lex Acker who is a chartered financial analyst with expertise in detecting fraud reports. The number of serious AEFIs were dramatically reduced in the report released to the public by manipulating the definition of a 'serious AEFI'.

Here is the definition that was used to reduce the number of serious AEFIs for release to the public...

Definitions
1. **Adverse event following immunization (AEFI)** - Any untoward medical event following immunization that is temporally (i.e., occurs within a biologically plausible timeframe after receipt of vaccine) but not necessarily causally associated.[8]
2. **Serious AEFI** - For the purpose of this report, a serious AEFI is one that resulted in hospitalization, permanent disability/incapacity, or death.

And here is the definition that had been used behind closed doors...

From:	Amos, Heather [BCCDC]
To:	Noftall, Kyle [BCCDC]
Subject:	RE: March 11 COVID19 AEFI Report
Date:	Monday, March 15, 2021 9:51:09 AM

Thanks!

From: Noftall, Kyle [BCCDC]
Sent: Monday, March 15, 2021 9:34 AM
To: Amos, Heather [BCCDC]
Cc: Naus, Monika [BCCDC]
Subject: RE: March 11 COVID19 AEFI Report
Hi Heather,

Today's report is attached (as you mention, the rates won't be accurate).

	Cumulative COVID19 Count	Cumulative COVID19 Rate (per 100,000)
Total AEFI	469	123.96
Serious AEFI	124	32.77
Anaphylaxis	79	20.88
Anaphylaxis Brighton levels 1/2/3	46	12.16
Other allergic	189	49.96

Serious AEFI defined as any of the following events: anaphylaxis, Bell's Palsy, cellulitis, seizure, encephalitis, transverse myelitis, GBS, intussusception, meningitis, ORS, paralysis, or thrombocytopenia; OR any of the following outcomes/recommendations: hospitalization, permanent disability/incapacity, death, or recommendation of no further immunizations.

Kyle Noftall, MPH
Communicable Disease Epidemiologist
Communicable Diseases and Immunization Service (CDIS)

...highlighted in purple are all the conditions that were removed from the definition. And this is how public health officials made problematic numbers magically disappear. Does anyone really think it is okay to remove things like inflammation of the brain (encephalitis) and paralysis from the definition of a serious side-effect?!? This is deceptive and hides the true potential harms of the COVID-19 shots.

Telling Bald-Faced Lies to Get Pregnant Women to Take the Shots

In Canada, members of the federal parliament are allowed to submit what are called order paper questions. Is it a way for them to obtain information from government agencies? As shown below, an order paper question that was posed was, "what is Health Canada's scientific basis for claiming safety of the XBB.1.5 mRNA product in pregnant and lactating women"?[9]

[9] https://uoguelphca-my.sharepoint.com/:b:/g/personal/bbridle_uoguelph_ca/EZIKzqFmYvxA sgwtS5nB_qsBSi38BNuSp8Xu3amSlFVXIw?e=hIQYYI

Government / Gouvernement
of Canada / du Canada

INQUIRY OF MINISTRY

...(g) what is Health Canada's scientific basis for claiming safety of the XBB.1.5 mRNA product in pregnant and lactating women; (h) what rigorous prospective studies, with active patient reporting and monitoring, is Health Canada relying upon to support their safety claims in the P&L population for the use of Omicron XBB.1.5 product?

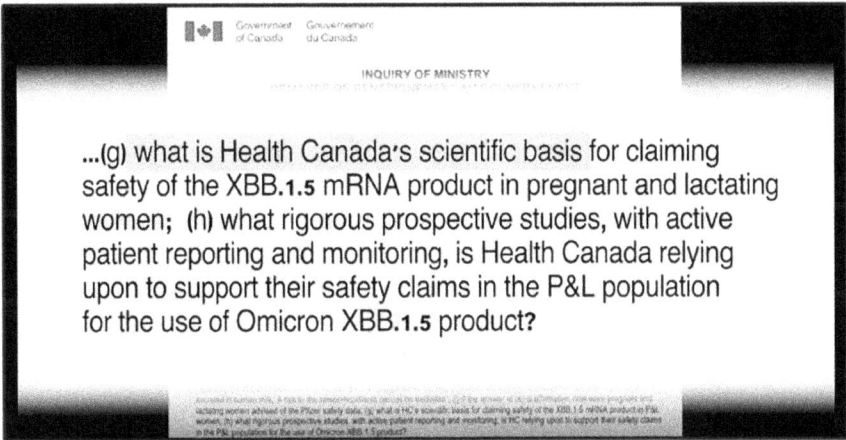

The answer was issued on December 13, 2023...

Government / Gouvernement
of Canada / du Canada

INQUIRY OF MINISTRY
DEMANDE DE RENSEIGNEMENT AU GOUVERNEMENT

PREPARE IN ENGLISH AND FRENCH MARKING "ORIGINAL TEXT" OR "TRANSLATION"
PREPARER EN ANGLAIS ET EN FRANÇAIS EN INDIQUANT "TEXTE ORIGINAL" OU "TRADUCTION"

QUESTION NO./Nº DE LA QUESTION	BY / DE	DATE
Q-2163	Mrs. Wagantall (Yorkton—Melville)	December 13, 2023

Reply by the Minister of Health
Réponse du ministre de la Santé

Signed by the Honourable Mark Holland

PRINT NAME OF SIGNATORY INSCRIRE LE NOM DU SIGNATAIRE	SIGNATURE MINISTER OR PARLIAMENTARY SECRETARY MINISTRE OU SECRÉTAIRE PARLEMENTAIRE

QUESTION

The answer was surprising considering public messages provided by officials as prominent as the province of Ontario's Minister of Health, Christine Elliot, more than two years earlier.

As can be seen and heard in a video produced by the Canadian Citizens Care Alliance[10], the Minister of Health stated the following with respect to COVID-19 shots in provincial parliament on November 30, 2021:

[10] https://www.youtube.com/watch?v=TBzoax4miXk&t=286s (accessed November 5, 2024)

"But it is also safe. It **has been tested. We are recommending that women who are pregnant do receive the vaccine** for the protection of themselves, protection of their baby as well. **It has been accepted by Health Canada**... Women who are pregnant, **it is entirely safe and recommended for them to receive the vaccine**." (bolding added for emphasis)
- Christine Elliot, Ontario Minister of Health -

But this was contradicted by product monographs provided by the manufacturers of the COVID-19 shots after these bold public claims were made by the minister. For example, here are relevant excerpts from the monograph for Pfizer/BioNTech's product, which had been updated on March 4, 2022[11]...

COMIRNATY®

COVID-19 Vaccine, mRNA

Suspension for Intramuscular Injection

Multiple Dose Vial

For 12 Years of Age and Older (after dilution each vial contains 6' doses of 0.3 mL)

For Age 5 Years to <12 Years (after dilution each vial contains 10* doses of 0.2 mL)

Active Immunizing Agent

BioNTech Manufacturing GmbH
An der Goldgrube 12
Mainz, Rhineland-Palatinate, Germany
55131

Date of Initial Authorization:
September 16, 2021

Date of Revision:
March 4, 2022

Imported and distributed by:
Pfizer Canada ULC
17,300 Trans-Canada Highway
Kirkland, Quebec, Canada H9J 2M5

Submission Control Number: 259675

---

[11] https://uoguelphca-my.sharepoint.com/:b:/g/personal/bbridle_uoguelph_ca/EQHWyjxOIKR OnnFKm__mw5cBiMiHqsks_tiL__ZGL50Qtw?e=awddby

7.1 Special Populations

7.1.1 Pregnant Women

The safety and efficacy of COMIRNATY in pregnant women have not yet been established.

Animal studies do not indicate direct or indirect harmful effects with respect to pregnancy, embryo/fetal development, parturition, or post-natal development (see 16 **NON-CLINICAL TOXICOLOGY**).

7.1.2 Breast-feeding

It is unknown whether COMIRNATY is excreted in human milk. A risk to the newborns/infants cannot be excluded.

The developmental and health benefits of breastfeeding should be considered along with the mother's clinical need for immunization against COVID-19.

Further, this is what Health Canada and the Public Health Agency of Canada said in the order paper...

Health Canada / Public Health Agency of Canada

(h) Health Canada has not approved any safety claims with regard to pregnant and lactating women.

...and...

Yet the minister had told everyone in the province, *"But it is also safe. It has been accepted by Health Canada... Women who are pregnant, it is entirely safe and recommended for them to receive the vaccine".*

This raises questions like why did officials make bold claims to the public that contradicted health regulatory agencies? Of equal importance, why did health regulatory agencies not endeavour to correct the public record? Both parties are guilty of allowing the public to be misled. With this kind of information coming to light it is unfathomable that pregnant and lactating women were coerced and mandated to take these shots.

Transparency and Integrity Should be Hallmarks of Public Health

Two of the three examples of public health deception presented here are from a Canadian context. However, the same playbook has been used around the globe. It highlights the need for people around the world to demand full transparency from their public health and health regulatory agencies that purport to have the best interests of people at heart. Ask where most of the money for their operating budgets come from. You may be surprised to learn that it is not from taxes, it is from fees paid by big pharma. This needs to change because one usually does not bite the hand the feeds.

It has been well over three years and deceptions by public health and health regulatory officials continue to be uncovered only through compelled release of information. The integrity of public health institutions has been shattered and there is no evidence that they intend to seek restitution. To restore faith in public health, those caught being deceitful need to be brought to justice.

Further, courts need to end the practice of granting judicial notice to regulatory agencies. Judicial notice assumes that statements made by health agencies are akin to the gospel truth and, therefore, regulators are not compelled to provide evidence to defend their statements in courts of law. This practice is nonsensical when health regulators are lying about and hiding information that would otherwise kill draconian policies.

Our public health institutions need to be torn down, rebuilt in ways to make them resistant to corruption, and then repopulated with experts that have a track record of integrity and transparency. Until this happens, the number of people who are hesitant to respond to public health messaging will continue to soar.

Finally, a moratorium needs to be placed on all RNA 'vaccines', including next-generation technologies like the self-amplifying RNA (replicon) vaccines. Academic censorship being done under the guise of 'combating misinformation' must end. And careers need to be restored for the scientists, health care providers, and many others who were 'left to the wolves' by negligent health regulators that sat on data that confirmed the concerns being expressed.

CHAPTER 5

A Kaleidoscopic Review of the COVID Craziness

Dr. Ramesh Thakur

Former United Nations Assistant Secretary-General

Dr. Ramesh Thakur is an Emeritus Professor in the Crawford School of Public Policy, The Australian National University. He is a former United Nations Assistant Secretary-General, and a Brownstone Institute Senior Scholar. Born in India and educated in India and Canada, he has held full time academic appointments in Fiji, New Zealand, Canada, and Australia and been a consultant to the Australian, New Zealand and Norwegian governments on international security issues. He has served on the international advisory boards of policy-oriented research institutes in Africa, Asia, Europe, and North America. He has written and edited more than 50 books.

The public policy madness of the COVID years seems less and less believable with each passing week and month. And yet, many incidents and scenes will be instantly recalled by most of us who lived through it all as soon as they are mentioned. This essay offers a few representative but not comprehensive snapshots of some of the more telling ones.

1 The Absurd, the Idiotic and the Farcical

To begin with, some were so absurd and farcical that, if presented in a work of fiction, they would be dismissed as too creative. There were photos of police tapes around rocks in public parks to warn people against sitting in case they got infected. There were photos of young children in primary school all masked up and anti-socially distanced, which was nothing less than child abuse. Sole occupant drivers were stopped by cops for being maskless. There were photos of election rallies in India with people crowding together, some masked, some with masks pulled below chins, some maskless.

Canada's chief medical officer advised people to put their masks on during sex. There were virus-free eating areas where a mask was not required when sitting but had to be worn when standing up or going to the lavatory. A lonely farmer operating his tractor in a paddock, miles from another human being, had to wear a mask. The supermarket had a check-out Plexiglas safety screen. The police, with tape measures in hand, enforced density limits for shops resulting in long queues.

And the winner is: South Australia's Chief Public Health Officer. She closed down the whole state based on a lie told by a man with COVID-19 about his link to a pizza shop. Nicola Spurrier speculated that COVID may have been transmitted via a highly infectious pizza box! She also advised footy fans to 'duck and do not touch' any errant football that came their way over the fence at Adelaide Oval because it might have been infected with the virus from Collingwood players coming from the plague state over the border. A COVID flunkey subsequently explained that her remark had been taken out of context and people could safely touch the ball if they used hand sanitiser.

You really could not make up any of this stuff in the pre-COVID era, before 2020.

2 The Many Faces of a Police State

Comical as these incidents were, the COVID excesses were no laughing matter. In many respects what we experienced was martial law dressed up as a medical emergency, a police state where far too many individual coppers were given free rein to indulge their inner bullies. And unfortunately, Australia led the world in this descent into authoritarianism, validating the *bon mot* from Clive James that its problem is not too many convict ancestors so much as too many prison guard ancestors.

Military joined the police to patrol our major cities. Heavily armed riot police in full battle gear and menacing-looking vehicles confronted peaceful protestors (but Black Lives Matter protests were okay because, well, racism is an even more lethal health risk). Rubber bullets were fired into crowds of protestors at Melbourne's Shrine of Remembrance. A young pregnant mother was arrested in her pyjamas in the presence of her shocked and distressed family for the crime of posting a link on Facebook about a peaceful protest with proper social distancing and masks. A man was dumped hard on the pavement while engaged in a conversation with another police officer. A woman on the beach was surrounded by five riot squad officers. Another sitting by herself on a bench in a park was accosted by two officers and told to move on. Riot police charged through Melbourne's Queen Victoria Market.

3 The Cruel and the Heartless

Unfortunately, the public health clerisy were determined to match police brutality with their own examples of cruelty and heartlessness. Examples that spring to mind begin with the heart-breaking image of the masked-up Queen sitting in a corner all alone in her grief at her beloved husband's funeral service. And the photo of the man in Milton Keynes, UK who went to comfort his mother during his father's funeral when an officious man interrupted the service to put him right. There were thousands who were forced to endure parents and grandparents dying lonely deaths in isolation wards,and loved ones with dementia looking out from behind glass windows with pain and confusion plainly written on their faces. There were missed family birthdays, anniversary reunions, wedding ceremonies.

Hospitals were closed because Queensland hospitals are for Queenslanders. There was the resulting death of one unborn twin because the paperwork and other red tape hassles in crossing from Ballina in NSW into Queensland and catching flights from Brisbane to Sydney caused too much wretched delay. There were poignant scenes of families reaching over the plastic barriers at the Tweed Heads (NSW) -Coolangatta (QLD) border. Australian citizens were prevented from returning home from India. There was the delay of a visit to Queensland by a California-based son to see his dying father, even though he had been allowed to enter Australia and was already in Sydney, willing to charter a private plane.

4 The Hypocrisy

What incensed the people even more was how the harshness and cruelty imposed on the general public was overridden by the elites when it came to their own behaviour. Sports and entertainment A-lister celebrities were exempt from many of the restrictions in order to give the public their weekly dose of bread and circuses. The Prime Minister made multiple overseas trips. A state chief public health officer exempted himself from travel restrictions he had laid down for everyone else in order to attend a function in Canberra where his contributions were honoured. Politicians in the U.S. enjoyed themselves in fancy French restaurants *sans* masks and in breach of physical distancing requirements, or in sunny locations mid-winter while exhorting their citizens to stay home. Many donned masks for photo-ops before returning to enjoy their group cocktails; look at the world's ruling elites at the G7 summit in Cornwall or Alexandria Ocasio-Cortez who danced merrily without a mask but put it on for a group photo. American politicians and celebrities mingled at ritzy functions without masks while the serving staff were forced to wear masks for fear of being fired.

5 Science and Data Illiteracy

Pandemics are relatively rare occurrences in history. Including COVID-19, there have only been five outbreaks since the First World War. Over that same period, advances in medical knowledge and technology have greatly expanded the toolkits of prevention, treatment and palliative care. There have also been major advances in medical education, training and research. Alongside these developments, countries learned from one another and cooperated to build national and international public health infrastructure to promote global health. In September 2019, the World Health Organisation (WHO) published a report that summarises the 'state of the art' policy advice for governments on health interventions to deal with pandemics. Many governments, including Australia, wrote their own pandemic preparedness plans that drew on a century of science, data and experience.

These were the best-practice contingency plans for the outbreak of pandemics as low-probability but high-impact 'black swan' events. Why were they abandoned just when most needed in early 2020? The science and evidence base did not change in that short timeframe.

Doctors combine their formal training, clinical knowledge, best available evidence, and familiarity with patients' medical history. Most importantly, they also take into consideration individual patient preferences and values in order to treat illness, manage risks, and relieve suffering. All this too was thrown out in favour of commands from centralised health bureaucracies. Why?

Modelling was all too often mistaken for scientific research and modelled scenarios for hard data and scientific conclusions. This was the basis for claiming that lockdowns, mask and vaccine recommendations-cum-mandates were based on science. A wide-ranging survey conducted by *TheTelegraph* and Census-wide, and published in *The Telegraph* on March 2, 2024 found that a third (33 percent) of scientists believe that officials had focused on only a minority of opinions, wrongly equating scientific scepticism with science denialism. Science is always work-in-progress, never an encyclopaedia of immutable facts. The sceptics had considerable tacit support in the scientific community. 'This was,however, muted by concerns about loss of patronage, access to research grants and difficulty in publication as the cost of speaking out', says Prof. Robert Dingwall.

6 Misinformation, Disinformation, Gaslighting

The threat from COVID-19 to the general population was greatly exaggerated. Between them, the real-life examples from the cruise ship the *Diamond Princess* and the US and French warships *Theodore Roosevelt* and *Charles de Gaulle* showed two things. In the first case, even under the worst possible conditions with mostly elderly people engaged in constant social interactions in close physical proximity, the mortality rate was quite low. In the latter two cases, involving healthy and fit mostly young men, the mortality risk was negligible. But to instil fear, the infection and case fatality rates, the distinction between dying with and dying from COVID, and that between absolute and relative risk reductions, were all blurred.

People were bombarded with slick propaganda messages saying that the threat was very grave for everyone. The effectiveness of interventions was exaggerated, the risk of collateral harms was seriously downgraded, the standard QALY (quality adjusted life years) metric for assessing the benefits of interventions were jettisoned, and the requirement for rigorous cost-benefit analyses was ignored. The media were bribed, bullied and otherwise co-opted into amplifying the pandemic fear porn.

Drug companies have a fiduciary duty to maximise returns for share-holders but no corresponding legal obligation to give the best treatment to citizens. The corporatisation of the healthcare sector has arguably compromised ethical standards. With rare exception, the results of pharmaceutical industry-sponsored clinical trials exaggerate the safety and benefits of their products, leading to lack of fully-informed consent. This is further compounded by the fact that because of commercial confidentiality, the raw data from clinical trials are rarely made available for independent analysis. Too many regulators of pharmaceutical products are dependent on the industry itself for their operating budgets and many of their personnel end up working for the drug manufacturers once they have served their term.

7 Harms

At the height of the pandemic, only a few dissenting scientific voices spoke out to highlight the health and economic risks from lockdowns, masks and vaccines. Now, *The Telegraph* poll cited earlier shows that 68 percent of British scientists believe more consideration should have been given to the fallout caused by shutting down the country. As national health services collapsed into *de facto* single service COVID-only health services, treatment of other illnesses was deferred and screening of detectable and treatable illnesses was postponed to an indefinite future. A study from University College London in February estimated that 12,000 quality adjusted life years had been lost in Britain and over 100,000 across Europe because of delays in diagnosing melanoma alone during COVID lockdowns.

Millions in the third world aspiring to join the lower middle class were instead flung back into harsh poverty. Financial strains and school closures put many children and women back into increased risk of domestic violence, child and sex trafficking. Hundreds of millions missed out on childhood immunisation with proven benefits and long-term safety profiles. Multiple studies have shown that lockdown increased developmental and learning delays. The vast amounts of money thrown at keeping individuals and businesses afloat through the shutdowns have pumped money into circulation to fuel inflation, add to the cost-of-living pressures, and rob today's children of secure debt-free futures.

Almost all highly-vaccinated countries have experienced high excess death rates that coincide with their vaccination campaigns. Yet, the general response from governing and public health authorities is that of the three wise monkeys: see no evil, hear no evil, speak no evil.

8 The Sinister

In the beginning many of us assumed that the institutional checks on abuse of power would come into play as self-correcting mechanisms, that the powers that be and the public would soon realise the error of their ways, and COVID-19 would be regarded by public health authorities and the people as just another endemic respiratory illness and infectious disease not meriting extraordinary interventions.

How wrong we were.

As weeks turned into months and months into years, what initially had seemed like well-intentioned incompetence and mistakes began to take on more sinister manifestations. The surprise at just how easy it had proved for governments to secure mass buy-in of the pandemic scare and near-universal compliance with lockdown, mask and vaccine diktats, turned into apprehension at the growing number of medical and human rights, civil liberties and political freedoms that were trampled.

Compliance with official regulations turned into the more sinister transformation of civil society into the snitch societies reminiscent of Stasi East Germany, Stalinist Russia and Maoist China, with citizens enthusiastically reporting possible breaches of the regulations by colleagues, neighbours and even family members. As vaccine apartheid took hold, many public commentators and intellectuals openly contemplated denying the unvaccinated jobs, entry into public spaces and even medical and hospital care for life-threatening illnesses.

Nor has the era passed of 'nudging' one's own citizens through techniques of behavioural psychological manipulation, compulsion and coercion. On the contrary, having learned how easily mass public opinion can be mobilised in service of the official narrative, there is every prospect of serial repeats of public emergencies across many sectors of human life. Meanwhile the WHO is preparing for a *de facto* coup to centralise unprecedented power and resources by means of a new pandemic treaty and amendments to the existing International Health Regulations. This is less of a globalist coup against sovereign states than a power grab by elites in collusion across state borders against the world's deplorables.

Perhaps the era of liberal democracy that underpinned growing prosperity and improved health outcomes for everyone has peaked and we have begun the descent into dystopia.

9 State Power and COVID Crimes

In effect we are witness to the culmination of a long-term trend since the Second World War. The Cold War saw the rise of the national security state. Then we had the growth of the administrative state with technocrats and bureaucrats being delegated more and more legislative, executive and judicial functions with correspondingly diminished public accountability. This was followed by the creation and spread of the surveillance state as governments harnessed the power of technology to spy on their own people, even more than on alleged enemies. Finally, during COVID we fell under the rule of the biosecurity state wherein citizens were regarded as disease-carrying biohazards. The national security elite entered into an active, mutually-beneficial partnership with the pharmaceutical, media, and technological leaders in society. The end result is not just the censorship industrial complex but the fusion of Big State, Big Pharma, Big Media and Big Tech to create an oppressive and suffocating ruling class.

10 What Is to be Done?

Has the public worm turned? A mere 3.3 percent of Australians aged 18-64 were 'fully immunised' by February 2024 and only a third (33.6 percent) of people over 75 have taken the recommended up-to-date booster.

If public disenchantment is replacing trust in the competence and good faith of the public health clerisy, it might be an opportune time to resurrect the campaign for a duly empowered Royal Commission, helmed by credible people with the appropriate mix of qualifications, experience, expertise and integrity, who are not tainted with conflicts of interest, to conduct an independent, impartial and rigorous inquiry.

In addition, those responsible for the extraordinarily damaging pandemic policies need to be identified, prosecuted, and, if convicted, punished. Only this can satisfy people's innate sense of justice, bring emotional closure to the victims and families of those who suffered grave harms, and act as an effective deterrent to comparable acts of malfeasance in the future.

CHAPTER 6

Integrity Under Fire

Dr. Charles Hoffe

General Practitioner and Emergency Room Doctor.

Dr Charles Hoffe is a South African trained general practitioner and emergency room doctor, who emigrated to Canada in 1990. He spent his career serving the First Nations people of Canada in small rural communities. As an early whistleblower he has been brutally persecuted by the Canadian medical authorities, for exposing the evidence of harm from Covid vaccines which occurred in his own patients. He is on trial for professional misconduct for alerting his community and the wider public to the safety signals and promoting the use of ivermectin to prevent or treat Covid. He has paid a heavy price, but his courage and integrity stand tall against the moral failures of the medical profession.

As 2020 dawned, the airwaves were filled with news of a terrifying new virus which had appeared in the city of Wuhan, China. The virus caused severe adult respiratory distress syndrome. It was lethal and highly infectious. Doctors and nurses were becoming infected and dying while trying to save the sick. The media showed constant photographs of medical personnel in hazmat suits and the hapless victims of the new disease on ventilators. The imminent risk to the global community and the threat of overwhelmed healthcare systems were the talk of the day. Sweeping new public health policies and restrictions based on computer modelling were rolled out in lockstep across the globe. The WHO named the new disease COVID-19 and declared a pandemic.

As an emergency room doctor in a small town in British Columbia, Canada, I was nervous. A work team arrived to divide our emergency department into two sections, Covid and non-Covid. They constructed a negative pressure room where victims were to be intubated and put on ventilators, pending transfer to an ICU. We ran drills to practise suiting up and suiting down in the correct sequence, donning hazmat suits to avoid contamination with the virus. I found working in a hazmat suit stifling and claustrophobic, and the limited visibility of goggles or a face visor made the delicate art of endotracheal intubation even more challenging. We were told that there was no treatment for this terrifying new disease, and that our only hope was to wait for a vaccine.

Meanwhile, in the alternative media, facts were gradually emerging which showed that the recovery rate from the new virus was in fact no worse than the seasonal flu, and like the flu, was only a significant risk to the frail elderly. Anyone monitoring it closely enough soon realised that all the fear, media hype and highly restrictive Covid mitigation measures made no sense whatsoever. Those who pointed out that absurdly restrictive healthcare policies were based on computer modelling rather than science, were slandered as being anti-science.

Meanwhile, innovative doctors around the world who developed early treatment protocols for COVID-19, using repurposed drugs, faced immediate opposition and ridicule from the media and public health. The government's response to their efforts to keep people out of hospital using safe, cheap and effective medication, showed once again that public health policy was not about safety.

Almost predictably, the pharmaceutical industry produced misleading scientific studies designed to show that ivermectin and hydroxychloroquine were ineffective and/or dangerous if used to treat COVID-19. These two drugs, which were pre-pandemic on the WHO list of essential medicines for their decades-long record of safety and efficacy, suddenly became 'dangerous' and 'ineffective' if used for COVID-19. Those who recommended them were ridiculed and slandered in the mainstream media.

The message from public health to the Covid infected was to isolate yourself at home and wait until you were critically ill before seeking help. To any clear-thinking healthcare professional, this was blatantly absurd. There are no respiratory infections that are untreatable. Early treatment is essential and lifesaving. Tragically, many lives were lost because of this cruel public health policy of actively withholding treatment. In Canada, where ivermectin had been a registered licensed prescription medication for decades, doctors were banned from prescribing it for Covid, despite 60 scientific studies showing its effectiveness and safety. Canada customs blocked all ivermectin shipments at the border, as though it had suddenly become a dangerous and illegal substance. So, many who were aware of its unique role in combating Covid, resorted to the use of veterinary ivermectin.

The announcement of new gene-based vaccines, which were supposedly coming to save us, was greeted enthusiastically by the media and the terrified masses. The world longed for something to keep them safe and bring an end to the pandemic. Klaus Schwab, leader of the World Economic Forum, announced: "No one is safe until everyone is vaccinated." Those who predicted that the vaccines would be mandated were ridiculed as conspiracy theorists. In the media, "fact-checkers" became the self-appointed experts and arbiters of truth. They served to slander, discredit, and ridicule anyone who contradicted the political narrative.

Yet, for those who knew that Covid was no more dangerous than the seasonal flu, and only a significant risk to the frail elderly, this was all quite clearly absurd.

I researched the history of experimental gene-based vaccines following the first SARS coronavirus epidemic in 2002/3. No successful coronavirus vaccine had ever been invented. So, scientists experimented with gene-based vaccines against SARS 1. In phase 1 trials, they inoculated laboratory animals with the new vaccine and found that they successfully developed antibodies. But when they exposed the laboratory animals to the virus several months later, many became extremely sick or died. The experimental vaccine was a failure. It made the laboratory animals more vulnerable to the coronavirus than if they had not been vaccinated.

Then came the Covid pandemic. It was portrayed as a dire global emergency. There was no time for animal trials. A sample of relatively healthy adults was selected to test the new vaccine, and after about three months, various vaccines were given emergency use authorisation. None of the usual safety protocols had been followed.

To any who understood the importance of correctly phased research trials to establish safety or efficacy of new treatments, this was lunacy. It takes five to ten years to establish the safety and effectiveness of any new treatment. Hence, it is impossible to establish the safety or effectiveness of a new treatment in two or three months. Nevertheless, despite the glaring lack of evidence, the medical profession and the public were blindly assured of the superb safety of the novel vaccines.

By the third month of the vaccine rollout, March 2021, 12 countries in Europe had shut down the Astrazeneca vaccine due to life-threatening blood clots. Nevertheless, Trudeau assured Canadians that it was quite safe, and Public Health continued to administer it as fast as possible.

In view of the serious lack of safety data, I expressed my refusal to participate in the vaccine rollout. However, I continued to get group emails to healthcare providers in our area on the progress of the roll-out. In March 2021, I sent an email to our group of 18 healthcare professionals – doctors, nurses and pharmacists, who were actively administering the injections – to alert them to the safety signal in Europe. In addition, I made them aware of their personal liability by administering a medical treatment without informing the recipients of the possible risks.

The response to my email was swift and harsh. Three days later, in a telephone meeting with a doctor from the regional health authority, I was given a stern reprimand. I was told that I was putting people at risk by creating vaccine hesitancy. I was forbidden from saying anything negative about the Covid shots in the course of my work in the ER. I was further instructed not to direct my questions or comments to my colleagues, but rather to the Medical Health Officer (MHO) in charge of the vaccine roll-out for our area, Dr Carol Fenton. I was also informed that my offending email had been sent to The College of Physicians and Surgeons of British Colombia as a complaint.

I accepted my reprimand with humility and agreed to comply with my gag order. But in the days that followed, I began to see an increasing number of alarming neurological problems in my own patients who had received their first dose of the Moderna vaccine. The evidence of harm from the gene-based vaccines was no longer just in Europe, it was happening to my own patients.

I sent a letter to the designated MHO to ask what these new medically induced diseases were, and how as a doctor I should treat them. I received no response, but instead, she sent my letter to the College of Physicians and Surgeons as a further complaint.

I had to find answers, and I needed to alert others. I drafted a letter to the Provincial Health Officer of BC, Dr Bonnie Henry, asking her the same questions. I also questioned the ethics of continuing to administer an experimental treatment that was clearly causing harm. This too, was sent to the College as another complaint.

I had been warned by a colleague that Dr Bonnie Henry does not reply to letters, and was told that, if I wanted any sort of response, it needed to be an open letter, which I duly wrote. In it, I recorded the number of my patients vaccinated, and the number of neurological injuries so far. The vaccine injury rate in my patients after their first Covid vaccine was 1 in 125, with one vaccine-induced sudden death. This was in stark contrast to the fact that not one single patient had been brought to our ER requiring care for Covid. Hence, by April 2021, it was clearly apparent to me that the vaccine was more dangerous than Covid.

Dr Bonnie Henry's response to my letter was to refer the matter to her top vaccine safety specialist, Dr Monica Naus, who offered me a telephone consultation. I asked her the same questions, namely the mechanism of injury, the suggested treatment, and whether it was ethical to continue the vaccine rollout in view of the evidence of harm. She had no answers.

However, Dr Naus confidently assured me that all of the vaccine injuries that I had seen in my patients were not vaccine injuries. She claimed, without any assessment of my patients, that their new signs and symptoms were either coincidences, or may have been caused by poor injection technique. I had been a family physician to these people for 28 years and knew them very well. There was no other medical explanation for their new medical problems. To call them coincidences was scientifically and logically absurd.

I told Dr Naus of my desperate efforts to find a neurologist who would urgently assess my six most badly injured patients. I had tried at three large tertiary hospitals, but whenever I mentioned the vaccine, the neurologist would go silent on the phone, and then tell me it was not their field. I could not find a single neurologist who would urgently assess my unfortunate patients to establish a diagnosis and give me guidance on how to treat them. Her advice, to overcome this resistance, was to simply not tell the neurologist that it was from the vaccine.

Clearly, the issue of the Covid vaccines is sacred ground where doctors feared to tread. I was on my own.

The only advice from Dr Naus was to submit vaccine injury reports. I asked her if this would trigger an investigation into the medical cause for these new diseases. She informed me that it would not, and that it was simply for statistical purposes. Clearly, public health had no interest in the alarming safety signal that I had seen in my own patients.

The irony of this was glaring. All the draconian Covid restrictions were done in the name of "safety". However, the absolute refusal of public health to acknowledge the safety signals from the novel vaccine showed that the public health measures were certainly not about safety. They were about enforcing compliance and control. They were simply determined to get as many people vaccinated as possible, in the shortest possible time, regardless of the human cost. Time and truth go hand in hand, and time will reveal the true motive.

My open letter to Dr Bonnie Henry, announcing the high rate of neurological injuries from the Moderna vaccine in my own patients, generated interest around the world. I appeared to be one of the first doctors to draw attention to this, and requests for interviews rolled in. My passion for advocating for the safety of my patients, regardless of the personal cost to me, clearly antagonised public health, who discovered that my moral integrity was stronger than their threats and warnings.

The first response of the College of Physicians and Surgeons to my open letter, announcing the vaccine safety signal in my patients, was to issue a warning to all doctors across Canada about spreading Covid misinformation. They appeared to consider any mention of vaccine injury, or early treatment options for Covid, to be misinformation. They warned that offending doctors would be investigated and might be disciplined. This threat was highly effective in creating an illusion of consensus in the medical community. Sadly, the majority of doctors failed to have enough courage or moral integrity to take a stand against falsehood in the face of opposition, and at the risk of personal loss.

Three weeks after my open letter, a vaccine injured patient came into our ER. I knew the patient well. I had been family doctor to her and her family for almost three decades. I knew that she and her family had all had Covid infections five weeks prior. Their Covid symptoms had been uniformly mild, but the Covid vaccine had made her significantly unwell, leading her to the ER. The fact that her Covid symptoms had been so mild showed that she had natural immunity. Clearly the Covid vaccine was more dangerous to her than Covid.

I informed the ER nurse of the research done at Duke University, Singapore, published in July 2020. When COVID-19 appeared, scientists had no idea how long natural immunity to this new virus might last, or how broad the protection against new variants might be. So, in 2020 scientists recruited people who had recovered from the first SARS in 2002/3, to see if they still had T-cell immunity 18 years later. Hallelujah, they did! They then tested to see whether that immunity would extend to SARS CoV-2, which was 20% different genetically. And again, they were immune. The relevance of this was that if natural immunity could protect us against a variant that was 20% different, it would have no difficulty protecting us against any of the known variants that were all less than 1% different from the original Wuhan strain.

I told the emergency room nurse to tell the vaccine injured patient, who had proven natural immunity, that she did not need her second shot. The nurse informed me that she was not allowed to tell anyone that they did not need a Covid shot.

The fallout of that conversation with the emergency room nurse was that I was fired from the emergency room, where I had served our community for almost three decades. I instantly lost 50% of my income. When I broke the shocking news to my wife and four children, they simply listened in silent disbelief. But the worst was still to come.

Fortunately, I still had a medical license and was therefore permitted to work in my private practice as a family doctor. As I dutifully submitted vaccine injury reports on my patients, the medical health officer, Dr Carol Fenton, to whom the reports were directed, held media briefings assuring the public that there were no significant vaccine injuries or evidence of harm. She claimed that my public announcements of vaccine injuries were unsubstantiated. This was hard to believe. I wondered why she ignored my vaccine injury reports, or why she refused to speak to either me, or my patients about their injuries. Instead, public health simply denied any evidence of harm.

After submitting 14 vaccine injury reports on my patients, and receiving 100% rejection from public health, I realised it was a futile exercise. Public health insisted that they were all coincidences. It became clear to me that the Canadian vaccine injury reporting system was censored. This enabled them to continue reassuring the public that the vaccine injuries were extraordinarily rare. I gave up trying to report any further vaccine injuries. Consequently, none of my 32 vaccine injured patients would ever qualify for government compensation.

My open letter announcing the vaccine injuries in my patients, had attracted the attention of doctors and scientists from around the world. I was invited to join a distinguished international group called "Doctors for Covid Ethics", with whom I had weekly zoom meetings. We tried to discover the nature of the injuries being caused by the Covid shots.

Dr. Byram Bridle had revealed the Pfizer bio-distribution study performed on laboratory animals, which had been published in Japanese. He had it translated into English. The study demonstrated that contrary to the claims of the vaccine manufacturers, the delivery system of the RNA vaccines (the lipid nanocapsule), enabled the vaccine to reach every part of the body.

Before the pandemic, lipid nanocapsules had been used as a delivery system for chemotherapy, since it penetrated every part of the human body, even the brain.

Dr. Sucharit Bhakdi theorised that since absorption from the bloodstream occurred predominantly in capillary networks, where blood circulation slows right down, it was entirely predictable that the majority of spike proteins would be formed in the cells surrounding the blood vessels, the vascular endothelium. Spike proteins are normally part of the viral capsule, so in a human cell they would become part of the cell wall. Vascular endothelium is supposed to be very smooth, for the unimpeded flow of blood. But once it contains spike proteins, the spikes would protrude into the vessel, creating a rough surface. The purpose of blood platelets is to adhere to rough surfaces in blood vessels, which the body interprets as a damaged vessel needing to be blocked, to stop bleeding from an injury. Therefore, it is inevitable that clotting will occur in any vessel lined by spike proteins. Because the majority of spikes will be formed in capillaries, the clots would be microscopic and scattered throughout the body, thus undetectable to medical imaging. So, how could this theory be tested?

The d-dimer test is performed in emergency rooms where suspicion of a blood clot exists. It does not tell you where the blood clot is, it simply indicates that a recent blood clot has formed. I began asking my patients who were shortly to receive their Covid shot if they would be willing to have their Covid shot monitored, to see if hidden microscopic blood clots were occurring. The plan was to check the d-dimer level before their shot, to establish a baseline for that patient, and then again four to eight days after the shot. Unfortunately, the majority of patients that I recruited had already had a shot in the previous eight days, so I nevertheless checked their d-dimer levels. All information could be useful.

By the time I received the results on the first eight people, five out of the eight had a positive d-dimer. I was horrified. In this small preliminary sample, 62% had evidence of clotting within eight days of their Covid injection. I had drafted letters that I sent to Doctors for Covid Ethics to try to recruit doctors from around the world to assist in this research, so that different vaccine types and batches could be compared, and a large number of subjects obtained. I had expected perhaps 5% evidence of clotting, but when it was 62%, I simply could not keep silent.

My frequent interviewers constantly asked about what I was seeing in my patients from the Covid shots. In a television interview with Laura Lynn Tyler Thompson, I told her about my findings and the proposed mechanism of injury that explained the neurological harm that I had seen. The evidence of micro clotting that I described immediately went viral around the world. That video was subtitled into numerous languages, and a documentary was made using my voice explanation taken from that interview.

The relevance of my findings was firstly, that the blood clots were not rare, but occurring in the majority of people vaccinated. However, because they were microscopic, they were hidden and obscured by a multitude of vague symptoms, depending on where the majority of the clots occurred. Secondly, these were not people with symptoms of vaccine injury. These were people who thought their shot was keeping them safe. They had no idea that they had been vaccine injured. Thirdly, the damage was permanent. Clotted vessels never return to normal. The damage is hidden, it is permanent, and it will accumulate with every shot.

In late June 2021, Western Canada sweltered in a record-breaking three-day heat wave. The small town of Lytton, BC, where I live and work, was frequently known as the hotspot of Canada. On June 29, 2021, the temperature peaked at 49.6°C, the hottest temperature ever recorded in Canada. The humidity was 9%. Everything was dried to a crisp.

The following day, June 30, the temperature dropped to a merciful 40°C. It was a Wednesday, and I was in my clinic. In the late afternoon something ignited a fire on the outskirts of town. It literally exploded as a fire storm, fanned by a 70 kph wind. In 23 minutes the entire town was engulfed in flames as burning tar shingles from roofs flew through the air like incendiary bombs, setting new fires wherever they landed. The occupants of the town fled in terror. Ninety percent of the town was eradicated, including my medical practice, the medical facility and the laboratory where the d-dimer tests were being done. I fled the burning building with my d-dimer research, and the records of my vaccine injured patients, but lost all else. By the grace of God, my home did not burn, as it was in a small subdivision upwind of the fire, which survived. But the loss of my medical practice, and the health facility where the d-dimer tests were being done, spelled the end of my vaccine surveillance efforts. My patients were scattered to the four winds and all those whose homes were not burned, were evacuated across a vast area.

In late 2021, after vaccinating most Canadian adults, the government announced their intention to vaccinate children down to six months of age. By that time, the Covid vaccines had broken all records for death and disability. Epidemiological data for COVID-19 showed that the risk to children was almost zero. Not a single healthy child or adolescent had died of Covid in Canada. Vaccinating children with the most harmful medical product ever rolled out upon humanity, to protect them against a disease that posed no risk to them, had no benign explanation. Again, I could not keep silent.

In December, 2021, I joined another BC family doctor, Dr Stephen Malthouse, and went on a series of speaking tours across western Canada trying to warn the public about the dangers to children. The College had already issued its warning to doctors regarding "Covid misinformation," and these speaking tours, which covered about 40 Canadian cities, clearly antagonised the authorities, who were desperately trying to conceal the risk of harm.

The Pfizer biodistribution study on laboratory animals revealed that the ovaries were amongst the top four destinations for vaccine deposition. When a baby girl is born, she has all of the eggs in her ovaries that she will ever have. If any are damaged or lost, they cannot be regenerated, therefore anything that damages ovaries will impair fertility. Since the spike proteins are known to cause clotting, bleeding, inflammation, and gene editing, having a large number in the ovaries would predictably reduce fertility.

In Canada, most university enrolment was dependent upon proof of vaccination; and participation in sport and school activities required vaccination. As vaccination did not stop transmission of the virus, and since Covid was almost zero risk to children, there was no benign explanation for the vaccine mandates for students. This clearly appeared to be a population control tactic.

In February 2022, I received a phone call from a Global News reporter in Toronto asking for comments on my citation. I was bewildered, and asked her to explain. She informed me that the College of Physicians and Surgeons of BC had issued a citation against me. I went to the College website and discovered that the College was accusing me of professional misconduct, for speaking about vaccine-related neurological injury, micro clotting, vaccine induced deaths, infertility, risks to children and the treatment of COVID-19 with ivermectin. They announced to the national media that I was under investigation for professional misconduct, and if guilty would be disciplined.

I was amazed that the College had chosen to broadcast their accusations in the national media without informing me. This appeared to be designed as yet another warning to all other doctors out there to obediently toe the party line, or face the consequences. Yet another threat to the medical profession to induce the illusion of consensus.

The relentless efforts of public health to conceal the evidence of harm by persecuting whistleblowers, threatening doctors, and censoring or ignoring vaccine injury reporting are still ongoing.

As my trial approaches, I have eight world-class doctors and scientists as expert witnesses to address each of the points of accusation against me. By the grace of God, they have all offered their expertise pro bono. They are Dr Peter McCullough, Dr Pierre Kory, Dr James Thorpe, Dr Claire Craig, Dr Jessica Rose, Dr Steven Pelech, Dr Eric Payne and Dr Kevan McKernan. The College of Physicians and Surgeons has chosen one expert witness, Dr Trevor Corneil, a family physician with a specialty in public health and epidemiology. My eight expert witnesses have submitted a total of 967 pages of testimony.

When the College saw the mountain of evidence stacked against them, they once again tried to bury the evidence. Nine days before the last scheduled date of trial, (which was subsequently adjourned), they applied for judicial notice, a legal tactic where a court declares certain facts to be irrefutable. The College asked for their list of "Facts" regarding safety and effectiveness of Covid vaccines to be declared irrefutable. If granted, this would prevent me from offering any defence, and would preclude my eight expert witnesses from testifying about the evidence of harm from the vaccines. This legal principle of judicial notice has been widely misused to pervert the course of justice during the pandemic.

A disciplinary hearing by the College of Physicians and Surgeons is a quasi-legal process. It carries legal weight in terms of evidence and punishment, but is judged by a disciplinary panel who are appointed and employed by the College. So, by their very nature, this may not be an impartial jury. They work for the College. It is therefore very encouraging that, by the grace of God, the disciplinary panel did not grant the wishes of the College to conceal the evidence of harm by granting judicial notice to the "Facts" of safety and effectiveness. The dishonesty of that application is just too blatant.

The College has sought to discipline me for revealing the evidence of harm from the Covid vaccines in my patients, and in the wider public. As an early whistleblower, I appear to be their chosen scapegoat, used to intimidate other doctors into silence and compliance. They have vast state-sponsored legal resources, while I must shoulder the cost of my own defence with the help of crowdfunding. This is David vs Goliath, and the personal cost has been enormous. Through all of this, I am banished from the emergency room after more than 30 years of dedicated service. My medical practice is burned, my marriage ended after 35 years and my children, estranged. I now face the possibility of losing my medical license and receiving a crippling fine by the College.

I have done what I have done as my duty, both as a Christian and a doctor. I cannot stand idly by and watch others being hurt. To do that, would be complicit in their harm. My patients are 70% Canadian First Nation people. They are beautiful, gentle, humble and simple folk who trusted the government and were betrayed. I have been their advocate and their defender. It has cost me much, but I have no regrets.

"All that it takes for evil to triumph, is for good people to do nothing." (Edmund Burke)

To God be the glory.

CHAPTER 7

The Psychology of Totalitarianism

From rationalism to mass formation and towards Truth speech

Professor Mattias Desmet

Professor of Psychology at Ghent University, Belgium.

Mattias Desmet is a professor of psychology at Ghent University, Belgium and author of The Psychology of Totalitarianism. He articulated the theory of mass formation during the COVID-19 pandemic. Desmet is the author of over one hundred peer-reviewed academic papers. In 2018 he received the Evidence-Based Psychoanalytic Case Study Prize of the Association for Psychoanalytic Psychotherapy, and in 2019 he received the Wim Trijsburg Prize of the Dutch Association of Psychotherapy.

At the end of February 2020, the global village began to shake on its foundations. The world was presented with a foreboding crisis, the consequences of which were incalculable. In a matter of weeks, everyone was gripped by the story of a virus—a story that was undoubtedly based on facts. But on which ones? We caught a first glimpse of "the facts" via footage from China. A virus forced the Chinese government to take the most draconian measures. Entire cities were quarantined, new hospitals were built hastily, and individuals in white suits disinfected public spaces. Here and there, rumors emerged that the totalitarian Chinese government was overreacting and that the new virus was no worse than the flu. Opposite opinions were also floating around: that it must be much worse than it looked, because otherwise no government would take such radical measures. At that point, everything still felt far removed from our shores and we assumed that the story did not allow us to gauge the full extent of the facts.

Until the moment that the virus arrived in Europe. We then began recording infections and deaths for ourselves. We saw images of overcrowded emergency rooms in Italy, convoys of army vehicles transporting corpses, morgues full of coffins. The renowned scientists at Imperial College confidently predicted that without the most drastic measures, the virus would claim tens of millions of lives. In Bergamo, sirens blared day and night, silencing any voice in a public space that dared to doubt the emerging narrative. From then on, story and facts seemed to merge and uncertainty gave way to certainty.

The unimaginable became reality: we witnessed the abrupt pivot of nearly every country on earth to follow China's example and place huge populations of people under de facto house arrest, a situation for which the term "lockdown" was coined. An eerie silence descended—ominous and liberating at the same time. The sky without airplanes, traffic arteries without vehicles; dust settling on the standstill of billions of people's individual pursuits and desires. In India, the air became so pure that, for the first time in thirty years, in some places the Himalayas became once more visible against the horizon.

It didn't stop there. We also saw a remarkable transfer of power. Expert virologists were called upon as Orwell's pigs—the smartest animals on the farm—to replace the unreliable politicians. They would run the animal farm with accurate ("scientific") information. But these experts soon turned out to have quite a few common, human flaws. In their statistics and graphs they made mistakes that even "ordinary" people would not easily make. It went so far that, at one point, they counted *all* deaths as corona deaths, including people who had died of, say, heart attacks.

Nor did they live up to their promises. These experts pledged that the Gates to Freedom would re-open after two doses of the vaccine, but then they contrived the need for a third. Like Orwell's pigs, they changed the rules overnight. First, the animals had to comply with the measures because the number of sick people could not exceed the capacity of the health care system (*flatten the curve*). But one day, everyone woke up to discover writing on the walls stating that the measures were being extended because the virus had to be eradicated (*crush the curve*). Eventually, the rules changed so often that only the pigs seemed to know them. And even the pigs weren't so sure.

Some people began to nurture suspicions. How is it possible that these experts make mistakes that even laymen wouldn't make? Aren't they scientists, the kind of people who took us to the moon and gave us the internet? They can't be that stupid, can they? What is their endgame? Their recommendations take us further down the road in the same direction: with each new step, we lose more of our freedoms, until we reach a final destination where human beings are reduced to QR codes in a large technocratic medical experiment.

That's how most people eventually became certain. Very certain. But of diametrically opposed viewpoints. Some people became certain that we were dealing with a killer virus, that would kill millions. Others became certain that it was nothing more than the seasonal flu. Still others became certain that the virus did not even exist and that we were dealing with a worldwide conspiracy. And there were also a few who continued to tolerate uncertainty and kept asking themselves: how can we adequately understand what is going on?

* * *

In the beginning of the coronavirus crisis I found myself making a choice—I would speak out. Before the crisis, I frequently lectured at University and I presented on academic conferences worldwide. When the crisis started, I intuitively decided that I would speak out in public space, this time not addressing the academic world, but society in general. I would speak out and try to bring to peoples' attention that there was something dangerous out there, not "the virus" itself so much as the fear and technocratic–totalitarian social dynamics it was stirring up.

I was in a good position to warn for the psychological risks of the corona narrative. I could draw on my knowledge of individual psychological processes (I am a lecturing professor at Ghent University, Belgium); my PhD on the dramatically poor quality of academic research which taught me that we can never take "science" for granted; my master degree in statistics which allowed me to see through statistical deception and illusions; my knowledge of mass psychology; my philosophical explorations of the limits and destructive psychological effects of the mechanist-rationalist view on man and the world; and last but not least, my investigations into the effects of speech on the human being and the quintessential importance of "Truth Speech" in particular.

In the first week of the crisis, March 2020, I published an opinion paper titled "The Fear of the Virus Is More Dangerous Than the Virus Itself." I had analyzed the statistics and mathematical models on which the coronavirus narrative was based and immediately saw that they all dramatically overrated the dangerousness of the virus. A few months later, by the end of May 2020, this impression had been confirmed beyond the shadow of a doubt. There were no countries, including those that didn't go into lockdown, in which the virus claimed the enormous number of casualties the models predicted it would. Sweden was perhaps the best example. According to the models, at least 60,000 people would die if the country didn't go into lockdown. It didn't, and only 6,000 people died.

As much as I (and others) tried to bring this to the attention of society, it didn't have much effect. People continued to go along with the narrative. That was the moment when I decided to focus on something else, namely on the psychological processes that were at work in society and that could explain how people can become so radically blind and continue to buy into a narrative so utterly absurd. It took me a few months to realize that what was going on in society was a worldwide process of *mass formation*.

In the summer of 2020, I wrote an opinion paper about this phenomenon which soon became well known in Holland and Belgium. About one year later (summer 2021) Reiner Fuellmich invited me onto *Corona Ausschuss,* a weekly live-stream discussion between lawyers and both experts and witnesses about the coronavirus crisis, to explain about mass formation. From there, my theory spread to the rest of Europe and the United States, where it was picked up by such people as Dr. Robert Malone, Dr. Peter McCullough, Michael Yeadon, Eric Clapton, and Robert Kennedy. After Robert Malone talked about mass formation on the Joe Rogan Experience, the term became a buzzword and for a few days was the most searched for term on Twitter. Since then, my theory has met with enthusiasm but also with harsh criticism. Despite this, I will continue to explore the concept of mass formation, apply it to contemporary phenomena, respond to criticism, and relate it to all kinds of other psychological phenomena.

What is mass formation actually? It's a specific kind of group formation that makes people radically blind to everything that goes against what the group believes in. In this way, they take the most absurd beliefs for granted. To give one example, during the Iran revolution in 1979, a mass formation emerged and people started to believe that the portrait of their leader—Ayatollah Khomeini—was visible on the surface of the moon. Each time there was a full moon in the sky, people in the street would point at it, showing each other where exactly Khomeini's face could be seen.

A second characteristic of an individual in the grip of mass formation is that they become willing to radically sacrifice individual interest for the sake of the collective. The communist leaders who were sentenced to death by Stalin—usually innocent of the charges against them—accepted their sentences, sometimes with statements such as, "If that is what I can do for the communist party, I will do it with pleasure."

Thirdly, individuals in mass formation become radically intolerant of dissonant voices. In the ultimate stage of the mass formation, they will typically commit atrocities toward those who do not go along with the masses. And even more characteristic: they will do so as if it is their ethical duty. To refer to the revolution in Iran again: I've spoken with an Iranian woman who had seen with her own eyes how a mother reported her son to the state and hung the noose with her own hands around his neck when he was on the scaffold. And after he was killed, she claimed to be a heroine for doing what she did.

Those are the effects of mass formation. Such processes can emerge in different ways. It can emerge spontaneously (as happened in Nazi Germany), or it can be intentionally provoked through indoctrination and propaganda (as happened in the Soviet Union). But if it is not constantly supported by indoctrination and propaganda disseminated through mass media, it will usually be short-lived and will not develop into a full-fledged totalitarian state. Whether it initially emerged spontaneously or was provoked intentionally from the beginning, no mass formation, however, can continue to exist for any length of time unless it is constantly fed by indoctrination and propaganda disseminated through mass media. If this happens, mass formation becomes the basis of an entirely new kind of state that emerged for the first time in the beginning of the twentieth century: the totalitarian state. This kind of state has an extremely destructive impact on the population because it doesn't only control public and political space—as classical dictatorships do—but also private space. It can do the latter because it has a huge secret police at its disposal: this part of the population that is in the grip of the mass formation and that fanatically believes in the narratives distributed by the elite through mass media. In this way, totalitarianism is always based on "a diabolic pact between the masses and the elite" (see Arendt, *The Origins of Totalitarianism*).

I second an intuition articulated by Hannah Arendt in 1951: a new totalitarianism is emerging in our society. Not a communist or fascist totalitarianism but a technocratic totalitarianism. A kind of totalitarianism that is not led by "a gang leader" such as Stalin or Hitler but by dull bureaucrats and technocrats. As always, a certain part of the population will resist and won't fall prey to the mass formation. If this part of the population makes the right choices, it will ultimately be victorious. If it makes the wrong choices, it will perish. To see what the right choices are, we have to start from a profound and accurate analysis of the nature of the phenomenon of mass formation. If we do so, we will clearly see what the right choices are, both at strategic and at the ethical levels. That's what my book *The Psychology of Totalitarianism* presents: a historical–psychological analysis of the rise of the masses throughout the last few hundreds of years as it led to the emergence of totalitarianism.

* * *

The coronavirus crisis did not come out of the blue. It fits into a series of increasingly desperate and self-destructive societal responses to objects of fear: terrorists, global warming, coronavirus. Whenever a new object of fear arises in society, there is only one response: increased control. Meanwhile, human beings can only tolerate a certain amount of control. Coercive control leads to fear and fear leads to more coercive control. In this way, society falls victim to a vicious cycle that leads inevitably to totalitarianism (i.e., extreme government control) and ends in the radical destruction of both the psychological and physical integrity of human beings.

We have to consider the current fear and psychological discomfort to be a problem in itself, a problem that cannot be reduced to a virus or any other "object of threat." Our fear originates on a completely different level—that of the failure of the Grand Narrative of our society. This is the narrative of mechanistic science, in which man is reduced to a biological organism. A narrative that ignores the psychological, spiritual, and ethical dimensions of human beings and thereby has a devastating effect at the level of human relationships. Something in this narrative causes man to become isolated from his fellow man, and from nature. Something in it causes man to stop *resonating* with the world around him. Something in it turns human beings into *atomized subjects*. It is precisely this atomized subject that, according to Hannah Arendt, is the elementary building block of the totalitarian state.

At the level of the population, the mechanist ideology created the conditions that make people vulnerable for mass formation. It disconnected people from their natural and social environment, created experiences of radical absence of meaning and purpose in life, and it led to extremely high levels of so-called "free-floating" anxiety, frustration, and aggression, meaning anxiety, frustration, and aggression that is not connected with a mental representation; anxiety, frustration, and aggression in which people don't know what they feel anxious, frustrated, and aggressive about. It is in this state that people become vulnerable to mass formation.

The mechanist ideology also had a specific effect at the level of the "elite"—it changed their psychological characteristics. Before the Enlightenment, society was led by noblemen and clergy (the "ancien régime"). This elite imposed its will on the masses in an overt way through its authority. This authority was granted by the religious Grand Narratives that held a firm grip on people's minds. As the religious narratives lost their grip and modern democratic ideology emerged, this changed. The leaders now had to be *elected* by the masses. And in order to be elected by the masses, they had to find out what the masses wanted and more or less give it to them. Hence, the leaders actually became *followers*.

This problem was met in a rather predictable but pernicious way. If the masses cannot be commanded, they have to be *manipulated*. That's where modern indoctrination and propaganda was born, as it is described in the works of people such as Lippman, Trotter, and Bernays. We will go through the work of the founding fathers of propaganda in order to fully grasp the societal function and impact of propaganda on society. Indoctrination and propaganda are usually associated with totalitarian states such as the Soviet Union, Nazi Germany, or the People's Republic of China. But it is easy to show that from the beginning of the twentieth century, indoctrination and propaganda were also constantly used in virtually every "democratic" state worldwide. Besides these two, we will describe other techniques of mass-manipulation, such as brainwashing and psychological warfare.

In modern times, the explosive proliferation of mass surveillance technology led to new and previously unimaginable means for the manipulation of the masses. And emerging technological advances promise a completely new set of manipulation techniques, where the mind is materially manipulated through technological devices inserted in the human body and brain. At least that's the plan. It's not clear yet to what extent the mind will cooperate.

* * *

Totalitarianism is not a historical coincidence. It is the logical consequence of mechanistic thinking and the delusional belief in the omnipotence of human rationality. As such, totalitarianism is a defining feature of the Enlightenment tradition. Several authors have postulated this, but it hasn't yet been subjected to a psychological analysis. I decided to try to fill this gap, which is why I wrote *The Psychology of Totalitarianism*. It analyzes the psychology of totalitarianism and situates it within the broader context of the social phenomena of which it forms a part.

It is not my aim with the book to focus on that which is usually associated with totalitarianism—concentration camps, indoctrination, propaganda—but rather the broader cultural–historical processes from which totalitarianism emerges. This approach allows us to focus on what matters most: the conditions that surround us in our daily lives, from which totalitarianism takes root, grows, and thrives.

Ultimately, my book explores the possibilities of finding a way out of the current cultural impasse in which we appear to be stuck. The escalating social crises of the early twenty-first century are the manifestation of an underlying psychological and ideological upheaval—a shift of the tectonic plates on which a worldview rests. We are experiencing the moment in which an old ideology rears up in power, one last time, before collapsing. Each attempt to remediate the current social problems, whatever they may be, on the basis of the old ideology will only make things worse. One cannot solve a problem using the same mindset that created it. The solution to our fear and uncertainty does not lie in the increase of (technological) control. The real task facing us as individuals and as a society is to envision a new view of humankind and the world, to find a new foundation for our identity, to formulate new principles for living together with others, and to reclaim a timely human capacity—Truth Speech.

A Note to Our Readers

Thank you for taking the time to read Canary In a (Post) Covid World: Money, Fear, and Power. Please help us spread the word, we'd be incredibly grateful if you could share your thoughts by leaving a rating and review on Amazon. Your feedback is our primary way of reaching new readers and helps others discover the book. Every review makes a big difference in spreading the word and encouraging more people to explore these important perspectives. Thank you for your support!

CHAPTER 8

Healing a Divided Nation: The Fight for Free Speech, Health, and Peace

Robert F. Kennedy Jr.

Environmental activist, attorney and advocate
for public health and civil liberties

Robert F. Kennedy Jr. is a renowned attorney, environmental activist, and advocate for public health and civil liberties. His legal career began in the early 1980s, but he rose to prominence in 1985 as an attorney for Riverkeeper, where his victories in environmental law helped protect the Hudson River. His work earned him accolades like TIME Magazine's "Hero of the Planet", and he co-founded the Waterkeeper Alliance, now the largest nonprofit devoted to clean water, mobilizing over a million volunteers across 47 countries.

Kennedy has spent nearly 40 years challenging corporate and government corruption, winning landmark cases against companies like General Electric and ExxonMobil. Beyond environmentalism, he is a leading advocate for vaccine safety, raising concerns about pharmaceutical influence on public health policies. As chairman of Children's Health Defense, he has been a vocal critic of the COVID-19 vaccine rollout, advocating for transparency and the rights of individuals to make informed medical decisions.

He is the son of Senator Robert F. Kennedy and the nephew of President John F. Kennedy, both of whom were assassinated while serving their country. A lifelong Democrat, Kennedy became estranged from the party in recent years, and in 2023, he announced his independent candidacy for President of the United States, driven by his commitment to freedom, accountability, and transparency.

Kennedy's dedication to civil liberties, medical freedom, and environmental justice continues to inspire those who believe in the importance of challenging powerful institutions and advocating for the public good.

This essay is based upon a speech given by Robert F. Kennedy Jr. on August 23rd 2024 announcing the suspension of his presidential campaign. It is included in this book thanks to the generosity and approval of RFK Jr.

In April of 2023, I launched my campaign for president of the United States. I began this journey as a Democrat, which is the party of my father, and my uncle. It is the party to which I pledge my own allegiance. Long before I was old enough to vote, I attended my first democratic convention at the age of six in 1960, and back then, the Democrats were the champions of the Constitution and of civil rights.

The Democrats stood against authoritarianism, against censorship, against colonialism, imperialism, and unjust wars. We were the party of labor, of the working class. The Democrats were the party of government transparency and the champion of the environment. Our party was the bulwark against big money interests and corporate power. True to its name, it was the party of democracy.

As you know, I left that party in October 2023 because it had departed so dramatically from the core values that I grew up with. It had become the party of war, censorship, corruption, Big Pharma, big tech, big ag and big money. When it abandoned democracy by canceling the primary to conceal the cognitive decline of the sitting president, I left the party to run as an independent.

The mainstream of American politics and journalism derided my decision. Conventional wisdom said that it would be impossible even to get on the ballot as an independent, because each state poses an insurmountable tangle of arbitrary rules for collecting signatures. I would need over a million signatures, something no presidential candidate in history had ever achieved, and then I'd need a team of attorneys and millions of dollars to handle all the legal challenges from the DNC.

The naysayers told us that we were climbing a glass version of Mount impossible. So the first thing I want to tell you is that we proved them wrong. We did it because beneath the radar of mainstream media organs, we inspired a massive independent political movement, more than 100,000 volunteers sprang into action, hopeful that they could reverse our nation's decline. Many work 10 hour days, sometimes in blizzards and blazing heat.

They sacrificed family time, personal commitments and sleep, month after month, energized by a shared vision of a nation healed of its divisions, they set up tables at churches and farmers markets. They canvassed door to door in Utah and in New Hampshire.

Volunteers collected signatures in snowstorms, convincing each supporter to stop in the frigid cold, to take off their gloves and to sign legibly during a heat wave in Nevada. I met a tall, athletic volunteer who cheerfully told me that he had lost 25 pounds collecting signatures in 117 degree heat.

To finance this effort, young Americans donated their lunch money, and senior citizens gave up their part of their social security checks. Our 50 state organization collected those millions of signatures and more. No presidential campaign in American political history has ever done that, and so I want to thank all of those dedicated volunteers and congratulate the campaign staff who coordinated this enormous logistical feat.

Your accomplishments were regarded as impossible. You carried me up that glass mountain. You pulled off a miracle. You achieved what all the pundits said could never be done. You have my deepest gratitude, and I'm never going to forget that, not just for what you did for my campaign, but for the sacrifices you made because you love our country.

You showed to everyone that democracy is still possible here, it continues to survive in the press and in the idealistic human energies that still thrive beneath a canvas of neglect and of official and institutional corruption.

Today, I'm here to tell you that I will not allow your efforts to go to waste. I'm here to tell you that I will leverage your tremendous accomplishments to serve the ideals that we share, the ideals of peace, of prosperity, of freedom, of health, all the ideals that motivated my campaign.

I'm here today to describe the path forward that you've opened with your commitment and with your hard labors. Now in an honest system, I believe that I would have won the election. In a system that my father and my uncles thrived in, a system with open debates, with fair primaries, and with a truly independent media, untainted by government propaganda and censorship, and a system of nonpartisan courts and election boards, everything would be different.

After all, the polls consistently showed me beating each of the other candidates, both in favorability and also in head-to-head matchups. But I'm sorry to say that while democracy may still be alive at the grassroots, it has become little more than a slogan for our political institutions, for our media and for our government, and most sadly of all for me, the Democratic Party.

In the name of saving democracy, the Democratic Party set itself to dismantling it, lacking confidence in its candidate that this candidate could win in a fair election at the voting booth.

The DNC waged continual legal warfare against both President Trump and myself. Each time our volunteers turned in those towering boxes of signatures needed to get on the ballot, the DNC dragged us into court, state after state, attempting to erase their work and to subvert the will of the voters who had signed those petitions. It deployed DNC-aligned judges to throw me and other candidates off the ballot and to throw President Trump in jail.

It ran a sham primary that was rigged to prevent any serious challenge to President Biden. Then when a predictably bungled debate performance precipitated the palace coup against President Biden, the same shadowy DNC operatives appointed his successor, also without an election. They installed a candidate who was so unpopular with voters that she dropped out in 2020 without winning a single delegate.

My uncle and my father both relished debate. They prided themselves on their capacity to go toe to toe with any opponent and the battle over ideas. They would be astonished to learn of a Democratic Party presidential nominee who, like vice president Harris, has not appeared in a single interview or an unscripted encounter with voters for 35 days.

This is profoundly undemocratic. How are people to choose when they don't know whom they are choosing? How can this look to the rest of the world? My father and my uncle were always conscious of America's image abroad because of our nation's role as the template for democracy, the role model for democratic processes, and the leader of the free world. Instead of showing us her substance and character, the DNC and its media organs engineered a surge of popularity for vice president Harris based upon nothing, no policies, no interviews, no debates, only smoke and mirrors and balloons in a highly produced Chicago circus.

In Chicago, the democratic speakers mentioned Donald Trump 147 times just on the first day of the convention. *Who needs a policy when you have Trump to hate?*

In contrast, at the RNC convention, President Biden was mentioned only twice in four days. I do interviews every day. Many of you have interviewed me. Anybody who asks gets to interview me. Some days, I do as many as 10. President Trump, who actually was nominated and won an election, also does interviews daily. How did the Democratic Party choose a candidate that has never done an interview or debate during the entire election cycle? We know the answer.

They did it by weaponizing the government agencies. They did it by abandoning democracy. They did it by suing the opposition and by disenfranchising American voters. What most alarms me isn't how the Democratic Party conducts its internal affairs or runs its candidates.

What alarms me is they resort to censorship and media control, and the weaponization of the federal agencies. When a US president colludes with or outright coerces media companies to censor political speech, it's an attack on our most sacred right, that of free expression, and that's the very right upon which all of our other constitutional rights rest.

President Biden mocked Vladimir Putin's 88% landslide in the Russian elections, observing that Putin and his party controlled the Russian press and that Putin prevented serious opponents from appearing on the ballot.

Here in America, the DNC also prevented opponents from appearing on the ballot. Our television networks exposed themselves as Democratic Party organs over the course of more than a year. In a campaign where my poll numbers reached at times in the high 20s, the DNC-allied mainstream media networks maintained a near perfect embargo on interviews with me during this 10-month presidential campaign. By comparison, in 1992 Ross Perot gave 34 interviews on mainstream networks. In contrast, during the sixteen months since I declared, ABC, NBC, CBS, MSNBC and CNN combined, broadcast only two live interviews with me. Those networks instead, ran a continuous deluge of hit pieces with inaccurate, often vile pejoratives and defamatory smears. Some of those same networks colluded with the DNC to keep me off the debate stage.

Representatives of those networks are in this room right now, and I'll just take a moment to ask you to consider the many ways that your institutions have abdicated this really sacred responsibility: the duty of a free press to safeguard democracy and to always challenge the party in power.

Instead of maintaining that posture of fierce skepticism toward authority, your institutions have made themselves government mouthpieces and stenographers for the organs of power. You didn't alone cause the devolution of American democracy, but you could have prevented it.

The Democratic Party's censorship of social media was even more of a naked exercise of executive power. A federal judge, Terry Doughty, upheld my injunction against President Biden calling the White House's censorship project, "The most egregious violation of the First Amendment in the history of the United States of America." ' [The] 155 page decision details how just 37 hours after he took the oath of office, swearing to uphold the Constitution, President Biden and his White House opened up a portal and then invited in the CIA, the FBI, and CISA, which is a censorship Agency.

It's the center of the censorship industrial complex, DHS, the IRS and other agencies. They censor me and other political dissidents on social media. Even today, users who try to post my campaign videos to Facebook or YouTube get messages that this content violates community standards. Two days after Judge Doughty rendered his decision, Facebook was still attaching warning labels to an online petition calling on ABC to include me in the upcoming debate. They said that violates community standards, their community standards.

The mainstream media was once the guardian of the First Amendment and democratic principles, and has joined this systemic attack on democracy. The media justifies their censorship on the grounds of combating misinformation, but governments and oppressors don't censor lies. They don't fear lies. They fear the truth, and that's what they censor. I don't want any of this to sound like a personal complaint, because it's not. For me, it's all part of a journey, and it's a journey that I signed up for. But I need to make these observations, because I think they're critical for us doing the thing that we need to do as citizens in a democracy, to assess where we are in this country and what our democracy still looks like, along with assumptions about US leadership around the globe. Are we living up to these assumptions?

Is this country still a role model for democracy, or have we made it a kind of a joke? Here's the good news; while mainstream outlets denied me a critical platform, they didn't shut down my ideas, which have flourished especially among young voters and independent voters, thanks to the alternative media. Many months ago, I promised the American people that I would withdraw from the race if I became a spoiler that would alter the outcome of the election, but had no chance of winning.

In my heart, I no longer believe that I have a realistic path to electoral victory in the face of this relentless, systematic censorship and media control. So I cannot, in good conscience, ask my staff and volunteers to keep working their long hours, or ask my donors to keep giving, when I cannot honestly tell them that I have a real path to the White House.

Furthermore, our polling consistently showed that by staying on the ballot in the battleground states, I would likely hand the election over to the Democrats with whom I disagree on the most existential issues; censorship, war and chronic disease.

I want everyone to know that I am not terminating my campaign. I am simply suspending it and not not ending it. My name will remain on the ballot in most states. If you live in a blue state, you can vote for me without harming or helping President Trump or vice president Harris and red states, just the same will apply. I encourage you to vote for me. If enough of you do vote for me and neither of the major party candidates win 270 votes, which is quite possible - in August 2024 our polling shows them tying at 269 to 269 - I could conceivably still end up in the White House in a contingent election.

But in about 10 battleground states where my presence would be a spoiler, I'm going to remove my name. I've already started that process and urge voters not to vote for me. It's with a sense of victory and not defeat that I'm suspending my campaign activities.

Not only did we do the impossible by collecting a million signatures, we changed the national political conversation forever; chronic disease, free speech, government corruption, breaking our addiction to war have moved to the center of politics.

I can say to all who have worked so hard, thank you for a job well done.

Three great causes drove me to enter this race in the first place, and these are the principal causes that persuaded me to leave the Democratic

Party to run as an independent, and now to throw my support behind President Trump. The causes were free speech, a war in Ukraine and the war on our children.

I've already described some of my personal experiences and struggles with the government censorship industrial complex. I want to say a word about the Ukraine war.

The Military Industrial Complex has provided us with a familiar comic book justification, as they do in every war. This one goes like this; the war is a noble effort to stop a super villain, Vladimir Putin, invading Ukraine, and then to thwart his Hitler-like march across Europe.

In fact, tiny Ukraine is a proxy in a geopolitical struggle, initiated by the ambitions of the US neocons or American global hegemony. I'm not excusing Putin for invading Ukraine. He had other options. The war is Russia's predictable response to the reckless neocon project of extending NATO to encircle Russia, a hostile act.

The credulous media rarely explained to Americans that we unilaterally walked away from two Intermediate Nuclear Weapons treaties with Russia and then put nuclear missile systems in Romania and Poland. This was a hostile act and the Biden White House repeatedly spurned Russia's offer to settle this war peacefully.

The Ukraine war actually began in 2014 when US agencies overthrew the democratically elected Government of Ukraine and installed a handpicked pro-Western government that launched a deadly civil war against ethnic Russians in Ukraine. In 2019 America walked away from a peace treaty, the Minsk agreement, that had been negotiated between Russia and Ukraine by European nations.

And then in April of 2022 we wanted the war. In April of 2022 President Biden sent Boris Johnson to Ukraine to force President Zelensky to tear up a peace agreement that he and the Russians had already signed. The Russians were withdrawing troops from Kyiv, Donbas and Luhansk.

And that peace agreement would have brought peace to the region, and would have allowed Donbas and Luhansk to remain part of Ukraine.

President Biden stated that month that this object in the war was regime change in Russia. His defense secretary, Lloyd Austin simultaneously explained that America's purpose in the war was to exhaust the Russian army, to degrade its capacity to fight anywhere else in the world.

These objectives, of course, have nothing to do with what they were telling Americans about protecting Ukraine's sovereignty. Ukraine is a victim in this war, and it's a victim of both Russia and the West.

Since then, we have forced Zelensky to tear up the agreement. We've squandered the flower of Ukrainian youth, as many as 600,000 Ukrainian kids and over 100,000 Russian kids, all of whom we should be mourning, have died. Ukraine's infrastructure is destroyed. The war has been a disaster for our country as well. We have squandered nearly $200 billion already; these are badly needed dollars in our communities, suffering communities all over our country.

The Nord Stream pipeline sabotage and the sanctions have destroyed Europe's industrial base, which form the bulwark of national security; a strong Germany with a strong industry is a much stronger deterrent to Russia. A Germany that is deindustrialized and turned into an extension of the US military base, means we push Russia into a disastrous alliance with China and Iran. This brings us closer to the brink of nuclear exchange than at any time since 1962. The neocons and the White House don't seem to care at all. Our moral authority and our economy are in shambles, and the war gave rise to the emergence of brics, which now threatens to replace the dollar as the global reserve currency.

This is a first class calamity for our country. Judging by her bellicose, belligerent speech in Chicago, we can assume that a President Harris will be an enthusiastic advocate for this and other neocon military adventures. President Trump says that he will reopen negotiations with President

Putin and end the war overnight as soon as he becomes president. This alone would justify my support for his campaign.

Last summer, it looked like no candidate was willing to negotiate a quick end to the Ukraine war, to tackle the chronic disease epidemic, to protect free speech, our constitutional freedoms, to clean corporate influence out of our government, or to defy the neocons and their agenda of endless military adventurism.

But now one of the two candidates has adopted these issues as his own, to the point where he has asked to enlist me in his administration. I'm speaking, of course, of Donald Trump.

Less than two hours after President Trump narrowly escaped assassination, Calley Means called me on my cell phone. I was then in Las Vegas. Calley is arguably the leading advocate for food safety, for soil regeneration and for ending the chronic disease epidemic that is destroying America's health and ruining our economy. Calley has exposed the insidious corruption at the FDA and the NIH, the HHS and the USDA that has caused the epidemic.

Calley had been working on and off for my campaign, advising me on those subjects since the beginning and those subjects have been my primary focus for the last 20 years. I was delighted when Calley told me that day that he had also been advising President Trump.

He told me, President Trump was anxious to talk to me about chronic disease and other subjects and to explore avenues of cooperation. He asked if I would take a call from the President. President Trump telephoned me a few minutes later, and I met with him the following day.

A few weeks later, I met again with President Trump and his family members and closest advisers in Florida in a series of long, intense discussions. I was surprised to discover that we are aligned on many key issues.

In those meetings, he suggested that we join forces as a Unity Party. We talked about Abraham Lincoln's Team of Rivals. That arrangement would allow us to disagree publicly and privately and furiously, if need be on issues over which we differ while working together on the existential issues upon which we are in concordance.

I was a ferocious critic of many of the policies during his first administration. There are still issues and approaches upon which we continue to have very serious differences. Still, we are aligned with each other on other key issues, like ending the Forever wars, ending the childhood disease epidemics, securing the border, protecting freedom of speech, unraveling the corporate capture of our regulatory agencies, getting the US intelligence agencies out of the business of propagandizing and censoring and surveilling Americans, and interfering with our elections.

Following my first discussion with President Trump, I tried unsuccessfully to open similar discussions with Vice President Harris. Vice President Harris declined to meet or even to speak with me.

Suspending my candidacy is a heart wreching decision for me. However, I'm convinced that it's the best hope for ending the Ukraine war and ending the chronic disease epidemic that is eroding our nation's vitality from the inside, and for finally, protecting free speech.

I feel a moral obligation to use this opportunity to save millions of American children, above all things. In case some of you don't realize how dire the condition is of our children's health and chronic disease in general, I would urge you to view Tucker Carlson's recent interview with Calley Means and his sister, Dr Casey Means, who was the top graduate of her class at Stanford Medical School.

This is an issue that affects ua all far more directly and urgently than any culture war issue and all the other issues that we obsess over that are tearing apart our country. This is the most important issue, therefore it has the potential to bring us together.

So let me share a little bit about why I believe it's so urgent today. We spend more on health care than any country on Earth; twice what they spend in Europe, and yet we have the worst health outcomes of any nation in the world.

We're about 79th in health outcomes behind Costa Rica, Nicaragua and Mongolia. Nobody has a chronic disease burden as we have in the US. During a covid epidemic, we had the highest body count of any country in the world. We had 16% of the covid deaths, and we only have 4.2% of the world's population. The CDC says that's because we are the sickest people on Earth. We have the highest chronic disease rate on earth, and the average American who died with covid had 3.8 chronic diseases. So these were people who had immune system collapse, who had mitochondrial dysfunction. Two thirds of American adults and children suffer from chronic health issues. Fifty years ago, that number was less than 1%.

We've gone from 1% to 66% . In America, 74% of Americans are now overweight or obese, and 50% of our children. A hundred and twenty years ago when somebody was obese, they were sent to the circus. They were literally case reports done about them. Obesity was almost unknown.

In Japan the childhood obesity rate is 3% compared to 50% in the United States. Half of Americans have pre-diabetes or type two diabetes. When my uncle was president, I was a boy, and juvenile diabetes was effectively non-existent. A typical pediatrician would see one case of diabetes during his entire career, a 40 or 50 year career. Today, one out of every three kids who walks through his office door is diabetic or pre-diabetic. The mitochondrial disorder that has caused diabetes is also causing Alzheimer's, which is now classified as diabetes, and it's costing this country more than our military budget. Every single year.

There's been an explosion of neurological illnesses that I never saw as a kid, ADD, ADHD, speech delay, language delay, Tourette's Syndrome, narcolepsy, ASD, Asperger's, Autism. In the year 2000, the Autism rate was one in 1500. Now, autism rates in kids are one in 36, according to CDC nationally. Nobody's talking about this.

One in every 22 kids in California has Autism. This is a crisis that 77% of our kids are too disabled to serve in the United States military. What is happening to our country, and why isn't this in the headlines every single day?

There's no other country in the world that is experiencing this. This is only happening in America. There has been no change in diagnosis, there has been no change in screening. This is a change in incidents. In my generation, 70-year-old men, the autism rates are about one in 10,000. In my kids' generation, one in 34. I'll repeat, in California, one in 22. Why are we letting this happen? Why are we allowing this to happen to our children? These are the most precious assets that we have. How can we let this happen to them?

About 18% of American teens now have fatty liver disease. That's like one out of every five that have the disease. When I was a kid, it only affected elderly, late stage alcoholics.

Cancer rates are skyrocketing, both for the young and the old. Young adult cancers are up 79%. One in four American women is on antidepressant medication. Forty percent of teens have a mental health diagnosis, and 15% of high schoolers are on Adderall. Half a million children on SSRIs.

So what's causing this suffering?

I'll name two culprits, first and the worst is ultra processed food. About 70% of American children's diet is ultra processed; that means industrial manufactured in a factory. These foods consist primarily of processed sugar, ultra-processed grains, and seed oils.

Laboratory scientists, many of them formerly worked for the cigarette industry, which purchased all the big food companies in the 1970s and 80s, deployed 1000s of scientists to figure out new chemicals to make the food more addictive. These ingredients didn't exist 100 years ago. Humans aren't biologically adapted to consume them. Hundreds of these chemicals are now banned in Europe, but ubiquitous in American processed foods.

The second culprit is toxic chemicals in our food, our medicine, in our environment, pesticides, food additives, pharmaceutical drugs and toxic waste. They permeate every cell of our bodies.

These assaults on our children's cells and hormones are unrelenting. To name just one problem, many of these chemicals increase estrogen. Because young children are ingesting so many of these hormone disruptors, America's puberty rate is now occurring between the ages of 10 to 13, which is six years earlier than girls were reaching puberty in 1900. Our country has the earliest puberty rates of anywhere on earth. And no, this isn't because of better nutrition, this is not normal.

Breast cancer is also estrogen driven, and now strikes one in eight women. We are mass poisoning all of our children and our adults. Considering the grievous human cause of this tragic epidemic of chronic disease, it seems crass to mention the damage it does to our economy, but I'll say it is crippling the nation's finances.

When my uncle was President, our country spent zero dollars on chronic disease. Today, government health care spending is almost all for chronic disease, and it's double the military budget. It's the fastest growing budget item in the federal budget. Chronic disease costs more to the economy as a whole - at least $4,000,000,000,000 - five times our military budget. That's a 20% drag on everything we do and everything we aspire to.

Minority communities suffer disproportionately. People who worry about Diversity Equity and Inclusion, or about bigotry of any kind, this dwarfs all of that. We are poisoning the poor. We are systematically poisoning minorities across this country.

Industry lobbyists have made sure that most of the food stamp lunch program, about 70% of food stamps and 70% of school lunches are processed foods. There's no vegetables. There's nothing that you would want to eat. We are just poisoning the poorest citizens, and that's why they have the highest chronic disease burden of anybody, any demographic, in our country, and the highest in the world.

The same food industry lobbied to make sure that nearly all agricultural subsidies are owed to commodity crops that are the feedstock of the processed food industry. These policies are destroying small farms, and they're destroying our soils. We give about eight times as much in subsidies to tobacco as we do to fruits and vegetables.

It makes no sense if we want a healthy country. The good news is that we can change all this. We can change it very, very quickly. America can get healthy again. To do that, we need to do three things.

First, we need to root out the corruption in our health agencies. Second, we need to change incentives in our healthcare system. And third, we need to inspire Americans to get healthy again.

Eighty percent of NIH grants go to people who have conflicts of interest. Joe Biden just appointed a new panel to NIH to advise on food recommendations, and they're all people from the industry, from the processed food companies. They're deciding what is healthy for Americans and the recommendations on the food pyramid; what goes into our school lunch programs, what goes to the Food Stamp programs.

They are all corrupted and conflicted individuals. These agencies—the FDA, USDA, and CDC—are all controlled by giant for-profit corporations. Seventy-five percent of the FDA funding comes from pharma. Pharma executives, consultants and lobbyists cycle in and out of these agencies.

With President Trump's backing, I'm going to change that. We're going to staff these agencies with honest scientists and doctors who are free from industry funding. We're going to make sure the decisions of consumers, doctors and patients are informed by unbiased science.

A sick child is the best thing for the pharmaceutical industry. When American children or adults get sick with a chronic condition, they're put on medications for their entire life.

Imagine what will happen when Medicare starts paying for Ozempic, which costs $1,500 a month. It's being recommended for children as young as six. To offer it for the condition of obesity that is completely preventable and barely even existed 100 years ago, is absurd. Given that 74% of Americans are obese, imagine the cost if all of them took an Ozempic prescription; $3 trillion a year. This is a drug that is made by Novo Nordisk, the biggest company in Europe. It's a Danish company, and the Danish government does not recommend it. It recommends a change in diet to treat obesity and exercise. In August 2024, we have a bill in front of Congress that is backed by the White House, backed by Vice President Harris and President Biden to allow Ozempic to be paid for by Medicare; this $3 trillion cost that is going to bankrupt our country.

For a fraction of that amount, we could buy organic food for every American family three meals a day, and eliminate diabetes altogether. We're going to bring healthy food back to school lunches. We're going to stop subsidizing the worst foods with our agricultural subsidies. We're going to get toxic chemicals out of our food. We're going to reform the entire food system, and for that, we need new leadership in Washington, because unfortunately, both the Democrats and the Republican parties are in cahoots with the big food producers, Big Pharma and big ag, which are among the DNC's major donors.

Vice President Harris has expressed no interest in addressing this issue. Four more years of Democratic rule will complete the consolidation of corporate and neocon power. Our children will be the ones who suffer most.

I got involved with chronic disease 20 years ago, not because I chose to or wanted to. It was essentially thrust upon me. It was an issue that should have been central to the environmental movement. I was a central leader at that time, but it was widely ignored by all the institutions, including the NGOs, who should have been protecting our kids against toxins.

It was an orphaned issue, and I had a weakness for orphans. I watched generations of children get sicker and sicker. I had 11 siblings and I have had seven kids myself. I was conscious of what was happening in their classrooms and to their friends. I watched these sick kids, these damaged kids in that generation, almost all of them are damaged, and nobody in power seemed to care or to even notice.

For 19 years, I prayed every morning that God would put me in a position to end this calamity. The Chronic Disease crisis was one of the primary reasons for my running for president, along with ending censorship and the Ukraine war, it's the reason I've made the heart-wrenching decision to suspend my campaign, and to support President Trump.

This decision is agonizing for me because of the difficulties it causes my wife and my children and my friends, but I have the certainty that this is what I'm meant to do, and that certainty gives me internal peace, even in storms.

If I'm given the chance to fix the Chronic Disease crisis and reform our food production, I promise that within two years, we will watch chronic disease burden lift dramatically.

We will make Americans healthy again. Within four years, America will be a healthy country. We will be stronger, more resilient, more optimistic and happier. I won't fail in doing this.

Ultimately, the future, however it happens, is in God's hands and in the hands of the American voters and those of President Trump.

If President Trump is elected and honors his word, the vast burden of chronic disease that now demoralizes and bankrupts the country will disappear. This is a spiritual journey for me. I reached my decision through deep prayer, through hard-nosed logic, and I asked myself, "What choices must I make to maximize my chances to save America's children and restore national health?"

I felt that if I refused this opportunity, I would not be able to look myself in the mirror, knowing that I could have saved the lives of countless children and reversed this country's chronic disease epidemic.

I'm 70 years old. I may have a decade to be effective.

I can't imagine that a president Harris, would allow me or anyone, to solve these dire problems. After eight years of a President Harris, any opportunity for me to fix the problem will be out of my reach forever.

President Trump has told me that he wants this to be his legacy. I'm choosing to believe that this time he will follow through, his biggest donors, his closest friends and all support this objective.

Ultimately, the only thing that will save our country and our children is if we choose to love our kids more than we hate each other.

That's why I launched my campaign to unify America.

My dad and uncle made such an enduring mark on the character of our nation, not so much because of any particular policies that they promoted, but because they were able to inspire profound love for our country and to fortify our sense of ourselves as a national community held together by ideals.

They were able to put their love into the intentions and hearts of ordinary Americans and to unify a national populist movement of Americans: blacks and whites, Hispanics, urban and rural Americans. They inspired affection and love and high hopes and a culture of kindness that continue to radiate among Americans from their memory.

That's the spirit on which I ran my campaign, and that I intend to bring into the campaign of President Trump. Instead of vitriol and polarization, I will appeal to the values that unite us, the goals that we could achieve if only we weren't at each other's throats.

A most unifying theme for all Americans is that we all love our children. If we all unite around that issue now, we can finally give them the protection, health, and the future that they deserve.

CHAPTER 9

Covid 19 Response and Excess Deaths

Andrew Bridgen

Four term British Member of Parliament (MP)

Andrew Bridgen is a former four-term British politician who served as the Member of Parliament (MP) for North West Leicestershire from 2010 until 2024. A vocal advocate for the rights of the vaccine-injured, Bridgen became a prominent figure in challenging the UK government's narrative on COVID-19 vaccines. His outspoken stance earned him a reputation as a courageous defender of those affected by vaccine side effects, giving a voice to the many who felt ignored by public health policies.

Bridgen's political career saw him win by overwhelming majorities, securing 44%, 49%, 58%, and 62% of the vote in successive general elections, before facing a dramatic drop in the 2024 general election as an independent candidate. His expulsion from the Conservative Party in April 2023, following the suspension of the party whip earlier that year, marked a turning point. Despite his political challenges, Bridgen remained steadfast in his advocacy, becoming a hero to many for his willingness to confront powerful institutions and question prevailing narratives.

In a time when political opposition to government policies on COVID-19 vaccines was rare, Bridgen stood out as a thorn in the side of the Conservative Party, and a true advocate for transparency, accountability, and the health of the public.

This essay is based upon a speech given by Andrew Bridgen in the UK House of Commons on April 18, 2024. It is included in this book thanks to the generosity and approval of Andrew Bridgen.

We are witnesses to the greatest medical scandal in this country in living memory, and possibly ever; the excess deaths in 2022 and 2023. Its causes are complex, but the novel and untested medical treatment described as a covid vaccine is a large part of the problem. I have been called an anti-vaxxer, as if I have rejected those vaccines based on some ideology. I want to state clearly and unequivocally that I have not; in fact, I am double vaccinated and vaccine-harmed. Intelligent people must be able to tell when people are neither pro-vax nor anti-vax, but are against a product that does not work and causes enormous harm to a percentage of the people who take it.

I am proud to be one of the few Members of Parliament with a science degree. It is a great shame that there are not more Members with a science background in this place; maybe if there were, there would be less reliance on Whips Office briefings and more independent research, and perhaps less group-think. I say to the House in all seriousness that this debate and others like it are going to be pored over by future generations, who will be genuinely agog that the evidence has been ignored for so long, that genuine concerns were disregarded, and that those raising them were gaslit, smeared and vilified.

One does not need any science training at all to be horrified by officials deliberately hiding key data in this scandal, which is exactly what is going on. The Office for National Statistics used to release weekly data on deaths per 100,000 in vaccinated and unvaccinated populations—it no longer does so, and no one will explain why. The public has a right to that data. There have been calls from serious experts, whose requests I have amplified repeatedly in this House, for what is called record-level data to be anonymised and disclosed for analysis. That would allow meaningful analysis of deaths after vaccination, and settle once and for all the issue of whether those experimental treatments are responsible for the increase in excess deaths.

Far more extensive and detailed data has already been released to the pharma companies from publicly funded bodies. Jenny Harries, head of the UK Health Security Agency, said that this anonymised, aggregate death by vaccination status data is "commercially sensitive" and should not be published. The public are being denied that data, which is unacceptable; yet again, data is hidden with impunity, just like in the Post Office scandal. Professor Harries has also endorsed a recent massive change to the calculation of the baseline population level used by the ONS to calculate excess deaths. It is now incredibly complex and opaque, and by sheer coincidence, it appears to show a massive excess of deaths in 2020 and 2021 and minimal excess deaths in 2023. Under the old calculation method, tried and tested for decades, the excess death rate in 2023 was an astonishing 5%—long after the pandemic was over, at a time when we would expect a deficit in deaths because so many people had sadly died in previous years. Some 20,000 premature deaths in 2023 alone are now being airbrushed away through the new normal baseline.

Shocking things happened during the pandemic response. In March 2020, the Government conducted a consultation exercise on whether people over a certain age or with certain disabilities should have "do not resuscitate" orders, known as DNRs, imposed upon them. A document summarising the proposals was circulated to doctors and hospitals; it was mistakenly treated as formal policy by a number of care homes and GPs up and down the country, who enacted it. At the same time, multiple hospitals introduced a policy that they would not admit patients with DNRs, because they thought that they would be overwhelmed. The result was that people died who did not need to die while nurses performed TikTok dances.

The average time to death from experiencing covid symptoms and testing positive was 18 days. It is a little-known fact that the body clears all the viruses within around seven days; what actually kills people is that some, especially the vulnerable, have an excessive immune response. Doctors have been treating that response for decades with steroids, antibiotics for secondary pneumonia infections and other standard protocols, but they did not do so this time. Even though the virus was long gone, doctors abandoned the standard clinical protocols because covid was a "new virus"—which it was not. They sent people home, told them to take paracetamol until their lips turned blue, and then when those people returned to hospital, they sedated them, put them on ventilators and watched them die.

The protocol for covid-19 treatment was a binary choice between two treatment tracks. Once admitted, ill patients were either ventilated in intensive care or—if they were not fit for that level of care—given end of life medication, including midazolam and morphine. The body responsible for that protocol, NG163, which was published on 3 April 2020, is called the National Institute for Health and Care Excellence, or NICE. Giving midazolam and morphine to people dying of cancer is reasonable, but there is a side effect, which is that those drugs have a respiratory depressant effect. It is hard to imagine a more stupid thing to do than to give a respiratory suppressant to someone who is already struggling to breathe with the symptoms of covid-19. But that is exactly what we did.

Why was midazolam removed from the same updated guideline NG191—the antecedent of NG163—on 30 November 2023? As it was removed, is it now considered and admitted that it was a mistake to ignore the warnings of so many experts about including that specific drug, midazolam, in NG163 when it was introduced? It has been confirmed in letters from Ministers to families whose loss of loved ones was down to this protocol that Ministers are now saying that doctors and nurses should have treated the individual patient with their own knowledge, rather than strictly following NICE guideline NG163. If legal cases for unlawful killing are brought, who is going to be taking the blame? Will it be NICE, will it be NHS England or will the individual doctors and nurses be held to account?

Interestingly, NICE has now removed these alternative protocols, including NG163, from its website, although every other historical protocol is still there for reference. Why NICE removed this protocol from its website? Is it ashamed of the harm it has caused? It certainly should be. What can we learn from this? We learn that very few doctors dare challenge what they are told. Protocols with no authors are distributed, and doctors fall into line.

There is a huge, stark contrast in how deaths and illnesses after vaccination have been recorded compared with those after covid. After a positive covid test, any illness and any death was attributed to the virus. After the experimental emergency vaccine was administered, no subsequent illness and no death was ever attributed to the vaccine. Those are both completely unscientific approaches, and that is why we have to look at other sources of data—excess deaths—to determine whether there is an issue.

First, however, I want to address the phrase "safe and effective". The fear deliberately stoked by the Government promoted the idea of being rescued by a saviour vaccine. The chanting of the "safe and effective" narrative began, and the phrase seemed to hypnotise the whole nation. "Safe and effective" was the sale slogan of thalidomide. After that scandal, rules were put in place to prevent such marketing in future by pharma companies, and they are prohibited from using "safe and effective" without significant caveats.

That did not matter this time because, with covid-19 vaccines, the media, the Government and other authorities turned into big pharma's marketing department, and it is very hard now to hear the word "safe" without the echo of the words "and effective." But they are not safe and effective. In March 2021, when the majority of UK citizens had already received these novel products, Pfizer signed a contract with Brazil and South Africa saying that "the long-term effects and efficacy of the Vaccine are not currently known and…adverse effects of the Vaccine…are not currently known." That is verbatim from the Pfizer contracts.

These so-called vaccines were the least effective vaccines ever. Is there anyone left under any illusion that they prevented any infections? When he was at the Dispatch Box for Prime Minister's questions on 31 January, even the Prime Minister, in answer to my question, could not bring himself to add "and effective" to his "safe" mantra. In his own words, he was "unequivocal" that the vaccines are "safe." The word "safe" means without risk of death or injury. Why is the Prime Minister gaslighting the 163 successful claims made to the vaccine damage payment scheme, totalling £19.5 million in compensation for harm caused by the covid vaccines? Have these people not suffered enough already? Those 163 victims are the tip of the iceberg, by the way. It also should be noted that the maximum payment is only £120,000, so each of those 163 victims got the maximum possible award, which should tell us something. The same compensation scheme paid out a total of only £3.5 million between 1997 and 2005, with an average of only eight claims per year, and that is for all claims for the entire country for all vaccines administered. So much for "safe."

How about effective? On 25 October 2021, the then Prime Minister— the Right Hon. Member for Uxbridge and South Ruislip, Boris Johnson— even admitted that the vaccine "doesn't protect you against catching the disease and it doesn't protect you against passing it on."

Looking at the levels of the virus found in sewage shows that the post-vaccine wave was of the same order of magnitude and duration as the previous waves. This proves that the vaccines changed nothing. They were not safe, and they were not effective.

Those who imposed these vaccines knew full well that they could never prevent infection from a disease of this kind. An injection in the arm cannot do that. Only immunity on the surface of the airways and the lungs can prevent viral infection; antibodies in the blood cannot. In Dr Anthony Fauci's words, "It is not surprising that none of the predominantly mucosal respiratory viruses have ever been effectively controlled by vaccines.

"This observation raises a question of fundamental importance: if natural mucosal respiratory virus infections do not elicit complete and long-term protective immunity against reinfection, how can we expect vaccines, especially systemically administered non-replicating vaccines, to do so?"

They knew that the so-called vaccines would never protect from infection, which explains why they never tested for protection from infection.

The Association of the British Pharmaceutical Industry rapped Pfizer on the knuckles for the sixth time, and said that its marketing practices had brought the industry into disrepute. It was asked to pay a paltry £30,000 in administrative expenses, with no fine on top. The person heading the ABPI at the moment is also the head of Pfizer UK. The Medicines and Healthcare products Regulatory Agency has a statutory duty to carry out this work, and it has handed its responsibility to the industry. This is an outrageous conflict of interest.

Let us turn back to excess deaths. The Australian Government has launched an inquiry into Australia's excess deaths problem. Australia is almost unique as a case study for excess deaths; it had the vaccine before it had covid. Its excess deaths are not so easily blamed on the long-term side effects of a virus. Like us in the UK, it saw a rise in deaths, which began in May 2021 and has not let up since. The impact was initially evident on the ambulance service. South Australia saw a 67% increase in cardiac presentations of 15 to 44-year-olds. That increase peaked in November 2021, before covid hit. We saw a similar, deeply worrying effect here. In the UK, calls for life-threatening emergencies rose from 2,000 per day to 2,500 per day in May 2021, and that number has never returned to normal.

By October 2021, despite it being springtime in Australia, headlines reported that ambulances were unable to drop off patients in hospitals, which were already at full capacity. Mark McGowan, Premier of Western Australia, said that he could not explain the overwhelmed hospitals: "Our hospitals are under enormous pressure. This has been something no one has ever seen before. Why it is, is hard to know."

In April 2022, Yvette D'Ath, Queensland's Health Minister, said about the most urgent ambulance calls, called "code ones": "I don't think anyone can explain why we saw a 40% jump in code ones... We just had a lot of heart attacks and chest pains and trouble breathing, respiratory issues. Sometimes you can't explain why those things happen but unfortunately, they do."

I think we could explain this if we were to look at the link to the vaccine roll-out. Omicron did cause some excess deaths in Australia from 2022 onwards. However, there was a huge chunk of excess deaths prior to that, which doctors have not been able to blame on the virus. Could those deaths be caused by the vaccine? Very few people dare even ask that question.

It is important to remember how the vaccines were made. Traditionally, the key to making a vaccine is to ensure that the pathological, harmful parts of the virus or bacteria are inactivated, so that the recipient can develop an immune response without danger of developing the disease. In stark contrast, the so-called covid vaccines used the most pathological or harmful part of the virus—the spike protein—in its entirety. The harm is systemic because, contrary to what everyone was told, the lipid nanoparticles, encapsulating the genetic material, spread through the whole body after injection, potentially affecting all organs. At the time, everyone was being reassured that the injection was broken down in the arm at the injection site. Regulators ought to have known that those were problems.

Furthermore, it is now plentifully evident that the drug results in continued spike protein production for many months—even years, in some people. The deaths thus far have been predominantly cardiac, but there may unfortunately be many more deaths to come from these novel treatments, which may induce extra cancer deaths. Dr Robert Tindle is the retired director of the Clinical Medical Virology Centre in Brisbane, and Emeritus Professor of Immunology. This month he published a paper highlighting the multiple potential harms from the vaccines, including harm to the immune system. As anyone who knows anything about biology will know, anything that disrupts the immune system can potentially increase the risk of cancer.

There are other reasons to be concerned about cancer being induced by these vaccines. Cancer is a genetic disease disorder that arises from errors in DNA, allowing cells to grow uncontrollably. Moderna has multiple patents describing methods for reducing the risk of cancer induction from its mRNA products. That risk comes from the material interrupting the patient's DNA. It turns out that an mRNA injection has very high quantities of DNA in it, which massively increases the risk of disturbing a patient's own DNA. Worse still, the DNA that was injected contained sequences that were hidden from the regulator. That is the SV40, or simian virus 40 promoter region, which has been linked to cancer and has been found in the Pfizer vaccines. That was no accident. Yet again, crucial information was hidden from the regulator and the public with absolute impunity. An independent study in Japan, published last week, has found links between increased cancer rates in Japan and those who took the first and subsequent booster vaccines. Perhaps that explains why Pfizer acquired a cancer treatment company for a reported $43 billion earlier this year.

In conclusion, the evidence is clear: these vaccines have caused deaths. Despite that, they have been described as safe and effective. However, for a proportion of people who took them, the vaccines have caused serious harm and death, and they will have raised the risk of cancer for many more. Nor are they effective. The vaccine does not prevent infection or transmission, and when the data is studied objectively, it shows that the vaccine does not prevent serious illness or death. Those are hard truths to face, but we must face them if we want to learn the lessons of the last few years. At some point we will have to face up to all the evidence that is building. It was fairly convincing 18 months ago when I first spoke out, but it is unequivocal now.

It is time to take the politics out of our science, and to put actual science back into our politics.

CHAPTER 10

Our Dystopian Present

HOW THE 'CONTROLIGARCHS' WEAPONIZED A VIRUS TO END PRIVACY & FREEDOM AS WE KNOW IT

Seamus Bruner

Researcher and best selling author

Seamus Bruner (@SeamusBruner) is the Vice President and Executive Director, Research at Peter Schweizer's Government Accountability Institute (GAI) and the author of three bestselling books, including Controligarchs: Exposing the Billionaire Class, their Secret Deals, and the Globalist Plot to Dominate your Life. He has worked with bestselling author Peter Schweizer since 2011 and GAI since 2013, providing research and support for numerous New York Times bestsellers—the last three landed the highly coveted #1 slot on the New York Times bestsellers list. Bruner's work helped kick off multiple FBI and Congressional probes into political corruption at the highest levels and has been featured on the front page of the New York Times, the Wall Street Journal, and the Washington Post, and has resulted in multiple 60 Minutes exposés. Bruner has discussed the results of his findings on national TV and radio.

When most people envision a dystopian future they imagine some post-apocalyptic fictional world—cities reduced to ash heaps, perhaps with hordes of marauding zombies—completely unrecognizable from our current reality. They typically do not think of a dystopia in the present tense. But Bill Gates, Jeff Bezos, Mark Zuckerberg and their ilk—the billionaires and bureaucrats who I call the "Controligarchs"—have built dystopia whether they appreciate it or not. And the COVID-19 pandemic accelerated our glidepath toward their full technocratic control.

We hear all the time that the pandemic is over and that we should move on, but nothing could be further from the truth. The pandemic was a blueprint for the future and proved that lockdowns were lucrative for those who control the data and the eyeballs. We also learned that most people would do as they are told, no matter the personal costs to themselves and their families, to achieve some elusive and ill-defined "greater good." People want to believe that we truly are in this together (that line was cooked up by Bill Gates who has multiple private jets and even a seaplane to spirit him away when the going gets tough).

Beyond the Great Reset

It was July 2020 when World Economic Forum (WEF) frontman Klaus Schwab declared the now-infamous "Great Reset," and announced the coming "digitalization" of everything. Digital IDs, digital vaccination passports, digital medical records, central bank digital currencies, an "internet of things" comprised of digital smart devices, and even Matrix-like digital realities composed by artificial intelligence (AI) would be essential, Schwab and the Controligarchs promised, to build back better after the pandemic. Eventually, Schwab says, digitalization of everything will lead to "a fusion of our physical, our digital, and our biological identities."[1]

The pandemic succeeded wildly in advancing these efforts. But the digitalization agenda of the Great Reset was accompanied by a pandemic response that was far less publicized: an angrier world.

"I don't know how it will play out in [the November 2020 US presidential election]," Schwab mused in his July 2020 Great Reset declaration broadcast on CNBC, "but what we know is that we will end up with many more unemployed." Schwab went on: "So, we will see definitively a lot of anger...because this crisis will be with us until we really have found a remedy. So, we must prepare for a more angry world." Four years later, it appears that Schwab was right. We do have an angrier world.

It's not just because the pandemic caused mass unemployment, as Schwab predicted, though. We see bloody conflicts on multiple continents, chaos, crime, and infighting in major world cities, traditions and values being eroded, and an interconnected global economy circling the drain as AI-driven job losses loom. A relatively harmless coronavirus that produced mostly flu-like symptoms did not cause this so-called "polycrisis." The

Controligarchs did. And in the background, their digitalization agenda marches us further into our dystopian present, which in turn will lead to more pain and anger.

One WEF visionary, Yuval Noah Harari, believes, like Schwab and the rest of the Controligarchs, that the pandemic presented a great opportunity to implement technocratic solutions to problems that no one knew existed. For example, few people are begging for biometric surveillance. But, according to Harari:

> Covid is critical because this is what convinces people to accept [and] to legitimize total biometric surveillance. If you want to stop this epidemic, we need not just to monitor people, we need to monitor what's happening under their skin.[2]

But sub-dermal microchips (things Bill Gates has patented and therefor hopes to profit from) are only the beginning. Harari believes that the entire human body will soon be hackable—that humans will be able to achieve immortality through biotechnological upgrades. For all human history, "death was the great equalizer," Harari claims. But a dystopian caste system is taking shape in which the poor still die but the rich, according to Harari "in addition to all the other things they get, also get an exemption from death."[3]

The identity of "the future masters of the planet," Harari told the current planetary masters in Davos, "will be decided by the people who own the data. Those who control the data control the future—not just of humanity but the future of life itself."[4]

It should come as no surprise that data hoarders and harvesters like Microsoft's Bill Gates, Google's Sergey Brin, Meta's Mark Zuckerberg, and Twitter's Jack Dorsey praise Harari and his visions.[5]

The Rise of AI

The WEF visionary seems particularly enthused about the rise of AI (which, Schwab says, has "accelerated" thanks to the pandemic, and Gates says will be essential to prevent the "next pandemic"). "We'll soon have the power to re-engineer our bodies and brains—whether it is with genetic engineering or by directly connecting brains to computers or by creating completely non-organic entities [like] artificial intelligence," Harari confidently predicted, adding that "these technologies are developing at breakneck speed."[6]

Schwab's visionary predicts that artificial intelligence and genetic engineering will "enable parents to create smarter or more attractive children." Aware of the eugenics implications, Harari acknowledges a new caste system arises when only the rich can genetically hack their biology and create new super-humans. He concedes that "biological inequality" could lead to more "inequality than in any previous time in history."[7]

"It's not just dystopian, it's also utopian," Harari says of biometric surveillance and AI-driven decision making that can "enable us to create the best healthcare system in history." Cooper: "What does Pfizer want the [biometric] data of all Israelis for?" Harari: "to develop new medicines, new treatments, you need the medical data... and, of course, it's not all bad!"[8]

Nonetheless, Harari expects that someday soon, humanity will face a crisis over what to do with non-Davos attendees. "The biggest question maybe in economics and politics in the coming decades will be *what to do with all these useless people* (emphasis added)."[9]

Unlike in Nazi Germany, the so-called "untermenschen" (or useless people) of the twenty-first century are not disabled or unfit, they are simply bored, and superfluous. Harari points out that modern day "bread and circuses" come in the form of dystopian drugs and digital entertainment:

The problem is more boredom, and what to do with people, and how will they find some sense of meaning in life when they are basically meaningless, worthless. My best guess at present is a combination of drugs and computer games as a solution for most...it's already happening.[10]

Harari cited Japan as an example of this dystopian present with its sharp rise in "virtual spouses" and "people who never leave the house and just live through computers."[11]

The Final Revolution

This vision of the future, filled with psychotropic placations, seems to mirror Aldous Huxley's *Brave New World* in which the fictional drug "Soma" made citizens love their servitude while pacified by a relentless stream of entertainment and pornography. At a 1961 San Francisco symposium titled *Man and Civilization: Control of the Mind*, Huxley elaborated on what he called "The Final Revolution":

> There will be in the next generation or so a pharmacological method of making people love their servitude and producing dictatorship without tears, so to speak. Producing a kind of painless concentration camp for entire societies so that people will in fact have their liberties taken away from them but will rather enjoy it, because they will be distracted from any desire to rebel by propaganda, or brainwashing, or brainwashing enhanced by pharmacological methods. And this seems to be the final revolution.[12]

In his book *New Bottles For New Wine* (1957), Aldous's brother Julian Huxley coined the term "transhumanism," which is still used as the all-encompassing term for the merger of man with machine today.[13]

The Huxley brothers' prophetic writings laid the groundwork for Schwab's Great Reset, the WEF's digitalization agenda, the Controligarchs' imminent plans to merge man with machine, and, ultimately, our dystopian present.[14]

Simply put, our dystopian present is a painless transhumanist concentration camp, like the one Huxley predicted nearly six decades ago, where all boredoms are amused, and all anxieties are tranquilized.

Many have long believed that Huxley's *Brave New World* imaginations might appear in the distant future. In a post-COVID world, however, that future feels like it is here. Big Brother, just like George Orwell imagined in his book *Nineteen Eighty-Four* (1949), was installed decades ago amid the rise of computers and the internet. And now with AI, Big Brother has matured to an omnipresent and inescapable force.[15]

A Transhuman Hellscape

The Big Tech Controligarchs' dystopian visions have obvious appeal to Schwab and his Davos patrons. They do not like fair and competitive playing fields and there are no competitors (in the conventional sense) at the architect level of dystopia, only partners and stakeholders. Facebook (Meta), Microsoft, and Google, for example, are not only building competing virtual and augmented reality products, but they are also in business with each other.[16]

And Harari is not just some fringe futurist. His books have sold more than 35 million copies worldwide and have been translated into sixty-five different languages. Barack Obama has promoted his work and CNN's Anderson Cooper calls Harari "one of the most popular writers and thinkers on the planet."[17]

The WEF visionary knows that some of their ideas seem off-putting. Harari rightly fears that the rise of AI is even more scary than computers gaining consciousness—the ability to feel pain and emotions like love and hate. Harari argues that AI will have no consciousness (nor conscience) and will therefor make decisions unburdened by human ethics. "And they will have power over us?" asked Cooper. "They are already gaining power over us," replied Harari. As an example, financial lenders use algorithms to make loans.[18]

The companies with the most data will control the world, according to the Schwab advisor, "Data is worth much more than money." Harari used Facebook's purchase of WhatsApp and Instagram for billions of dollars as an example. Why would they do this? Because data is power. Biometric data is the crown jewel and Harari envisions a day when biometric data harvesters are implanted beneath the skin.[19]

In one lecture, Harari summed up the future envisioned by the Controligarchs perfectly:

> "Netflix tells us what to watch, and Amazon tells us what to buy. Eventually within ten or twenty or thirty years, such algorithms could also tell you what to study at college, and where to work, and whom to marry, and even for whom to vote."[20]

Seems like at least some of that is happening *presently*, no?

"It's not just dystopian, it's also utopian," Harari says of biometric surveillance and AI-driven decision making that can "enable us to create the best healthcare system in history." Cooper: "What does Pfizer want the [biometric] data of all Israelis for?" Harari: "to develop new medicines, new treatments, you need the medical data... and, of course, it's not all bad!"[21]

Much like Schwab and other fans of global governance who attend Davos, Covid-19 was extremely convenient for their plans. "We are at the point when we need global cooperation," Harari claims. "You cannot regulate the explosive power of artificial intelligence on a national level."[22]

And to any useless peasants contemplating revolt, think again because resistance is futile, says Harari:

> We are used to thinking about the masses as powerful, but this is basically a nineteenth-century and twentieth-century phenomenon... I don't think that the masses even if they somehow organize themselves stand much of a chance, we are not...in nineteenth-century Europe.[23]

* * *

So many people are always looking for a silver bullet—a panacea of some kind—or some white knight to ride in and save the day. But perhaps the most concerning aspect of our increasingly dystopian present is our own complicity in it. It is easy to surrender control and outsource decision making They make it so easy to say, "hey Alexa, play classical music." Or "ok google, start the dryer." It's easy. And that's the hard part. Because the convenience is the thin end of the wedge. It is like slipping into a warm bubble bath of tyranny.

Sadly, I do not know the answer to holding the apparently lawless Controligarchs accountable. But I do know that we can win the fight for humanity and for our country with the passion and energy I see all around the country. But we've got to unite—not on this specific issue per se—but against our common enemies: the Controligarchs and their puppets. And as my dear colleague Peter Schweizer likes to say—*we need to throw them all out.*

[1] Pin Lean Lau, "3 Issues to Address Before We Dive into the Metaverse," World Economic Forum, February 7, 2022, https://www.weforum.org/agenda/2022/02/metaverse-legal-issues; Stefan Bramilla Hall and Moritz Baier-Lentz, "3 Technologies That Will Shape the Future of the Metaverse—And the Human Experience," World Economic Forum, February 7, 2022, https://www.weforum.org/agenda/2022/02/future-of-the-metaverse-vr-ar-and-brain-computer; "Fourth Industrial Revolution," World Economic Forum, accessed December 1, 2022, https://www.weforum.org/focus/fourth-industrial-revolution; Klaus Schwab, "KLAUS SCHWAB: Revolution Will Lead to a Fusion of our Physical, Digital, and Biological Identity," II Teatro della Politica, November 10, 2020, YouTube Video, 00:1:09, https://www.youtube.com/watch?v=t1SpC3B1KyM.

[2] Yuval Noah Harari, "Yuval Noah Harari: Panel Discussion on Technology and the Future of Democracy," October 4, 2020, YouTube Video, 00:32:40 to 00:33:00, https://www.youtube.com/watch?v=JfyIW9wRvB4.

[3] "Yuval Noah Harari: The 2021 60 Minutes Interview," 60 Minutes, October 31, 2021, YouTube Video, 00:09:15, https://www.youtube.com/watch?v=EIVTf-C6oQo&t; Yuval Noah Harari and Daniel Kahneman, "Death Is Optional," Edge, March 4, 2015, video, 00:41:54, https://www.edge.org/conversation/yuval_noah_harari-daniel_kahneman-death-is-optional; Yuval Harari, "Read Yuval Harari's Blistering Warning to Davos in Full," World Economic Forum, January 24, 2020, https://www.weforum.org/agenda/2020/01/yuval-hararis-warning-davos-speech-future-predications.

[4] Yuval Noah Harari, "Will the Future Be Human?—Yuval Noah Harari," World Economic Forum, January 25, 2018, YouTube Video, 00:03:25 to 00:03:43, https://youtu.be/hL9uk4hKyg4.

[5] Yuval Noah Harari (@yuval-noah-harari), "Bill Gates has been a fan of Yuval Noah Harari's work for several years," Instagram, August 25, 2018, https://www.instagram.com/p/Bm5lGRsltpT; "Bill Gates, Mark Zuckerberg, and Barack Obama are Fans. Meet Yuval Noah Harari," ABC News, September 4, 2018, https://www.abc.net.au/triplej/programs/hack/meet-yuval-harari-superstar-historian-to-mark-zuckerberg/10200906; Nick Romeo, "Yuval Harari's New Book Feeds the Tech Czar's God Complex," The Daily Beast, updated May 23, 2017, https://www.thedailybeast.com/yuval-hararis-new-book-feeds-the-tech-czars-god-complex.

[6] Schwab and Malleret, Covid-19: The Great Reset; Gates, How to Prevent the Next Pandemic (New York: Alfred A. Knopf, 2022); "Yuval Noah Harari: The 2021 60 Minutes Interview," 00:01:03 to 00:01:30.

[7] "Yuval Noah Harari: The 2021 60 Minutes Interview," 00:01:48 to 00:02:15.

[8] Ibid.

[9] "WEF Advisor Says Global Elite 'Don't Need the Vast Majority of the Population' to Live," American Faith, August 12, 2022, https://americanfaith.com/wef-advisor-says-global-elite-dont-need-the-vast-majority-of-the-population-to-live; Ian Sample, "AI Will Create 'Useless Class' of

Human, Predicts Bestselling Historian," *The Guardian*, May 20, 2016, https://www.theguardian.com/technology/2016/may/20/silicon-assassins-condemn-humans-life-useless-artificial-intelligence.

[10] Harari and Kahneman, "Death Is Optional."

[11] Ibid.

[12] Kate Whiting, "6 Dystopian Novels That Resonate Today," World Economic Forum, October 23, 2019, https://www.weforum.org/agenda/2019/10/6-dystopian-novels-that-resonate-today; Regents of the University of California, "Aldous Huxley Speaking at 'Man and Civilization' Symposium," Photograph Collection, E—Events and Awards, Symposium Man and Civilization, photograph, 1961, accessed December 1, 2022, https://calisphere.org/item/cabf65fd-7830-4c66-906f-0602140887b6; "Aldous Huxley: 'Facts Do Not Cease to Exist Because They Are Ignored'—Top 10 Quotes," Radio Butut, November 21, 2022, YouTube Video, 00:02:34, https://www.youtube.com/watch?v=RqbpzWMHPGk; Sienna Mae Heath, "How We Win 'The Final Revolution (Part 1),'" Medium, December 31, 2020, https://medium.com/illumination-curated/how-we-win-the-final-revolution-part-1-f86f3421d80d.

[13] Julian Huxley, *New Bottles for New Wine* (London: Chatto & Windus, 1957), 13, https://archive.org/details/NewBottlesForNewWine/page/n15/mode/2up.

[14] Andrew Miller, "Immortal Cyborgs: Is this Humanity's Future?" TheTrumpet.com, April 21, 2017, https://www.thetrumpet.com/15703-immortal-cyborgs-is-this-humanitys-future; Renata Silva Souza, Edna Alves de Souza, Tatiane Pereira da Silva, and Maria Eunice Quilici Gonzalez, "The Transhumanist Conception of Body: A Critical Analysis from a Complex Systems Perspective," *Natureza Humana* 22, no. 1 (June 2020): 17–33, http://dx.doi.org/10.17648/2175-2834-v22n1-431; Valerie Christopherson, "Communicating Futuristic Concepts: Perception is Everything," Forbes, September 9, 2022, https://www.forbes.com/sites/forbesagencycouncil/2022/09/09/communicating-futuristic-concepts-perception-is-everything; Daniel Y. Teng, "Zuckerberg's Metaverse a Gateway to 'Transhumanism,' Gettr CEO Warns," The Epoch Times, October 3, 2022, https://www.theepochtimes.com/zuckerbergs-metaverse-a-gateway-to-transhumanism-gettr-ceo-warns_4770484.html; Steve Mollman, "Jeff Bezos and Bill Gates are Making Bets on Brain Interface Company Synchron as Elon Musk's Neuralink Faces Controversy and a Federal Investigation," *Fortune*, December 15, 2022, https://fortune.com/2022/12/15/jeff-bezos-bill-gates-invest-brain-computer-interface-startup-synchron-amid-elon-musk-neuralink-controversy; Alex Knapp, "Elon Musk Sees His Neuralink Merging Your Brain with A.I.," Forbes, July 17, 2019, https://www.forbes.com/sites/alexknapp/2019/07/17/elon-musk-sees-his-neuralink-merging-your-brain-with-ai.

[15] Mike Elgan, "Big Brother is Watching You—And He's a Computer," Computerworld, June 22, 2007, https://www.computerworld.com/article/2542177/big-brother-is-watching-you----and-he-s-a-computer.html.

[16] Charlie Bell, "The Metaverse is Coming. Here are the Cornerstones for Securing It," Microsoft (blog), Microsoft, March 28, 2022, https://blogs.microsoft.com/blog/2022/03/28/the-metaverse-is-coming-here-are-the-cornerstones-for-securing-it; Kali Hays, "Meta Competed Fiercely with Google and Microsoft for Years. Now It's Working with Former Rivals as CEO Mark Zuckerberg Pushes for an 'Open' Metaverse," Business Insider, October 11, 2022, https://www.businessinsider.com/facebook-youtube-vr-app-quest-headset-microsoft-metaverse-2022-10; "Meta Announces New Quest Pro Headset, Microsoft Partnership," Yahoo! Finance, October 11, 2022, YouTube Video, 00:03:32, https://www.youtube.com/watch?v=5pzEM9KyRzI.

[17] "Yuval Noah Harari: The 2021 60 Minutes Interview," 00:00:15 and 00:12:54.

[18] Ibid.

[19] Ibid.

[20] Ibid.

[21] Ibid.

[22] Ibid.

[23] "Yuval Noah Harari ve Daniel Kahneman Söyleşisi," Kolektif Kitap, May 20, 2015, YouTube Video, 00:29:54 to 00:31:16, https://www.youtube.com/watch?v=-3aPT8MuH_E.

CHAPTER 11

The larger agenda: COVID restrictions as a precursor to '15-minute cities,' CBDCs and digital ID

Michael Nevradakis, Ph.D.

Journalist and senior reporter for the
Defender and CHD TV host.

Michael Nevradakis, Ph.D., based in Athens, Greece, is a senior reporter for The Defender, published by Children's Health Defense (CHD), and part of the rotation of hosts for CHD.TV's "Good Morning CHD." For 10 years, he produced and hosted the "Dialogos" radio program and podcast, and he has previously been published by The Guardian, the Huffington Post, the Daily Kos, Truthout, Mint Press News and other outlets. He completed his Ph.D. in media studies at the University of Texas in 2018 and holds a masters degree in public policy from Stony Brook University. He is an instructor in communications and journalism and has taught at various institutions of higher education in Greece and the U.S.

It was a Monday morning in Athens, Greece, in early March 2020, a few days before COVID lockdowns were imposed. I had just walked to a local pharmacy, one that I had also been to two days prior. Upon arrival though, I noticed that a new door had been installed: a glass door with a round slot that could open from the inside. That door had not been there on Friday. As it turned out, that door was installed to serve customers without them having to go inside, due to social distancing rules. Yet, that door was installed, apparently on a weekend (in a country where barely any such work takes place on weekends), *before* the lockdowns and social distancing policies were introduced. Many other pharmacies had done the same thing, begging the questions: what did they know, when did they know it and who did they learn it from?

A week or so later, just ahead of lockdown, which I saw coming and which I knew would not be "just for two weeks to flatten the curve," I 'dared' to set foot on an airplane and travel back to the U.S. to spend time with my parents in rural New York, so that they wouldn't be by themselves during this period. Sitting on the couch one evening, I attempted to think through the then-current state of play and to figure out where 'the powers that be' were going with this. What I did know is that the reaction to COVID-19 very early on seemed incredibly over-the-top and coordinated—from the dancing and remarkably well-choreographed TikTok nurses (shouldn't they have been busy in 'overwhelmed' ICUs?), to one celebrity after the other coming out and proclaiming that they had COVID (at a time where case numbers were in the low thousands worldwide—what are the odds?), to the remarkably similar and near-simultaneous pronouncements and rhetoric used—and measures enacted or promoted—by politicians, public health officials and media mouthpieces globally. What occurred to me is that such a degree of coordination couldn't possibly have been about a "novel virus" that would surely have caught the world off-guard. It was more a case of 'the ends justify the means.'

This chapter examines those 'ends'—and how COVID is linked to a broader global agenda that could broadly be defined as the "Great Reset" and "Fourth Industrial Revolution"—both concepts introduced by the World Economic Forum (WEF) and promoted heavily by this organization in the ensuing years. This agenda encompasses measures proposed in the name of climate change, digital currency and digital ID, all with the goal of altering human habits and to benefit a small coterie of powerful 'private' corporations. Widely promoted to the public as 'stakeholder capitalism' and 'ESG' (the 'environmental, social and governance investment principle), this agenda has little to do with a 'free' market or protecting the environment or public health—and much more to do with consolidating power within a new technocratic control grid. This is equally true for Western governments and states, and those which supposedly represent a new 'multipolar world order,' who also have embraced, for instance, the COVID-19 lockdown and vaccine agenda and central bank digital currencies (CBDCs). Aside from limiting freedom and personal liberties, these policies and concepts share an additional common denominator: they are all touted as being 'for our own good.' Or as French philosopher Albert Camus once said:

"The welfare of the people in particular has always been the alibi of tyrants, and it provides the further advantage of giving the servants of tyranny a good conscience."

'15-minute cities'

In several countries during the COVID-19 lockdowns, particularly in Europe, citizens' freedom of movement was restricted not just to a small list of 'essential' reasons, such as going to the supermarket or pharmacy or walking your dog, but also to a small radius around one's residence. In France, for instance, citizens were typically restricted to a one-kilometer radius around their homes and had to carry with them a complex paper form containing details such as their name, address, and their 'reason' for being out. Greece took things a step further. While citizens were 'allowed' to travel a relatively generous two-kilometer radius around their homes, they were obliged to first send a text message to a special government number with their name, address and a number from 1 to 6, representing one of six valid 'reasons' for going out. In both countries, those violating these restrictions were subject to fines and harassment from the police.

Now consider the example of Oxford, England, which in 2023 began to pilot so-called "traffic filters" as part of the city's 2040 development strategy. According to this plan, the city was divided into six districts, and residents of any given district could 'freely' drive anywhere within that district but would need to apply for a permit to drive to any other district— but even then, they would only be allowed to do so for 100 days per year.

This plan is an example of the so-called '15-minute cities' concept. Defined by Reuters as "urban planning model that envisions an environment where people can access amenities within a 15-minute walk, bike ride, or public transport journey from their homes," this concept is heavily promoted by entities such as the WEF and the C40 Cities Climate Leadership Group, which has brought together the mayors of 96 prominent cities "that are united in action to confront the climate crisis."

In 2022, C40 announced a partnership with real estate investment firm NREP to "deliver proof of concept for '15-minute city' policies." Notably, billionaire philanthropist and former mayor of New York City Michael Bloomberg, now the United Nations Secretary-General Special Envoy for Climate Ambition and Solutions, is president of the board of directors of C40, while Antha Williams, head of Bloomberg Philanthropies' Environment Program, is also a member of the C40 board.

At this point, one might say that the '15-minute city' concept sounds nice conceptually: having vital services, shopping and public transportation available to you within a short distance is indisputably not a bad thing. And Reuters vehemently denies that the concept is related to a desire to impose future lockdowns, stating that it "found no evidence that the concept promotes or equates to a lockdown, as many people have claimed online." But as the examples of Oxfordshire and of COVID-era lockdowns indicate, the right to freedom of movement is far from a 'given,' and this right can be taken away in the name of 'public health'—or in the name of 'protecting the environment.' After all, thinking back to COVID-era movement restrictions of one or two kilometers, it bears noting that it takes the typical person 10-12 minutes to walk one kilometer.

CBDCs, digital money and programmable currency

Like '15-minute cities,' CBDCs, digital money and 'cashless' societies have their proponents—and efforts to dissuade the public from using physical currency were readily apparent during the 'COVID era.' In April 2020, the Centers for Disease Control and Prevention (CDC) published a guide to "Running Essential Errands." One of the recommendations this guide advised the public to, "If possible, use touchless payment (pay without touching money, a card, or a keypad)." And a November 2020 Bank of England report stated that while "the risk of transmission via banknotes is low," the pandemic "the way people use cash has changed, with less being used for transactions," in part due to "concerns about the risk of banknotes transmitting the virus." And in May 2020, the Associated Press noted that "many businesses worldwide have banned cash transactions and governments are taking extra precautions."

Even though such practices were proven to be useless in a 2022 Brigham Young University microbiology study, the damage was done. According to a November 2023 report by the Federal Reserve Bank of Boston, the use of cash declined dramatically early during the pandemic, and while it levelled off, it has not recovered.

Of course, it did not take COVID-19 for anti-cash narratives to begin circulating (pun intended). For instance, a 2018 study concluded that "Cashless payments hinder tax evasion because they build a trail for the underlying transactions." In Greece, a country where tax evasion is said to be rampant, the use of cards and electronic payments is popularly understood as a way of 'fighting' tax evasion—although this trope lets the wealthy, who are able to stash their assets in offshore tax havens and are thus responsible for a significant amount of actual tax evasion—off the hook. Notably, Greece prohibited cash transactions exceeding 500 euros in December 2023, with fines of up to twice the value of the transaction. In 2020, Greece required 30% of people's purchases to be made using a debit or credit card, with fines for non-compliance. Greece also had the strictest COVID-19 restrictions in Europe, according to Oxford University's Government Response Tracker. See a pattern?

Of course, CBDCs take things a step—or more—further than conventional credit or debit cards and electronic payments, as they create the groundwork for any country's central bank to eliminate physical cash from circulation. A 2017 WEF article states that the "gradual obsolescence of paper currency" is one of the "characteristics of a well-designed CBDC." But that's not all. In October 2020, for instance, Agustín Carstens, general manager of the Bank of International Settlements, said "general use" of CBDCs would have a "huge difference" from cash. What sort of difference? According to Carstens, "For instance, with cash, we don't know who is using a $100 bill today. A key difference with the CBDC is the central bank will have absolute control on the rules and regulations that will determine the use of that expression of central bank liability [cash], and also, we will have the technology to enforce that."

These "rules and regulations" may include programmable digital money. "Programmable money offers a broad range of new use cases that include spending restrictions, triggers and limits," KPMG blandly states in a 2022 report, while in a 2023 report, global security technology firm Giesecke+Devrient spells it out more explicitly, stating that "CBDC smart wallets could be used to promote policies that help meet sustainability objectives, e.g. by issuing a 'green' wallet that would be a stimulus for consumers to buy environmentally friendly products and services." The same report also states that conditions of use of a digital wallet could be set "on behalf of customers at the issuance level, e.g. a wallet designed solely for use by a company's employees for the purchase of healthy food." In a merger of two goals—going 'green' and going cashless—a 2019 WEF video suggests that, in the future, humans could have the privilege of enjoying "one beef burger, two portions of fish and one or two eggs per week" in order to "save the planet." It's likely not far-fetched to surmise that programmable digital currency could be used to restrict spending on more than one's allocation of, say, beef, just like it could potentially be used to restrict transactions outside one's '15-minute' zone.

Further illustrating this point, in 2019, Swedish fintech company Doconomy introduced the 'DO Card.' Backed by MasterCard, the DO Card tracks the carbon emissions of goods that are purchased and sets a "climate impact cap" for each user of the card. That year, the WEF praised the initiative, stating that "While many of us are aware that we need to reduce our carbon footprint, advice on doing so can seem nebulous and keeping a tab is difficult. DO monitors and cuts off spending, when we hit our carbon max." In 2021, Doconomy teamed up with another Swedish fintech firm, Klarna, to provide 90 million consumers with "carbon footprint insights" by calculating the "climate impact" of each transaction completed through the Doconomy service. In 2024, Greece's Piraeus Bank, in collaboration with Visa, offered its customers the option of enrolling in its "Carbon Footprint Calculator." Described as "The green banking solution for sustainable goals," this service provides information "about the carbon footprint corresponding to the products and services you consume" and issues "advice and informative messages with practices for reducing it." And a 2021 article in the journal Nature cited "the need for a low-carbon recovery from the COVID-19 crisis," arguing that this, along with "recent advances in AI for sustainable development," has opened "a new window of opportunity for PCAs"—personal carbon allowances.

Of course, even good ol' traditional bank accounts are not immune to the whims of governments and banking institutions for people who run afoul of the 'rules'—as evidenced by the examples of participants and supporters of the Canadian Freedom Convoy in 2022, who opposed restrictive COVID-related measures and mandates and whose bank accounts were frozen. But CBDCs and programmable money will not only facilitate such 'punishments' but could also extend to restricting or prohibiting transactions for any reason, including in the name of the environment or public health.

Digital health 'passports' necessary to 'move around'?

Both '15-minute cities' and CBDCs require a technological system of credentials to be fully deployable at scale—just as the enforcement of COVID-era restrictions and, in particular, vaccine mandates did. Enter digital ID. Seen during the pandemic under the guise of so-called 'vaccine passports,' digital ID is now being touted for its convenience—as the primary component of 'digital wallets' that include our drivers' licenses, for instance—and, especially in poorer countries, it is being presented as a means of inclusion in the economy. Indeed, one of the UN's Sustainable Development Goals—Target 16.9—calls for the provision of a digital legal identity for all, including newborns, by 2030, on the basis of guaranteeing said 'inclusion.'

Why such 'inclusion' can't be achieved through any other means or why such exclusion exists in the first place under the governance of the same politicians and officials now promising 'inclusion' is, of course, not typically discussed.

The United States, of course, did not have a national, digital vaccine passport, much as there is no national ID card, digital or otherwise. This is an anomaly in the global context, as national ID cards that are separate from one's, say, drivers' license are standard in most countries. Several U.S. states, however, developed their own 'voluntary' digital vaccine passports using the SMART Health Card standard—backed by the likes of Amazon Web Services, Microsoft, Apple, Google and Mitre—the latter described by *Forbes* as a "cloak-and-dagger R&D shop" that "runs some of the U.S. government's most hush-hush science and tech labs."

Another similar example, The Good Health Pass, was launched by ID2020 as a collaborative effort between Mastercard, the International Chamber of Commerce and the WEF and the endorsement of embattled former U.K. Prime Minister Tony Blair—whose name has been floated as a possible successor to WEF founder and executive chairman Klaus Schwab. Mastercard is a partner of the Good Health Pass Collaborative, while Microsoft is a founding member of the ID2020 Alliance, as are the Bill & Melinda Gates Foundation, the World Bank, the Rockefeller Foundation and Gavi, The Vaccine Alliance—which in 2018 partnered with the WEF's Center for the Fourth Industrial Revolution.

And the European Union's 'Green Pass'—or digital vaccination certificate—which was first proposed at the EU level by Greece—was subsequently adopted by the World Health Organization (WHO) in June 2023 as the global standard for digital health credentials. This partnership is under the auspices of the WHO's Global Digital Health Certification Network (GDHCN). One outcome of the EU-WHO-

GDHCN partnership is the European Vaccination Card, which began being piloted in five EU member states—Belgium, Germany, Greece, Latvia and Portugal—in September 2024 and whose development is being coordinated by the University of Crete in Greece. It was during the 2022 meeting of the B20—bringing together business representatives from the G20 countries—that Indonesia's health minister (and Gavi board member) Budi Gunadi Sadikin revealed plans to launch the GDHCN and called upon the G20 to adopt a "digital health certificate acknowledged by the WHO" that would allow the public to "move around."

Notably, Gates—a known advocate of universal vaccination who recently has promoted and funded 'climate change' vaccines for livestock— is a particularly ardent proponent of digital ID, as evidenced, for instance, by his support for government-backed digital ID for newborns in Kenya, the UN's "50-in-5" digital ID campaign, and for India's nationwide biometric digital ID, Aadhaar, which has been beset by security breaches and other controversies, but which nevertheless was subsequently linked to a digital health ID system the Indian government launched in 2021.

One possible endgame of digital ID and digital health certificates? Restricting movement, just as we've seen with the ideas for '15-minute cities' and 'personal carbon allowances' tied to bank cards or programmable digital currency. At a panel discussion during the WEF's 2024 annual meeting, Queen Máxima of the Netherlands said that digital ID is "very necessary" for the provision of a range of public services—and suggested that it can be used to track the unvaccinated. She said digital ID "is very necessary for financial services [and] is also good for school enrollment, it is also good for health — who actually got a vaccination or not."

Manipulating the human desire to do good

Ultimately, the 'public health' measures adopted during the years of COVID can be viewed as a microcosm of the broader goals of 'stakeholder capitalism,' epitomized by '15-minute cities,' CBDCs and universal digital

ID. During the pandemic, we were asked to wear masks, socially distance, to refrain from visiting family members or friends, to stay home or remain within a close radius to our residences, and, of course, to get the shot. In other words, we were asked to change our behavior and to give up our bodily autonomy, all in the name of the 'greater good.'

The innate, for many, desire to contribute toward the 'greater good' helped contribute to wide acceptance of COVID restrictions and served as the basis for behavioral psychology tactics such as 'nudging' to encourage compliance and shame non-compliers. Such 'nudging' is already viewed as a means toward attaining other 'ends,' such as reduced meat consumption and eating insects instead. For instance, a 2020 study gauging public interest in consuming insects as a source of protein suggested that "As humans are a particularly social species, leveraging the social nature may prove particularly useful."

Interestingly, a form of nostalgia for the days of lockdown and restrictions appears to have also set in for some. A July 2024 Facebook thread I came across can serve as an indicative example. With the caption "Can you believe it's been 4 years since the world stood STILL" posted alongside photos of grounded aircraft and an eerily empty Times Square, comment after comment waxed nostalgic about the good old days of spring 2020 and about the 'green' virtues of ceasing practically all human activity. "*I loved Lockdown! I wish we could have one every few years!*" one user wrote, apparently unironically. "*It was so peaceful, beautiful all you could hear were the birds singing,*" wrote another. "*During our daily hour of freedom my husband and I went for a bike ride... we live in a coastal town so we went to the sea front and I swear we could hear the earth and sea sighing in relief at the peace around us,*" another user wrote, apparently missing the irony of being permitted a "daily hour of freedom." If nothing else, these comments indicate how easily—and indeed willingly—many people change their behavior, when told it is for the 'greater good.'

Similarly, plans for '15-minute cities,' digital ID, digital wallets, CBDCs and 'personal carbon allowances' also aim to change human habits: asking us to reduce our mobility, to drive less, travel less, consume less meat (and perhaps more insects), alter our spending and consumption habits and make 'sacrifices for the greater good,' whether that 'greater good' is protecting public health, saving the climate, or stamping out tax evasion.

This idea of the 'greater good' is also supposedly embedded into the concept of 'stakeholder capitalism'—defined as "a system in which corporations are oriented to serve the interests of all their stakeholders"—with "customers, suppliers, employees, shareholders, and local communities" as potential stakeholders. But are some stakeholders 'more equal than others?' If you ever wondered why large corporations, supposedly motivated only by a capitalist profit motive, all went along so eagerly with COVID lockdowns and restrictions instead of 'letting the free market decide,' the answer might become clearer when considering that Amazon posted record profits during the first year of the pandemic and that, globally, billionaires' wealth increased by $3.9 *trillion* just between March and December 2020, according to a 2021 Oxfam report.

And if the words of an infamous 2016 WEF video predicting that, by 2030, "You're going to own nothing [and] you'll be happy" seem far-fetched, consider the move away from the ownership of physical media (and consumer devices that can play such media) and toward streaming and subscriptions, or HP's new printer subscription plan, with a monthly fee to print a limited number of pages on your 'own' device. Or consider large investment funds such as BlackRock and Vanguard— who are also each other's biggest shareholder—cornering the residential real estate market or Bill Gates becoming the largest owner of farmland in the U.S. To paraphrase George Carlin, the 'stakeholder' club is a big one—and you ain't in it!

CHAPTER 12

Weaponized Fear Corrupts the Human Operating System

The Restoration Involves Self-Healing and Social Connection

Meredith Miller

Holistic coach, author and speaker

Meredith Miller is a holistic coach, author and speaker. Her mission is bridging the gap between trauma and purpose. She helps people transmute the past into gold and transform their wounds into a legacy of light so they can step into their Divine purpose and make a difference in the world around them. Meredith is passionate about helping people liberate themselves and evolve so they can live as free, empowered, responsible, awakened, purposeful and actualized human beings who contribute to the liberation and evolution of others in their own unique ways.

If we want to learn, heal and evolve from what happened since 2020, it's important to start with the question: Who or what was powerful enough to get the entire world to shut down?

Was it the federal or local governments? The WHO? The WEF? The NHS or NIH? The corporations? The media? The coronavirus?

It was actually none of the above.

If we look at the bigger picture, it was fear that shut down the world.

It was fear that drove billions of people to stay home and choose not to see their loved ones for months or years.

It was fear that caused people to comply with increasingly insane rules created by hypocritical public figures who were often caught disregarding those very same rules.

It was fear that drove people to roll up their sleeves and participate in a medical experiment—either voluntarily because they feared sickness and death for themselves and others, or involuntarily by coercion or force because they feared losing their jobs, educational opportunities, seeing loved ones, enjoying events, concerts, restaurants, travelling or otherwise participating in society.

It was fear that blinded people from seeing the manipulation and deception in the propaganda.

It was fear that drove people to hate one another.

Biological fear is a natural survival mechanism built into the nervous system. When fear alerts us of a threat in the environment, the defence system automatically gets activated so we can fight or flee from the danger.

However, fear can become a formidable weapon when it's used to manipulate a person's perception and drive their behaviour.

Weaponized, prolonged fear corrupts the human operating system.

This kind of fear becomes the gateway to hatred, anger, rage, violence, false guilt, compliance, powerlessness, helplessness, hopelessness, apathy, toxic shame, chronic illness and suicide.

Fear is the glue of the trauma bond in abusive relationships. The relentless progression of fear bombardment is alternated with moments of perceived kindness and hope. This psychological and neurological programming is why victims stay and why they keep returning to abusers, or falling for new ones, again and again.

Fear is the ammunition for Divide & Conquer in an abusive system such as a family, workplace or society. Fear interrupts our ability to create secure emotional attachments and healthy social bonds.

Prolonged fear programming locks us in lower states of consciousness where we don't have access to our higher human faculties such as creativity, insight, intuition, critical thinking, imagination and self-healing.

After working with hundreds of survivors of psychologically abusive relationships and family systems, I discovered that each situation was unique, yet the core pattern was always the same: Fear is the currency of control.

Eventually there comes a time in some abusive relationships when the target's denial is pierced by the disruptive truth. I say *some* because most people who are victims of psychological warfare in their partnerships, friendships, family, workplace or society don't realize they're being deceived, manipulated and abused.

After the false security bubble of denial is pierced, a newly awakened mind doesn't know what to believe any more. Once everything collapses, it feels like there's no solid ground upon which to stand. That can be extremely destabilizing and disorienting.

A person lacking a healthy support network of trusted loved ones can end up feeling alone and crazy. Those feelings can quickly escalate to suicidal thoughts. We need to be able to verify reality together.

That's one of the reasons why social connection is so important to our sanity and wellbeing—and that's exactly what the fear disrupts. This is why abusers instinctively know they must isolate their targets in order to keep them in the trance.

Scientific studies done before and during 2020 clearly show how fear and isolation can be used to influence perception and behaviour.

They sure did *follow the science.*

The fear and isolation tactics deployed to sell all things COVID to the public are the same ones that will be used against us in ongoing manipulation campaigns about climate, war, economy, food, energy, elections, etc.

1. Use of fear appeals for persuasion.

Appealing to Fear: A Meta-Analysis of Fear Appeal Effectiveness and Theories (2015)

This 2015 study concluded the following, paraphrased here in plain language:

1. Appealing to fear is effective for influencing attitude, intentions and behaviour.
2. There are very few circumstances in which the fear appeals aren't effective.
3. There are no circumstances in which the fear appeals backfire and lead to undesirable outcomes.
4. Efficacy statements increase the effectiveness of the fear appeals.

Fear can be used to modify perception and behaviour. It's part of the basis for the marketing slogan: *safe and effective*. The use of the word "effective" increases the success of the persuasion in the fear-based messages to get people to take the experimental injections. "Safe" is a carrot of hope dangled as promised relief from the relentless fear bombardment.

2. Dose the masses with hope.

Uplifting Fear Appeals: Considering the Role of Hope in Fear-Based Persuasive Messages (2019)

In this 2019 study, it was discovered that an element of hope can be introduced in order to increase the success of the fear appeals used to coerce people into certain behaviours.

The dosing of hope is a tactic employed by all psychological manipulators to numb the target's critical mind, gain compliance and keep the target in the abuse cycle. Hope causes people to work harder and invest more in that relationship or situation, despite all the harm being done.

This was the basis of Google's marketing campaign, *Get back to what you love,* the same slogan used in YouTube's Vaccine Confidence Project. The Economist magazine cover of November 2020, *Suddenly, hope* was a powerful image for the launch of the jab.

After the relentless fear bombardment, many were desperate to get back to the people, events and activities that they loved and missed. The injections were positioned as the hope and only escape from that nightmare.

3. Use people as vectors to spread fear and isolation.

COVID-19 Vaccine Messaging, Part 1 (2020)

In 2020, Yale University did a study of 10 different messages to sell the jab to the public. These fear-based messages appealed to personal freedom, economic freedom, self-interest, community interest, economic benefit, guilt, embarrassment, anger, trust in science and bravery.

The study states five primary and secondary outcome measures, para-phrased here in plain language:

1. Get people to get vaxxed.
2. Get people to trust the vax.
3. Get people to get other people to get vaxxed.
4. Get people to fear the unvaxxed.
5. Get people to socially judge the unvaxxed based on the following parameters: trustworthiness, selfishness, likeableness and competence.

All of these fear-based messages were used by the media, corporations, organizations, politicians, philanthropaths and influencers, then spread by the masses across social media and society. An abuser would be powerless without enablers. It's the enablers who maintain an abusive system. This is why they had to get the people to do their bidding.

Some messages were clearly more effective than others. Those became the standard talking points of the narrative as well as the knee-jerk social reactions to anyone questioning the narrative.

Community interest was used in messages like "we're all in this together," and "do your part."

Trust in science appeared in slogans like "follow the science," and was combined with embarrassment in ad hominem attacks such as "you're anti-science."

Guilt was the manipulation in curses such as "You're going to kill grandma."

4. Gaslight the public about the health consequences of prolonged isolation and loneliness.

An Overview of Systematic Reviews on the Public Health Consequences of Social Isolation and Loneliness (2017)

In 2017, this study revealed some of the devastating consequences of morbidity and mortality, particularly on cardiovascular and mental health, due to prolonged social isolation and loneliness. The science clearly showed what would happen as a result of social distancing.

The isolation that people experienced was physical (stay home, keep six feet apart, wear a mask, fear other people as vectors of the virus) as well as psychological, which is equally devastating.

Psychological isolation means that a person feels alone in their perception of reality even when in contact with others, whether in person or online. This mainly happens through information control and gaslighting. Censorship and propaganda on social media platforms was vital for spreading the fear-based narrative as well as silencing and smearing people, including doctors, who dared to challenge it.

Isolation is the first parameter of Stockholm Syndrome. Physical and/or psychological isolation is necessary for the fear bombardment to work, and in order to create a trauma bond.

We are currently seeing the downstream effects of isolation and loneliness in society. While these devastating trends are partially being acknowledged now in mainstream media, it's being wrapped in the gaslighting of justification that it was necessary to save lives. In other words, they're saying they had to sacrifice lives to save lives.

There will be long-term consequences on the physical and mental health of individuals and society. Perhaps decades from now this period of time in history will be known as the epidemic of isolation, disconnection and loneliness.

Fear and isolation were the main tools weaponized against us.
Social connection is a biological imperative in mammals, including humans. That's why a person awakening from an abusive relationship needs social support in order to heal from the trauma. It's the same

reason why people need allies now as we're waking up to the massive lies and manipulation.

Neuroscientist, Dr. Andrew Huberman cites in his podcast that there's a "tremendous literature on the biology of social isolation and all of the terrible things that happen when animals or humans are socially-isolated."

Huberman explains how the chronically-elevated stress hormones caused by forced isolation also create an additional problem. It changes the nature of the brain and body such that it makes social connection more challenging. After prolonged social isolation, people become more irritable and aggressive. This shows up particularly when people are given the chance to socialize again. That's why there are increasing news headlines about violence and aggression.

This trend is also visible in online dating. During the peak fear days of the plandemic, people were more willing to connect and meet in person than nowadays. Due to the post-trauma of fear bombardment and isolation, people are more defensive now. Even when people do meet IRL, their unresolved trauma is often triggering each other's defence mechanisms, which shuts down the mammalian attachment system, inhibiting a healthy and secure connection.

When the defence system is engaged, the attachment system is offline.

The defensive system is the stress response of fight, flight, freeze and fawn. This happens when the Autonomic Nervous System detects cues of danger or life threat. The defensive reactions are survival mechanisms. However, these states interfere with social bonding.

The fight response to the fear has been incredibly obvious online and in person, further fomenting the polarization in families, social groups and society.

When we are stuck in seemingly inescapable situations, we might adapt by fawning. This means compliance and people-pleasing. A person gets programmed, often starting in childhood, that it's safer to do what the abuser and enablers want in order to maintain the peace, get rewarded or temporarily avoid the abuse. Most people complied with the mandates. But compliance never ends the abuse cycle—it only prolongs it.

Survivors of childhood trauma often get neurologically programmed to freeze or shut down because fighting back is dangerous and there's no escape. The freeze state is only meant to be a last-ditch survival mechanism because vital organ systems such as digestion, heart rate and respiration are shutting down in order to feign death.

When we have to cope with overwhelming fear and intensely stressful experiences that endure over time, humans adapt to the freeze state by dissociating. This is a form of flight. It means we zone out—doing nothing or engaging in activities like fantasy, TV, smartphone scrolling, porn, numbing through alcohol, over-eating and substance abuse, as well as other dysfunctional behaviors.

Gen Z is raising awareness online about the "functional freeze state" that many people of all ages are experiencing more now than ever. The younger generations, who are the future of humanity, have been the most devastated by the fear and isolation that took place during key developmental stages of their lives.

In a defensive state, and even when interacting with others, the nervous system senses disconnection, which it reads as cues of danger or threat because our species needs secure connection for survival. When we are anxious or afraid, we trigger each other's nervous systems to react in defence. Defensiveness becomes contagious, and isolation persists.

Humans experience social homeostasis through connection.
We need each other to keep ourselves sane and healthy. With each ongoing anti-life campaign launched against the public in this New Normal world, we are going to see escalating devastation done to the physical, mental

and spiritual health of individuals as well as our collective ability to form healthy social connections as a society.

It's essential that we develop the skills and fortitude to self-regulate as responsible individuals so we can co-regulate together with presence and attunement.

It's important to create social containers where we can talk about what happened, then digest and process the feelings emerging so we can heal and move forward. If not, we will continue in the repetition compulsion of the unresolved trauma at the individual level, and history will keep repeating itself due to the trauma frozen in the collective consciousness. It will become the burden of future generations.

We can start to reverse the damage by observing our thoughts, beliefs, behaviors, choices and perceptions of reality. We ought to ask ourselves where those are coming from, whether internally from authenticity and discernment or from an outside entity, program or peer pressure.

As we discover distorted belief programs, we can unsubscribe from the lies and fear as well as anything else that's not aligned with what we really want to create.

The manipulators aim to use us as enablers to co-create a twisted reality in the world where corruption is rewarded. In fact, they need us to do so because they cannot do it without our participation. Our choices are where we find our power.

The Powers That Shouldn't Be are counting on us reacting automatically to their Problem > Reaction > Solution trick instead of consciously choosing our response to life. Responding instead of reacting is how we take our power back.

We ought to reclaim autonomy and sovereignty over our body, mind and spirit. Fear programming is a form of control that corrupts our human consciousness. It locks us in a state of psychological, neurological and spiritual captivity. Liberation means facing reality, setting boundaries, reprogramming ourselves and grieving what happened so we can heal the trauma.

Together we can witness and grieve what's happened. The post-trauma isn't caused by what happened but rather the loneliness of being unmet by existential empathy, when there's no one there to mutually witness reality. The worst part is the isolation.

Social connection is the antidote to the fear and isolation epidemic and it's exactly what abusers fear the most. Yet our attempts to connect are sabotaged by our defence mechanisms, which get automatically activated when triggered by the trauma programming. This is why the collective work starts within each individual's commitment to the responsibility of self-healing. As we heal ourselves, we can connect and heal together, contributing to a healing world.

1. https://pubmed.ncbi.nlm.nih.gov/?term=Tannenbaum+MB&cauthor_id=26501228
Appealing to fear: A meta-analysis of fear appeal effectiveness and theories Melanie B
Tannenbaum 1, Justin Hepler 2, Rick S Zimmerman 3, Lindsey Saul 4, Samantha Jacobs 4,
Kristina Wilson 1, Dolores Albarracín 1. November, 2015.
2. https://pubmed.ncbi.nlm.nih.gov/29313717/
Uplifting Fear Appeals: Considering the Role of Hope in Fear-Based Persuasive Messages Robin
L Nabi 1, Jessica Gall Myrick 2, April, 2019.

3. https://clinicaltrials.gov/study/NCT04460703
Yale University, updated May 2022

4. https://pubmed.ncbi.nlm.nih.gov/28915435/
An overview of systematic reviews on the public health consequences of social isolation and
loneliness
N Leigh-Hunt 1, D Bagguley 2, K Bash 3, V Turner 4, S Turnbull 5, N Valtorta 6, W Caan 7,
September, 2017.

CHAPER 13

The Upside Down World of Pandemic Science: The Case of Fisman's Fraud

Dr. Regina Watteel

PHD in statistics and author of Fisman's Fraud.

Regina Watteel is a Canadian statistician and bestselling author. She holds a PhD in Statistics from the University of Western Ontario as well as an MSc in Statistics and a BSc in Mathematics & Physics from McMaster University. She has been an outspoken critic of the fraudulent modeling and misleading statistics that fueled the Canadian government's destructive pandemic response. Currently, Regina is focused on exposing provable acts of scientific fraud in order to hold influential researchers and institutions accountable for the harms caused by their actions. Lightly edited excerpts from the book "Fisman's Fraud: The Rise of Canadian Hate Science" by Dr. Regina N. Watteel, RainSong Books, November 2023.

Before April 25th, 2022 I had little to no knowledge of David Fisman. I say "little to no knowledge" instead of "no knowledge" because, in all likelihood, his name had come up on the radio or in news articles that I'd stumbled upon without taking much notice. With so much profound upheaval over the course of the pandemic, bigger problems were top of mind. Well, all that changed one afternoon in spring after encountering numerous headlines warning of the risk of mixing with the "unvaccinated."

Instinctively and scientifically, I knew the headlines to be false, and so ignored them at first. I assumed the media was just sensationalizing yet another garbage study, one of many that had been published throughout the pandemic. But the headlines kept popping up everywhere, and the timing seemed suspicious given the politics at play. So, I pulled up the actual study to see first-hand how the researchers possibly could have arrived at such a backwards conclusion.

Utter disgust. That is the feeling that best sums up the experience.

Disgust as a mathematician and statistician. Disgust as a mother. Disgust as a Canadian. Disgust as an honest and decent human being.

I couldn't believe what I was reading, initially flooded with so many thoughts and emotions. The nonsense of it all was dizzying. I had to walk away from the so-called "study" several times, midstream, just to clear my head. Appalling on so many levels, I haven't been able to let it go. Straight-away, I recognized the societal discord it was meant to sow and the hateful policies it was attempting to legitimize. I had become all too familiar with them. There was no way I could hold my tongue on this one. How could anyone?

Compared to the assessments I had done in the past, the general risk analysis for COVID-19 was straightforward and the results markedly clear: the very elderly and those with comorbid conditions were at highest risk; healthy, working-aged individuals were at fairly low, manageable risk; while children and young adults had almost no risk of serious COVID-19 complications — less than the seasonal flu. Moreover, the risk between the oldest age group and the youngest changed by a factor of about a thousand. Based on this early assessment, my focus turned to my aging parents and my two siblings who worked in the health care sector. I kept track of the changing dynamics, government responses, emerging scientific findings as well as vaccine progress. When the clinical trial reports and assessments became available, I was quick to study them.

Things didn't add up right from the beginning. At every stage in the pandemic the government appeared to act nearly opposite to what the data indicated should be done, at least from a risk mitigation perspective. And when the vaccines rolled out, my concerns multiplied.

During the spring of 2021, I became increasingly concerned about the use of the novel vaccines on children and healthy young adults given the absence of long-term safety data or any clear benefits to them. In addition, concerns of myocarditis in youths had also been raised in the medical community. That summer, there was talk of mandatory vaccination for in-person university courses, health care workers and federal employees.

From a risk-benefit perspective, I understood this to be a very dangerous precedent. So, when the 2021 federal election was called, in a protective impulse I threw my hat into the ring to oppose the mandates. Desperate times call for desperate measures, so the saying goes. I had no shot at winning, but I gave it my all, nonetheless, just to get the message out.

Canada had entered into a truly dark period. PM Trudeau's shocking remarks in a French-language TV interview during his election campaign illustrate the country's downward spiral:

> Yes, we will emerge from this pandemic through vaccination. We know people who are still making up their minds and we will try to convince them, but there are also people who are vehemently opposed to vaccination. They do not believe in science, who are often misogynists, often racists, too; it is a sect, a small group, but who are taking up space, and here we have to make a choice, as a leader, as a country. Do we tolerate these people?
> —Prime Minister Justin Trudeau, September 2021
> (translated from French)

Sadly, the mandates came to pass. Hard months followed. The unvaccinated were barred from international travel, yet the Omicron variant made its way to Canada all the same. Unvaccinated Canadians weren't permitted to travel within their own country by plane or train, but cases surged across the provinces anyway. Workplaces that had purged their premises of unvaccinated workers saw an unprecedented rise in COVID-19 cases amongst their vaccinated workforce. COVID-19 cases rose to record heights, dwarfing all pre-vaccination peaks. Canadian COVID-19 hospitalizations under the milder cold-like variant more than doubled previous records. It became impossible to hide the complete failure of the vaccines to curtail community transmission, and equally difficult to interpret the segregation of the unvaccinated as anything but unfounded discrimination. Provinces soon abandoned their vaccine passports and by spring of 2022 it seemed the federal restrictions were ready to topple... That is, until Fisman's "study" miraculously appeared and gave the feds one last gasp for air.

The Fisman Flip

On April 25th, 2022 a research study appeared in a respected Canadian medical journal claiming justification and strong support for federal and provincial restrictions based on vaccination status. It was David Fisman and his two colleagues, Afia Amoako and Ashleigh R. Tuite, to the federal government's rescue.

In essence, the researchers overwrote the Omicron surge with a fake simulation showing disproportionately greater infection rates amongst the unvaccinated — a trend opposite reality — in an attempt to scapegoat the unvaccinated for: 1) SARS-CoV-2 transmission, 2) vaccine failure, and 3) poor public health care decisions. But the research trio went even further.

The three career mathematical modellers proceeded to pass off the fabricated results as fact despite no real data being used, no hypothesis being tested and no model validation of any kind. Under the guise of "science" the researchers claimed the results supported the governments' harsh vaccine restrictions. When called out by droves of researchers from around the world for the flawed modelling and deceptive findings, the researchers refused to correct the record. Instead, the main author doubled-down on his divisive rhetoric and support of punitive measures against the unvaccinated.

Figures 4 & 5 compare the incident cases fabricated using Fisman, Tuite and Amoako's contrived model to the actual incident cases observed in Ontario during the Omicron surge. Note that the baseline conditions used in Fisman's simulation were matched to the conditions in Ontario at the emergence of Omicron. In Fisman's reality, the epidemic wave was driven by incident cases amongst the unvaccinated, as shown in Figure 4 (taken directly from the journal publication). However, the official government of Ontario data — posted on the government's website and readily available to the researchers and the public at the time — showed the opposite trend (Figure 5).

Figure 4: COVID-19 Incident Cases
Fisman et al.'s Simulated (FAKE) Scenario

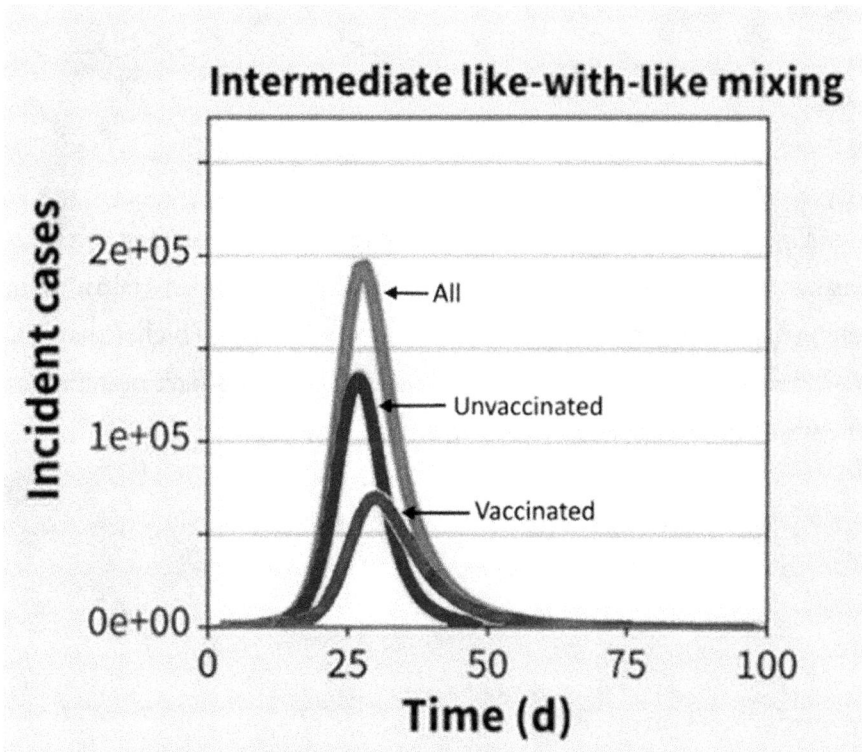

Figure 5: COVID-19 Incident Cases
Ontario (REAL) Data: (Nov. 28, 2021 - Feb. 25, 2022)

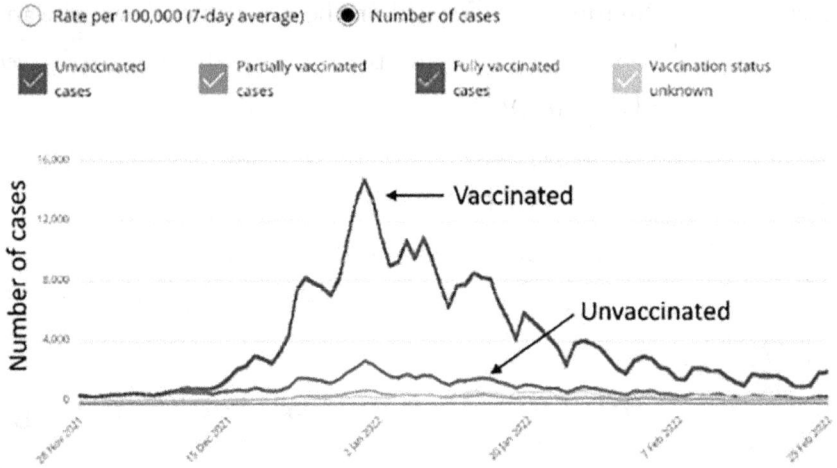

Figures 6 and 7 provide a comparison of incident rates between Fisman's simulation and real-world observations. In Fisman's fabrication, the unvaccinated incident rates were disproportionately higher than the vaccinated — again, opposite reality. Many researchers have pointed out the study's contradictions to reality.

Figure 6: COVID-19 Incident Rates

Fisman et al.'s Simulated (FAKE) Scenario

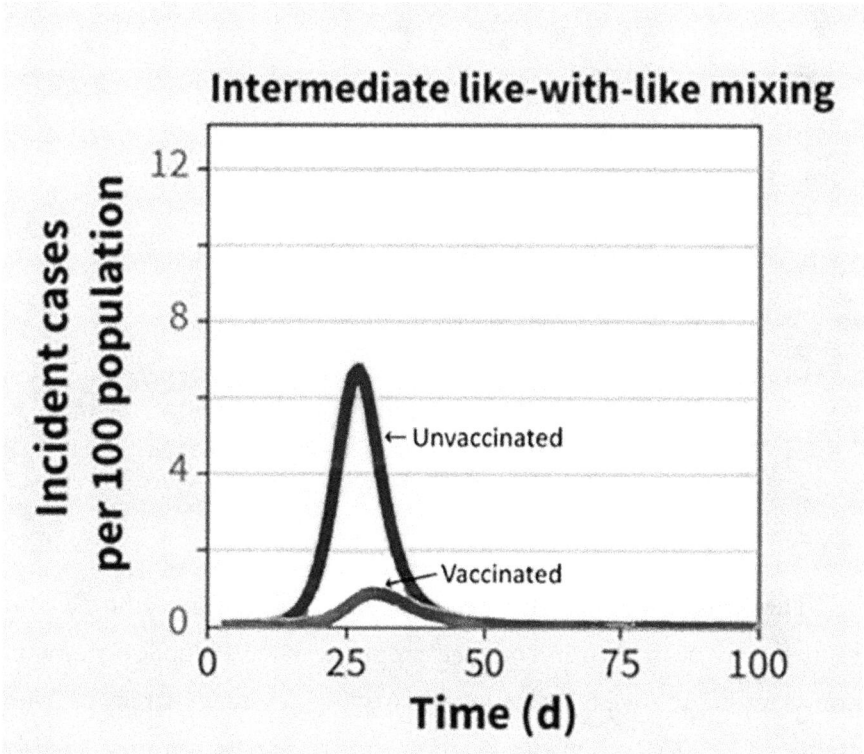

Figure 7: COVID-19 Incident Rates
Ontario (REAL) Data: Dec. 24, 2021 to Jan. 22, 2022

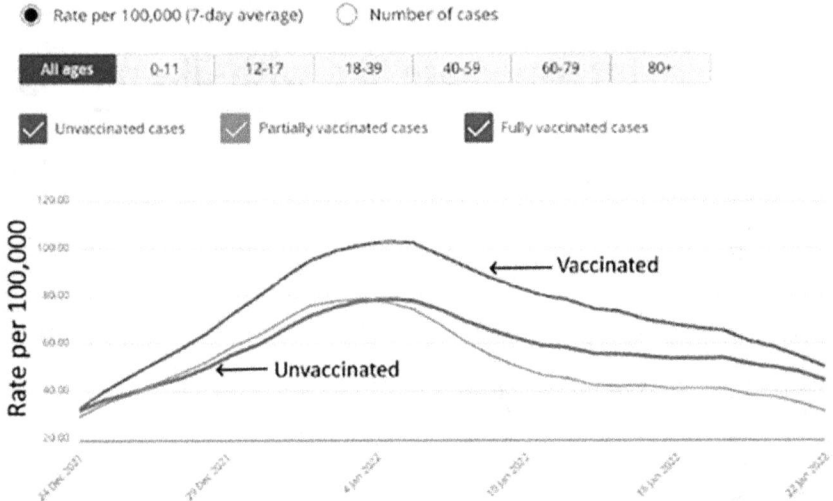

The divisive study took Canada by storm. Its main author, David Fisman — an outspoken and partisan supporter of harsh public policy with numerous ties to the pharmaceutical industry — claimed that people who decline COVID-19 vaccination put the vaccinated at disproportionate risk.

Within hours of the study's official publication, articles in dozens of top newspapers and magazines flooded the nation, warning of the dire risks of merely "hanging out" with unvaccinated people. The vaccine was touted as powerful at stifling COVID-19, yet, it was incapable of protecting the population so long as the unvaccinated were present. Somehow, the absurd notion spread like wildfire.

Those who refused to accept the genetic injections were vilified as selfish souls. Numerous podcasts, interviews and articles citing Fisman's paper compared the unvaccinated to carriers of syphilis and reckless drivers.

A few days later, the news even entered into Canadian parliamentary proceedings. A timely development — the Trudeau government was in desperate need of "scientific" justification for extending their federal vaccine mandates and travel restrictions, irrespective of the vaccines' utter failure to curb Omicron.

> "Vaccinated individuals have a right not to have their efforts to protect themselves undermined," Fisman said, stressing that the (study) findings are "very supportive" of vaccine mandates for flights and trains. — Forbes, April 25, 2021

It became abundantly clear that this fraudulent activity needed to be addressed. The study's potential to influence public policy and set an unacceptable precedent in the production, distribution and ultimate consumption of degenerate science had to be curtailed.

I reached out to the Canadian Medical Association Journal (CMAJ) — the journal that published the study.

I wrote them ONCE. I wrote them TWICE. I wrote them THREE TIMES!

I reached out to the University of Toronto (U of T) — the institution where the research was carried out.

ONCE. TWICE. THREE TIMES!

I reached out to The Canadian Institutes of Health Research — the federal institution that funded the study.

AM I INVISIBLE?

Deny. Deflect. Dismiss.

So, I wrote to the Ontario Provincial Police (OPP).

I requested an investigation and sent them a 150-page evidential report.

I wrote to the Ontario Premier's office.

I asked that they support an OPP investigation.

Lip service.

The Players & the Politics

My efforts to have the Fisman paper retracted and the record corrected revealed a web of complicity and self-serving interests. Incriminating changes made to the Fisman paper as it propagated through the CMAJ peer
review process indicate that the journal was actively involved in the evolution of the deceptive and defamatory content. Perhaps the most striking
revisions involved efforts to present the illusion that the simulated trends
were based on real people as opposed to predetermined results concoct-
ed by the researchers. With the elimination of modelling jargon together
with repeated insertions of the word "people" — used only once in the
preprint but appearing 76 times in the final publication — it's little wonder laypersons mistook the fake study for one grounded in reality.

The inclusion of unwarranted and derisive comparisons in the CMAJ
publication was jarring for what should have been an objective scientific
paper. Fisman, the lead author, subsequently engaged in numerous interviews, podcasts, and social media exchanges where he continued to exploit
the fraudulent study and defame individuals. The defamatory statements
included: casting the unvaccinated as casual spreaders of disease who constitute an unacceptable risk to other people; comparing the decision to not
take the COVID-19 vaccines to reckless behavior such as driving under
the influence of alcohol and other intoxicants, or driving at 200 km/hr for
fun; and, insinuating that the unvaccinated were largely responsible for
overburdening hospitals and causing the cancellation of elective surgeries
for cancer and cardiac disease patients.

The defamatory statements were a clear effort to tarnish the character and reputation of the unvaccinated, to influence policy makers, and to seek public buy-in for punitive measures against the unvaccinated. I was shocked to discover that, far from screening out such statements, a number of them actually had been added during the peer review process.

There's little doubt that the modifications made to the preprint helped spur the media's sensationalized headlines. It is rare for academic papers to get such mainstream publicity. The publication's online engagement represented CMAJ's second most highly engaged article, as tracked by Altmetric Digital Science, since tracking began in 2011. It scored in the top 0.01% of all online research outputs across all sources. I submitted a formal complaint to U of T calling for an investigation into allegations of research fraud. The allegations included fabrication and falsification of data and results; specific text-book incidents of the scientific fraud were highlighted. I followed U of T's process for dealing with such allegations. Their framework promises a thorough process to address and resolve all questions raised by the complaint.

The university had no interest whatsoever in investigating the misconduct. After a few back-and-forth letters prompting them to reconsider, U of T closed the file without addressing a single concern. In April 2022, just weeks before Fisman's paper was released, U of T had announced a partnership with Moderna Inc. to advance research in RNA science and technology. The university supported COVID-19 vaccine mandates and restrictions throughout the pandemic and had, like many universities across the country, been granted large financial incentives from the Government of Canada to address "vaccine hesitancy" and other related matters. The Canadian Institutes of Health Research (CIHR) funded the Fisman study. CIHR is Canada's federal funding agency for health research; it is accountable to Parliament through the Minister of Health. The fraudulent study had been cited in Parliament by the Parliamentary Secretary to the Minister of Health as justification for retaining travel restrictions against the unvaccinated. I informed CIHR of the transgression, provided solid proof and substantiation, and I asked that they set the record straight. The Agencies Presidents voted against my request.

In short, the Government of Canada funded a fraudulent study that was subsequently used to provide justification for its coercive measures at a time when there appeared to be no real justification.

It is clear that individuals who chose to forgo COVID-19 vaccination have been subjected to extreme animosity and discrimination without due justification. In the case of Fisman's study, he and his two colleagues were willing to commit fraud to scapegoat the unvaccinated for product failure. Though Fisman's faux study sets a new low in research ethics and integrity, it did not occur out of the blue. It followed a series of systemwide failures that were exploited during the pandemic. The abandonment of fundamental practices in science, health care, democratic governance and law have led to the collapse of long-established safeguards to protect the health, well-being and civil liberties of Canadians. The results have been devastating.

What Sets This Case Apart

One might argue that during the COVID-19 pandemic, deception and misinformation ran rampant, leaving no shortage of individuals to investigate for potential acts of fraud. So why focus resources on a few mathematical modelers?

There are five main reasons why this particular case of scientific misconduct requires attention: (1) the researchers' clear intent, (2) the crucial role they played in deceiving the public, (3) the far-reaching impact of their fraudulent activity, (4) the willful backing by the establishment, and (5) the potential for future harm.

Faux mathematical modeling has become the nucleus of the "follow the science" scheme.

The Omicron variant changed the playing field. Real-world data could no longer support the mass COVID-19 vaccination strategy and no amount of data manipulation could salvage it. The final tool in the "science" arsenal was to abandon reality completely and simply contrive models to support the storyline and provide the results wanted. All that was needed were willing researchers to create the faux models and lend their credentials to the cause, along with an incentivized media to propagate the findings.

By calling out the faux models and publications for what they are — fraudulent — and holding the researchers legally responsible for their activity, the scheme collapses.

The fraudulent modeling doesn't get more clear-cut than the Fisman, Tuite and Amoako case. Their actions and intent were undeniable. Their language was clear; their timing suspicious.

A strong deterrent against this activity is needed or it will propagate. Fisman et al. crossed the line into overt fraud and hate science. Prosecuting the fraud provides an opportunity to expose the danger of mathematical modeling as a means of deception and its harmful impact, not only on health, but in promoting a morally degenerate society that embraces discrimination. Holding these researchers (and publishers) legally accountable would serve as a warning to all scientists tempted to commit these opportunistic crimes. Without complicit researchers like Fisman, the fraudulent "follow the science" scheme cannot be sustained.

***Lightly edited excerpts from the book "Fisman's Fraud: The Rise of Canadian Hate Science" by Dr. Regina N. Watteel, RainSong Books, November 2023.

CHAPTER 14

Modern Medicine's Great Controversy

Dr. Peter McCullough

Practising Internist and Cardiologist

Dr. Peter McCullough is a prominent internist, cardiologist, and epidemiologist, holding degrees from Baylor University, University of Texas Southwestern Medical School, University of Michigan, and Southern Methodist University. He is widely recognized for his expertise in managing cardiovascular complications, infectious diseases, and vaccine-related injuries.

Dr McCcullough has broadly published on a range of topics in medicine with more than 1000 publications and over 685 citations in the National Library of Medicine. His works include "Pathophysiological Basis and Rationale for Early Outpatient Treatment of SARS-CoV-2 (COVID-19) Infection" - the first widely utilized treatment regimen for ambulatory patients infected with SARS-CoV-2 in the American Journal of Medicine and subsequently updated in Reviews in Cardiovascular Medicine. He later published the first detoxification approach titled "Clinical Rationale for SARS-CoV-2 Base Spike Protein Detoxification in Post COVID-19 and Vaccine Injury Syndromes" in the Journal of American Physicians and Surgeons and the PUBMED indexed journal CUREUS. He has dozens of peer-reviewed publications on the infection and has commented extensively on the medical response to the COVID-19 crisis in The Hill, America Out Loud, and on FOX NEWS Channel. Dr. McCullough testified multiple times in the US Senate, US House of Representatives, Texas Senate Committee on Health and Human Services, Arizona Senate and House of Representatives, Colorado General Assembly, New Hampshire Senate, Pennsylvania Senate, South Carolina Senate and the EU Parliament concerning many aspects of the pandemic response. He has had years of dedicated academic and clinical efforts in combating the SARS-CoV-2 virus and in doing so, has reviewed thousands of reports, participated in scientific congresses, group discussions, press releases, and has been considered among the world's experts on COVID-19.

Dr. McCullough is co-author of the best-selling book "The Courage to Face COVID-19: Preventing Hospitalization and Death While Battling the Biopharmaceutical Complex," by John Leake & Peter McCullough, MD, MPH. New York: Skyhorse Publishing, 2022.

The Bio-Pharmaceutical Complex is using censorship, propaganda and manipulation to keep people living in fear. But what we need now is courage.

Do you remember loved ones in the hospital? Do you remember being told that all we can do is wait for a vaccine? Do you remember being told there's nothing that can be done? They told us; just wait for the government to tell us what to do in the setting of an emergency. The most interesting thing about this crisis is how simultaneous it was and how coordinated worldwide. It was truly extraordinary.

All of us have now become closet virologists. Even the average person on the street knows what the nucleocapsid and spike protein are in the structure of SARS-CoV-2. The spike protein is the engineered part of this chimeric virus. It was engineered collaboratively and organized by Dr. Anthony Fauci. The chief scientist was Dr. Ralph Baric at the University of North Carolina, Chapel Hill. The person who coordinated this across the globe was Peter Daszak at EcoHealth Alliance. And then the person who actually physically did the work in her team was Dr. Shi Zhengli at the Wuhan Institute of Virology. This is now all fully understood, exposed in the Covid House Select Committee investigations led by Representative Brad Wenstrup.

Recently, I testified on Capitol Hill just two days after Fauci was there, questioned by the same group who questioned Fauci. Fauci conceded that the creation of this virus was for the purposes of making a vaccine. That's what it was all about. That is what disease X is all about. There is a worldwide scientific agenda to create biological threat after biological threat.

The United States has been preparing for this for years. We have the 2005 CARES act that said, there will be biological threats and there will be government countermeasures, which are vaccines. That was written by HHS in Congress in 2005. This has been planned for a long time.

As citizens and as doctors and health care professionals and mothers and fathers, we have to defend the issue of public safety. For new biologic products, we have to demand safety, safety, safety. We've got a consumer product safety issue on our hands of massive proportions.

In the first year of the pandemic, Dr. Scott Atlas and I were writing op-eds in *The Hill*, which is read by the White House, the House of Representatives and the Senate. Scott was focusing on masks and lockdowns. I was focusing on early treatment and what was going to be required to prevent hospitalizations and deaths.

This vaccine program was a gamble. It was a gamble for all time with humanity. Doctor Karina Acevedo-Whitehouse in Mexico has done a wonderful job in explaining in the peer-reviewed literature that the genetic vaccines are the messenger RNA vaccines. They are the genetic code for the spike protein, which was engineered in the Wuhan Institute of Virology. The spike protein is the lethal part of the virus. The genetic code is injected in the human body and there's no off switch. Some people invariably are going to produce too much spike protein for too long in the wrong parts of the body, and it's going to be fatal. All of this could have been easily predicted ahead of time.

There were only a few of us anywhere in the world questioning this in writing. Why wouldn't we question the notion of injecting the genetic code for the lethal part of the virus?

We followed up with a paper pretty quickly in May 2021, outlining an enormous number of concerns. Titled, "SARS-CoV-2 mass vaccination: Urgent questions on vaccine safety that demand answers from international health agencies, regulatory authorities, governments and vaccine developers," was published in preprint at Researchgate.net. This paper was sent to every single government in the world. Roxana Bruno gets a great amount of credit for this. We had a litany of questions regarding these vaccines. Where are they going to go? How do we ensure safety? How are we going to protect populations who could be harmed by the vaccines? Where's the risk stratification in terms of who really would need a vaccine if it indeed worked?

What's come out in paper after paper - and it's only the tip of the iceberg because there's so much bias against any manuscript questioning the vaccines - is that shedding is happening. This is inadvertent vaccination of people who really are not recipients directly of the vaccine. For example, adverse events are happening in babies who are breastfed by vaccinated mothers. It is nothing short of astounding. It is really the medical story of our lifetime.

The story of the mRNA is a continuing one. A paper from Stanford by Roltgen et al found the mRNA is still present in lymph nodes at 60 days. In a cohort of hepatitis C patients, researchers found the messenger RNA circulating in blood 28 days after injection. It may have been longer, but that's as long as they measured it in their study.

People who took these shots simply took them on faith. No one could have known what was going to happen once they got an injection of a brand new technology messenger RNA loaded on a lipid nanoparticle.

There's mRNA in breast milk. Remember, if a drug gets into breast milk, it's a big deal for a lactating woman. Now the vaccine is getting into the placenta. Pregnant women and women of childbearing potential were specifically excluded from the clinical trials. Therefore they should never have received an experimental genetic vaccine with coding for the lethal part of the virus because there's two patients, the mother and the baby. They were also at lower risk; studies showed pregnant women have better outcomes than non-pregnant women with COVID-19. They're the lowest at risk population. Yet when the shots came out in the first week of the vaccine campaign, over 3,000 pregnant women were vaccinated. They were not excluded. In fact, the American College of Obstetrics and Gynecology said in an unprecedented manner that pregnant women should take the vaccine at any time during pregnancy. Remember, the first trimester is organogenesis. That's when the baby is forming. That was unprecedented, to show absolutely no concern for the mother or the baby. Now the results of the first randomized trial of pregnant women taking the vaccine shows a 4 to 1 increase in the rate of birth defects in the babies in Pfizer's own study, which they cut short.

The next issue is contamination of the vaccines. Two papers have found the Simian Virus 40 in vaccines. It's a known proto-oncogene activator, the origin of antibiotic resistant genes. But the contamination of vaccines is very old news. Over a hundred years old. The smallpox vaccine was grossly contaminated in the late 1800s and early 1900s. We had no way of purifying it. It was coming literally from the juices of cows or horses, or human-to-human and arm-to-arm vaccination. It was grossly contaminated with staphylococcus and streptococcus and tetanus and syphilis and foot and mouth disease. People died of the smallpox vaccine in large numbers. What was the government response? Mandatory vaccination, taking kids out of school. Putting people in jail. Corporal assault and vaccination with smallpox. That's what happened in the U.S., in the UK and in Europe. That was 120 years ago, and it's as if we've learned nothing. The smallpox vaccine failed miserably. It didn't stop smallpox. And just like Doctor David Brownstein (West Bloomfield, MI) showed, smallpox faded out of existence not because of the vaccine, but because we had improved hygienic measures (washing bed sheets and personal hygiene).

Another example of contaminated vaccines is the polio vaccine. An Institute of Medicine report on the polio virus vaccine contamination with SV-40. Between 1954 and 1963, 98 million Americans received the polio vaccine contaminated with a carcinogenic monkey virus, SV-40. The Institute of Medicine has reviewed this. We can't know how much cancer today is really due to the fact that children were vaccinated against smallpox using this faulty vaccine. There is a history of willful blindness to vaccine safety issues, because vaccines fall into what's considered an ideology. It's like a religion. And vaccines are accepted as an article of faith.

Some of my colleagues have had the courage to reach back and communicate with me over the last four years, and one of them from Johns Hopkins asked me, "don't you believe in vaccines anymore?" In medicine we don't believe in things or not. We actually evaluate them. We have a scientific evaluation, a clinical understanding, and we're constantly reviewing the literature. I can tell you the safety review on these vaccines is an absolute catastrophe. If any candidate running for office is willfully blind to what's going on and they are not openly campaigning on this, it's a tragedy.

The Vaccine Adverse Event Reporting System (VAERS) numbers went through the roof when the COVID vaccines came out. The CDC has fully vetted and accepted 18,655 Americans and growing, who have died due to the vaccine, reported by doctors like me, who believe the vaccine is the cause of death. 1150 people died on the same day they took the shot, 1225 died the day after the shot. The CDC has the patient's name, email, phone number, family members' numbers, the clinical vignette. Hundreds of papers have been written and analysed from these, including the vignettes. I've read them. The vaccine looks like it's the direct cause of death. VAERS can be used to ascertain the cause of death. We simply read the clinical vignettes and we adjudicate in clinical research.

Prior to the rollout of the COVID vaccines, the highest number of deaths that has ever been recorded in this system over the last 30 years was 150 in a single year. Now it's 18,655. But there's a significant underreporting factor in VAERS due to the complexity of submitting a report.

It is estimated that this is by a factor of 30. This would make the true number closer to 559,650 American deaths to date.

We have candidates running for office who do not acknowledge this catastrophe. This is worse than the Civil War. This vaccine campaign has created a biological safety catastrophe. In Texas, the vaccines are so dangerous that we had to ban any mandate because we couldn't mandate someone to take a lethal vaccine. They're lethal in so many people.

Nick Hulscher, MPH, from University of Michigan, has led the most important sets of studies. He's shown that broadly 73.9 percent of all the deaths that occur after a vaccine that come to autopsy, are directly due to the vaccine.

The next person you hear of who dies with no antecedent illness, with no apparent reason to die - it is the vaccine until proven otherwise. That's a conservative safety approach. Until proven otherwise.

A few years ago, we'd hear about correspondents and others dying right after they took the vaccine. Now the vaccine is being expunged from any press reports. People now simply die of "unknown" or "natural causes" with no antecedent illness. What you're being told and what you're witnessing is a safety cover up.

Fortunately, a large number of people look like they're fine. Thirty percent of people have no side effects whatsoever. Not even a sore arm. Nothing appears to happen. Just under two thirds take a vaccine and they have some minor side effects. But approximately 4.2 percent of people who take a shot get in trouble. It's called hot lots. The explanations are that maybe some of the vials have too much mRNA or are excessively contaminated with DNA process-related impurities (SV-40). There have been visible contaminants in the vaccines.

The vaccines have never been inspected for the quantity of messenger RNA. Of the 75 percent of Americans who took a shot, 94 percent of them took a mRNA vaccine. Fortunately, 25 percent of Americans, according to the COVID States Program report, did not take a COVID-19 vaccine. But in a Danish study, it was 4.2 percent of people who are in trouble. According to the CDC V-safe data - which the CDC refused to release to the public until forced to do so by a court order - it's 7.7 percent of Americans who are in trouble after taking a COVID vaccine. We are seeing cardiovascular, neurologic, hematologic and immunologic problems everywhere.

After the vaccine, my clinic and Dr. Brownstein's clinic was like a war zone of blood clots, heart damage, amputations, and heart failure. Many people are absolutely miserable now with deep regret. And every single one of them has said, "you know, I won't go to the doctor who told me to get the vaccine. I don't see that doctor anymore." So, there are doctors who actually are not seeing *any* of the vaccine complications, because the patients, those five to 10 percent of patients who are really damaged, never go back to them.

A major area of concern is cancer. A paper from Angus and Bustos at the University of Oregon indicates that there are multiple mechanisms by which the vaccines could cause cancer. The spike protein inhibits tumor suppressor systems p53 and BRCA. The messenger RNA itself impairs DNA repair. We now have great concerns that the Pfizer and Moderna vaccines could be accelerating cancer. Since 2021, every cancer registry in the world is on the way up. What most people need to know is we're talking largely about solid organ cancers like lung cancer, kidney cancer, etc.. From the time a cancer begins to the time it's clinically recognized, it's typically five years. But these vaccines have potentially accelerated the course of the cancer. The term is turbo cancer.

When I testified on Capitol Hill recently, I explained that the FDA says that the risk period for gene transfer technology products - the messenger RNA vaccines (Pfizer and Moderna) and the Adenoviral vaccines (Janssen and AstraZeneca) - is between five and 15 years of concern, observation and worry. Family members took these vaccines. How long are you going to worry about them? The FDA says from five to 15 years.

People always ask me, when is it over with? My reply is, "not for a long time, because we don't know. The genetic code is long lasting. The spike protein in the body is even more long lasting." There are probably hundreds of thousands of manuscripts out there regarding serious safety syndromes that cannot get into the peer reviewed literature.

There is a paper from Harvard showing the messenger RNA is getting into the heart muscle, causing inflammation damage and edema of cells. Thirty days later when people die it is found at autopsy. That means all mRNA vaccines will probably physically be in the heart, causing heart damage.

This means that Moderna's other RNA-based vaccines such as their influenza vaccine and their respiratory syncytial vaccine will also be found in the heart. They've already halted their trials. So the Epstein-Barr virus vaccine will also likely cause myocarditis. Get used to saying myocarditis. We'll see a lot of it if messenger RNA technology is advanced, because spike protein, produced by mRNA, is toxic to human heart cells.

Yet the vaccines were rolled out. A study done by Nakhara et al, at the University of Texas at Houston, showed that the vaccinated have markedly abnormal cardiac PET scans positron emission tomography compared to the unvaccinated. Also, cancers do that. Everybody who took a vaccine, whether they look healthy to you or not, should be cause for concern. We are seeing cardiac arrests where we don't have classic myocarditis present. But we know from the University of Texas study, that the cardiac PET scans are abnormal. We don't know the implications of this, but we do know that those who had a sore arm had more intense cardiac PET findings.

A paper from Harvard published by Yonker et al in Circulation, the best cardiac research journal, showed that young boys hospitalised at Massachusetts General Hospital who had myocarditis had circulating spike protein, and the antibodies were not neutralising the spike protein. Research now shows that with repeated vaccines, the body shifts to relatively useless forms of antibodies, so-called IgG subclass four. They don't bind the spike protein. Now, the boys who were fine with no myocarditis also had spike protein, but the antibodies were appropriately blocking the spike protein. We have no way of predicting who the next person is, who takes a shot, who's going to have unopposed spike protein circulate in their body and cause heart damage.

I worked on a paper with Dr. Jessica Rose which extrapolates from the studies available right now, that there is a measurable mortality rate with myocarditis that ranges from 1 to 4 percent even in the first few months. Myocarditis is not transient, it's not self-limited, and it's not benign. We have no idea how large this problem is. What I'm telling you is the tip of the iceberg.

There are just so many stories of heart failure following the fatal Pfizer vaccine. In a study published by Choi and colleagues, a 22-year-old man goes to a Korean hospital five days after the first shot of Pfizer. He dies seven hours later with full CPR, full ICU, full everything. His heart biopsy necropsy at the time of autopsy shows his heart is rotted out with inflammation from the vaccine. Fatal Pfizer myocarditis cannot be saved.

In Connecticut, two boys aged 16 and 17, days three and four after their Pfizer shots, are found dead in bed. No chance for CPR, no chance to be saved. An autopsy was performed and scientists from the University of Michigan and the University of Connecticut were called in to help the coroner. The conclusion? Fatal Pfizer COVID-19 vaccine induced myocarditis.

Parents should be outraged. Parents should be pressing candidates running for office to the wall on this. Why are our young children dying of the vaccine, proven in autopsy confirmed studies? The willful blindness of our candidates is shameful. Honestly, this should be an outrage. If people are outraged about a single life being lost due to a murder by a migrant, why aren't they worried about two boys who die after taking a vaccine where it's so clear cut?

Oscar Cabrera admitted he didn't want to take the shots. He tweeted, "I don't want to take these shots." He was from the Dominican Republic, he played in the European basketball leagues, and he had to take the shots. He had a cardiac arrest on the floor, and he was revived and he tweeted, "I had this cardiac arrest because of these shots." Two years later, he was trying to make a comeback. He was doing a medical grade stress test and he died on the treadmill, two years after his initial myocarditis. I'm telling you, it's not over after a few days after these shots. We are seeing cardiac arrest now occurring years after taking these vaccines.

Nic Hulscher's paper outlines the mechanism of what's going on. The shots are taken into the body. There are probably risk factors. About half the time there are symptoms. The other half of the time there are no symptoms. The cardiac MRI lights up like a Christmas tree in severe cases, typically the inferior lateral wall. And it's typically the outer part of the myocardium adjacent to the pericardium. We have blood tests and things we can do; maybe we can intercept people as high risk before they get the shot.

Doctor Brownstein talked about using an advanced EKG as a technique. The MRI is not foolproof. The MRI can only take slices at certain distances. And we're seeing the MRI does not completely diagnose all the cases. When a surge of adrenaline occurs, then the fatal arrhythmia kicks off.

A paper titled "Autopsy findings in cases of fatal COVID-19 vaccine-induced myocarditis" by Hulscher et al., has received more downloads and reads than any paper now for years. It's the number one paper on the entire preprint server system. Now we are responding to letters to the editor where people are trying to take shots at this. We've just simply described a couple dozen people who died after the vaccine. And the autopsies are conclusive. They have fatal vaccine induced myocarditis. Pfizer knew about 1223 deaths within 90 days of their vaccine. Pfizer refused to release the data, and they were forced to do so under court order. The FDA protected Pfizer and tried to keep this data from you, the reader, for 55 years.

Now, remember our FDA reports to HHS, and then HHS to cabinet. We have had two presidents now who have allowed this to happen. Both parties are involved here. There's plenty of blame to go around both to Democrats and Republicans.

The FDA is covering up safety data on a vaccine that was essentially forced on Americans. It's not safe anywhere. The World Council for Health, which is a worldwide body, said to pull them off the market in 2022. The Association of American Physicians and Surgeons, myself and many of the doctors here belong to that group and in 2023 we all said pull them off the market. Tons of data suggest they're not safe for human use. I made the call in 2022, to the European Parliament and the US House of Representatives. They're not safe for human use anywhere in the world.

You know, there's not a single chief of medicine in the country who has come out and expressed their concern about the vaccine. Not a single chief of infectious disease, not a single dean. But we have about 200 state and federal officials right now who have come to the point where they're saying, "listen, these aren't safe." For further information on this on the internet, follow Dr. Mary Talley Bowden in Houston. She is keeping track of this.

So what did the vaccine actually do? There were multiple false claims. They never prevented infection with the current strains. They don't stop transmission. They don't reduce hospitalization and death. Not a single randomized trial showed they reduce hospitalization and death. These were false claims. The consent form shows the only theoretical benefit claimed is the vaccines have been shown - past tense - to prevent COVID-19 infection. The consent form does NOT say COVID-19 vaccination reduces transmission, severity, hospitalization, or death. If the consent form doesn't say this, why would our FDA, CDC, NIH, and medical associations promote the vaccine like this? Why would Pfizer and Moderna promote the vaccine like this? We never promote things beyond the claims made in a consent form. It's fraudulent promotion; false drug advertising done on a massive scale to push the vaccines. Four years later, we still have cases of COVID-19 in the fully vaccinated.

As mentioned, we've had failed vaccines before. The smallpox vaccine was probably the greatest example, a failed vaccine. There are peer reviewed papers demonstrating hundreds of thousands, if not millions of cases of smallpox in people vaccinated against the disease. It's obvious the vaccine didn't work. It simply did not work. This was 100 years ago. And yet it became mandated. It became part of vaccine ideology. Why? Why does this happen?

The Omicron variant blew through natural immunity is blowing through the vaccine immunity. The newer versions of the vaccines are so outdated by the time new variants come up. It's obvious now in any study that has fair access to vaccination status that the vaccines are failing grossly, just like the 19th century smallpox vaccine. Approximately 75 percent of people in the UK hospitalized or dead with COVID-19, are fully vaccinated. In the Cleveland Clinic data the best performing group is the unvaccinated with natural immunity. They have the lowest risk and those who keep taking the shots, they're getting sicker and sicker and sicker with recurrent COVID-19 illness.

This has been a financial bonanza for these companies. John Leake, my co-author in *The Courage to Face COVID-19* was right when he said it's a crime. You know, a blockbuster drug used to take 20 years to develop and cost between $500-million and $1-billion. Then, in its first year on the market, it could potentially earn back that $1-billion. For Pfizer, that was Lipitor. Did you know that Pfizer and Moderna have made tens of billions of dollars without the development, sales or marketing costs for their COVID vaccines? These were pre-purchased without any public oversight or consent.

As Doctor Brownstein pointed out, whether they're vaccinated or not, some people need early treatment. We do not have large randomized trials to hand us the answer. As doctors we need to use clinical judgement. Let's find drugs that have acceptable safety and signals of benefit. Use them in combination. Make careful observations and let's figure out what works because early in the pandemic, lives were at stake and academic medical centres were frozen in fear with no protocols for outpatients and preoccupied with very late and ineffective treatment in those hospitalized with acute COVID-19.

We treated and shared information the best we could at the time. We understood that the infection had a viral proliferation phase, an inflammation phase, and then in the end, thrombosis or blood clotting.

There are plenty of places in the world where they never even treated the virus with antivirals. They just treated the inflammation and treated the blood clotting, and patients avoided hospitalization and death. Doctor Chetty in South Africa demonstrated these principles in his protocol from South Africa. Doctor Eugenia Barrientos in El Salvador separately had a similar risk stratified protocol with similar success rates. Dr. Sean Downing, did this in Sarasota, Florida with his protocol that did not employ antivirals (ie no hydroxychloroquine or ivermectin) he just treated the inflammation and the blood clotting and people got through the illness.

I've been impressed with the clinical impact of nasal washes and gargles, unknown to me prior to the pandemic. The quality of these clinical trials and the results are astounding. With just 1 percent povidone iodine, a couple of drops of iodine in some saline, by day three positivity rates have plummeted.

Masks didn't stop the infection. Vaccines didn't stop the infection, social distancing and lockdowns didn't stop the infection. This was the answer; nasal sprays and gargles shut down transmission of the virus. This was the answer, had we only used nasal sprays and gargles, we would have dramatically reduced transmission.

I think everybody would have gotten the illness eventually, but we would have markedly reduced the number of people getting very sick all at one time. And this was something we could have used up front. We could then turn to additional drugs or therapies later on. There's data from 20 studies, 17 randomized trials that show a 53 percent lower risk of adverse outcomes with viricidal / static nasal sprays and gargles (dilute povidone iodine, xylitol).

When Representative Nancy Mace discovered this, she was extremely frustrated; "why isn>t our federal government trying to message this to people?" she asked.

Did you know that the Federal Trade Commission, the FDA, and other government agencies tied up every single company making a nasal spray or gargle and sued them and did not let them pursue their research? Every single product we tried, Hydroxychloroquine, Ivermectin, Colchicine, Prednisone, Monoclonal antibodies, Aspirin, nasal sprays and gargles was impeded by the federal government. It was not just hydroxycholoquine and ivermectin, but in fact all components of the McCullough Protocol were undermined. High-tech, expensive, Operation Warp Speed monoclonal antibodies were safe and effective, yet the FDA pulled them off the market within a matter of weeks after their market entry for theoretical concerns over viral resistance. I think it was a vaccine-only strategy worldwide from the beginning; no therapeutic was going to steal the stage from mass genetic vaccination, the real aspiration of the Bio-Pharmaceutical Complex.

CEPI, (Coalition for Epidemic Preparedness and Innovation) has said that there will be a series of pandemics and this is a business opportunity; mass vaccination over and over again. We've already seen this with COVID and COVID vaccines. Don't forget also that we have had a worldwide and national declared monkeypox crisis and the launch of monkeypox vaccines. We are in the midst of a respiratory syncytial virus bonanza, where every person my age is supposed to get an RSV vaccine. All pregnant women are supposed to get RSV vaccines in the third trimester. All newborns should be getting monoclonal antibodies (Beyfortis) against RSV. This is being done with no data or concerns over long-term safety.

Something has happened. Something in the human medical mind has clicked in a very distorted, unnatural, reckless way. There's simply no attention to safety now. Look at the data on Xylitol. This is my number one prevention strategy. This isn't a vaccine. This isn't a drug. This is a xylitol nasal spray, shown in a double blind, randomized, placebo controlled trial to have 71 percent efficacy. You could buy it at any pharmacy, it's a simple nasal spray. Why wouldn't we message this to everybody? Use your nasal spray as a bit of prevention, whether it's COVID, influenza, the common cold. Protect yourself.

Why did we use hydroxychloroquine, Aspirin, Ivermectin, Prednisone, colchicine, low-molecular weight heparins? Because we're supposed to do what the FDA says, and it's stated right on their website. When we're faced with an unmet need, we should be using drugs off their original advertising label. That's what we do in medicine. The FDA fully supports the use of off-label prescribing.

Due to a court action settlement, the FDA was forced to take down all of its distorted, deceptive statements on ivermectin. Ivermectin has been in the Association of American Physician and Surgeons Home Treatment Guide since August of 2020.

Those aligned with the Frontline Critical Care Consortium have been working with ivermectin in the same time frame. We've used it now for four years. It's safer than Tylenol. I think it's one of the most effective drugs we have. We knew by December of 2020, that there was clear and convincing evidence that early treatment was dramatically reducing the risk of hospitalization and death. To this day, we could have saved about two thirds of those lives that were lost. We could have spared all those hospitalizations, but we were impeded by every government agency out there. This happened all over the world, all at once.

Now we're faced with this issue of long COVID or patients who've had the vaccine. There are millions and millions of Americans who don't feel well. They have fatigue, neuropsychiatric, cardiovascular, respiratory symptoms.

In a paper from Germany (Diexer et al), we have learned that about 70 percent of long COVID is really due to the vaccine because people have been loaded with the spike protein. So, when you read a manuscript about long COVID, look at the date. If it's from 2020, it could be long COVID. If it's 2021 and beyond, it's likely the vaccine.

Dr. Peter Parry from Australia has appropriately positioned this as spike-opathy. The malaise is due to the spike protein in the human body.

Many medical centres see patients and make no assessment for the spike protein either directly or by antibody measurement. Some long-COVID clinics actually give additional vaccines, loading the body with even more spike protein and making patients much worse. That's how perverted this is.

Brogna and colleagues found that about half of the subjects who take a vaccine have the circulating Pfizer or Moderna spike protein in the bloodstream for six months. No wonder people feel bad after the vaccine. They have the protein that was engineered in the Chinese biosecurity lab in their bloodstream circulating for months. This is the worst idea in the history of medicine. This was what I was envisioning in August 2020 when I wrote a paper and pointed out that nobody had a clue of what might happen when we install the genetic code for the potentially-lethal Wuhan spike protein.

The spike protein comes from the infection and from the vaccine. The spike protein is in plasma attached to red blood cells, within tissues, blood clots, and is the cause of long-COVID and vaccine injury syndromes. The spike protein levels are many orders of magnitude higher from the vaccine, than in those who have had natural infection. Because the vaccine doesn't work, most people who've been vaccinated have had COVID as well. So they've actually been double or triple dosed on spike protein. I think one of the growing problems is going to be quantitative exposure. What the regulatory agencies in Canada and the United States have not done are cumulative toxicity studies. We should see what the side effects are at one shot, two shots, three shots, four shots, five shots. Is there cumulative toxicity?

We are working like crazy to come up with approaches to try to rid the body of the spike protein. One is the McCullough Protocol Base Spike Protein detoxification. What we've proposed is three natural substances; nattokinase starting dose 2000 units twice a day, bromelain 500mg a day, and curcumin 500mg twice a day. Nattokinase and bromelain enzymatically dissolve the spike protein in pre-clinical models. We don't know what happens therapeutically in the body at this point. It has been shown that curcumin in human randomized trials definitely reduces spike protein inflammation. So this is the proposal until large, prospective, double-blind placebo controlled randomized trials can be completed.

The Biden administration has spent $1 billion on the long COVID question. The result has been no proposals, no new drugs, no protocols, nothing. Academic medical centres took all this money and they blew it. At ClinicalTrials.gov there's not a single large randomized trial testing this yet.

So what have we've done? We've made careful observations in our clinic. We have thousands of people doing this. We've advanced the doses. We add other drugs depending on what the syndrome is. We've held teleconferences and calls. I've talked to doctors across the U.K. who are doing this. We believe it helps people get better from long COVID and vaccine injury syndromes, but it's slow. It could take three, six, nine, twelve months. People have been sick now for a couple of years. They're not going to get better in a couple of days. This is a base trio.

On the question of natural immunity after SARS-CoV-2 infection, the best paper to read is by Chin and colleagues in the New England Journal of Medicine, October 2022. It took a look at the US prison system; 59,000 prisoners, 16,000 staff. In a nutshell, the important thing to learn is that if a person had been infected with the Delta or Omicron variant, and they got COVID again, there was zero risk of hospitalization and death. Consider that these are people who are motivated to get out of prison and be hospitalized. Previous COVID infection is the lowest risk for serious illness thereafter.

The vaccine was irrelevant in the Chin study. The vaccine doesn't reduce anyone's risk of getting C or change their natural history. But prior infection does. Natural immunity protects, it makes the symptoms milder every time.

A recent paper in JAMA demonstrated that trust in physicians and health systems is rock bottom low. It's under 50 percent. I think we're in for about a 20 year course of reckoning. The reason why I say this in my book, *Courage to Face Covid-19,* is that I tell the story from the mid 19th-century, when Ignaz Semmelweis had the data showing that doctors should wash their hands, otherwise they'll spread infection among pregnant women and cause fatal postpartum sepsis. He was castigated, he was censored, he was kicked aside. It was 20 years later that the medical community said, "oh, we were wrong. We should have. We should have been washing our hands. Semmelweis was right." Rosen Hill, around 1950, proposed that smoking caused lung cancer. Doctors and nurses and health administrators were advertising cigarettes. They were smoking in the operating rooms. Twenty years later, the Surgeon General reported smoking causes lung cancer. Now it's the opioid pandemic; Purdue Pharma. The doctors prescribed these opioids. "They won't be addictive," they said. Now, 20 years deep, everyone's recognizing that we have an opioid crisis.

It's typically a 20 year corrective course. It's almost as if large numbers of people need to be retired or terminated. There has to be a house cleaning because the regulators, the medical professionals who endorsed this, can't come back from this. They advised the vaccines. They took the vaccines themselves. They mandated them on their employees. We haven't seen anybody come out and say, "I'm sorry." I don't expect we will see that. Unfortunately, that's not human nature. When people are too deep into it, they essentially have to retire, go away or be terminated. Then a new group comes in and recognizes that we've got a major problem.

I want everybody reading this to understand that the moment for you is now. There is no time that's more decisive. Don't look for an elected official to save you. Save yourself and your family, save your friends and make your community as wide and broad and healthy as you possibly can. Armed with the knowledge about what happened during the pandemic and with the principles of early treatment and detoxification for long-COVID, get organized. Another Disease X from the Bio-Pharmaceutical Complex is a certainty in our immediate future.

Baumeier, C.; Aleshcheva, G.; Harms, D.; Gross, U.; Hamm, C.; Assmus, B.; Westenfeld, R.; Kelm, M.; Rammos, S.; Wenzel, P.; et al. Intramyocardial Inflammation after COVID-19 Vaccination: An Endomyocardial Biopsy-Proven Case Series. *Int. J. Mol. Sci.* 2022, *23*, 6940. https://doi.org/10.3390/ijms23136940

Rose J, Hulscher N, McCullough PA. Determinants of COVID-19 vaccine-induced myocarditis. Ther Adv Drug Saf. 2024 Jan 27;15:20420986241226566. doi: 10.1177/20420986241226566. PMID: 38293564; PMCID: PMC10823859.

Hulscher N, Hodkinson R, Makis W, McCullough PA. Autopsy findings in cases of fatal COVID-19 vaccine-induced myocarditis. ESC Heart Fail. 2024 Jan 14. doi: 10.1002/ehf2.14680. Epub ahead of print. PMID: 38221509.

McCullough PA, Alexander PE, Armstrong R, Arvinte C, Bain AF, Bartlett RP, Berkowitz RL, Berry AC, Borody TJ, Brewer JH, Brufsky AM, Clarke T, Derwand R, Eck A, Eck J, Eisner RA, Fareed GC, Farella A, Fonseca SNS, Geyer CE Jr, Gonnering RS, Graves KE, Gross KBV, Hazan S, Held KS, Hight HT, Immanuel S, Jacobs MM, Ladapo JA, Lee LH, Littell J, Lozano I, Mangat HS, Marble B, McKinnon JE, Merritt LD, Orient JM, Oskoui R, Pompan DC, Procter BC, Prodromos C, Rajter JC, Rajter JJ, Ram CVS, Rios SS, Risch HA, Robb MJA, Rutherford M, Scholz M, Singleton MM, Tumlin JA, Tyson BM, Urso RG, Victory K, Vliet EL, Wax CM, Wolkoff AG, Wooll V, Zelenko V. Multifaceted highly targeted sequential multidrug treatment of early ambulatory high-risk SARS-CoV-2 infection (COVID-19). Rev Cardiovasc Med. 2020 Dec 30;21(4):517-530. doi: 10.31083/j.rcm.2020.04.264. PMID: 33387997.

Hulscher N, Procter BC, Wynn C, McCullough PA. Clinical Approach to Post-acute Sequelae After COVID-19 Infection and Vaccination. Cureus. 2023 Nov 21;15(11):e49204. doi: 10.7759/cureus.49204. PMID: 38024037; PMCID: PMC10663976.

CHAPTER 15

The Cost of Ignoring Science: Dr. Angus Dalgleish's Stand Against the COVID Vaccine Strategy

Angus Dalgleish

Professor Emeritus of Oncology at
St George's, University of London

Angus Dalgleish MD FRCP FRACP FRCPath FMedSci. Foundation Professor of Oncology at the University of London, now Emeritus. Principal of the Institute of Cancer Vaccines and Immunotherapy. Angus trained in medicine at UCL and UCH London achieving an intercalated BSc(hons) in Anatomy. Following house jobs he became a flying doctor in Mt. Isa, Queensland. He then trained in Internal medicine and Radiotherapy in Queensland before moving to Sydney to do Medical Oncology. He did his MD with Prof Robin Weiss at the ICR and RMH discovering the HIV receptor as well as its epidemiology in Africa. He was an MRC Senior Clinical scientist and honorary Consultant in Internal medicine, medical oncology , immunology and Virology. He has pioneered cancer immunotherapy and vaccines for HIV and cancer. He received the Joshua Lederberg award for his role in developing Thalidomide analogues leading to Lenalidomide and Pomalidomide .

In spite of these achievements he was completely ignored by Chris Whitty, Patrick Vallance and SAGE in the United Kingdom when he pointed out that COVID arose after a GOF lab leak and that the genetically altered spike protein would be highly dangerous if used as a vaccine.

My first experience of being a Canary in a Covid World was when my long-term research colleague, collaborator and friend, Birger Sorenson, called me from Norway after the SARS-2 sequence had been released in the scientific journal Nature.

We had previously developed a very good and effective HIV vaccine, which produced remarkable results in HIV chronically infected patients. It was far more effective than any of the mainstream vaccines, which had been extremely well-funded and pursued by NIH and big pharma. Birger and I agreed that all attempts to make a vaccine based on the approach taken by NIH and big pharma were doomed to fail as it had too many antigens and would cause too much noise in the immune system for it to recognise any achilles heel of the virus. We both agreed that a similar approach to COVID-19 vaccines, using the spike protein would cause marked auto-immune effects, particularly with regard to clotting and neurological damage.

On further analysis, it became clear that this was no ordinary virus. Birger is a biochemist and biophysicist and as such spotted what seems to have been ignored by all my classical immunological and virological colleagues. He noted that the virus had a charge of over eight, when most natural viruses rarely go above six in this class of coronavirus. In layman's terms, this means it was markedly more virulent than most natural viruses. Further analyses revealed six inserts with higher than expected charge, which had been placed there deliberately. There was evidence in the literature that this had been the goal of a team in the Wuhan lab. We also noted a furin cleavage site on this virus, which bizarrely was not commented on by the team who published the sequence, even though we strongly suspect that they had previously inserted it in experiments performed many months before this virus appeared.

In short, we felt that this was positive proof that the virus had been engineered in the laboratory and that it had almost certainly escaped. We tried to publish this and could get nowhere, even when the infamous study by Kirsten Anderson on the proximal origins of SARS-2 was published in Nature, we were unable to get our criticism of this paper published on the grounds that it was not in the public interest and the rejections came fast from major science journals; The Lancet, Science, Journal of Virology, all with exactly the same wording.

Even I, a virologist who had discovered the CD4 receptor for HIV and spent two years doing in-depth research on this interaction, could see that Anderson's paper was absolutely nonsensical. I tried to point this out on many occasions and was warned of committing slander or libel. It is now well established this paper was promoted by Fauci so he could use it as proof that the virus was natural, even when it was obvious to everybody at the time that this was no natural virus and it had most likely escaped. I wrote a summary of all these events and the details in a book called '*The Origin of the Virus*' by Paolo Barnard, Stephen Quay and myself, and it is of great interest that Stephen Quay's Bayesian analysis completely fits with our sequential analyses and comes to the same conclusion.

The Appearance of a Respiratory-Like Virus in the U.K.

It was obvious in retrospect that this virus was present in England and the U.K. as early as November 2019 and possibly earlier. However, it did not really cause the first wave until the first quarter of 2020 when the hospitals were overwhelmed enough for the Government to introduce a lockdown in March 2020. My professional colleagues who were used to dealing with respiratory epidemics were horrified at this prospect. It was clear that although the hospitals were overwhelmed and there was initially a high death rate, this was all due to complete incompetence, as opposed to hospitals being overwhelmed. To be perfectly clear, my colleagues and I pointed out that this was a respiratory virus of unknown origin and the classical approach would be to use a first aid line approach.

It is clear from analyses of the literature that 'flu and all other viruses are much worse in people with low Vitamin D levels and that this is endemic in the U.K. I therefore proposed that everybody be given high doses of Vitamin D and classical approach for a respiratory tract infection, which includes gargling with Aspirin, mouth washes, intranasal interferon, which was known at the time as 'First Defence', Becotide and steroids if there was evidence of inflammation, along with antibiotics. I knew of many patients and friends who suffered from 'flu symptoms, all of whom benefitted from this regime and did not go to hospital. We questioned why people should do nothing until they were so ill that they had to call an ambulance to go to hospital, where they had a high chance of being admitted and put on a ventilator, the last thing that should happen to patients with an inflammatory pulmonary condition. The ventilators were actually causing more harm than good. It took some time before this became so obvious that ventilators were gradually relegated to those with conditions that really needed them, but not before many thousands of useless ventilators had been ordered, and the first of billions of dollars wasted. This, along with the outrageous personal protective equipment, hastily ordered because there were no emergency supplies, despite so-called pandemic preparedness.

We challenged the lockdown on the grounds that this was a respiratory virus and only people who should be considered very vulnerable should be withdrawn from the environment. I wrote many articles in the mainstream media, particularly in the Daily Mail, on this subject and received tremendous backing from the editorial staff on the madness of lockdowns, particularly when no quarantine had been applied. We ended up with the farcical situation whereby the population was locked down for three weeks whilst planes were still flying in from Wuhan!

We made a very loud noise that natural immunity was the one thing that would save us all and the Great Barrington Declaration was given wide publicity, but completely shouted down on no scientific basis whatsoever by Matt Hancock and other ministers. Had they paid attention, recommendations from The Great Barrington Declaration could have saved the country at least half a trillion pounds. This figure will certainly rise as the damage that we predicted to ongoing health management, particularly long term mental health issues, education and the economy, would be greater than could possibly be calculated. We also pointed out that there must be no comparison of the benefits and otherwise of lockdowns. I and others praised Angers Tegnel, the CMO of Sweden, who persisted in spite of criticism from 2,000 colleagues in defending an open policy and avoiding lockdown. It is well worth pointing out that Sweden had the lowest death rate from COVID in the western world, even though it committed that same sin as the U.K. did by pushing the infected elderly from hospitals into care homes. Apart from that, the subsequent death rate was far lower in Sweden and continues to be so.

The Coming of the Vaccine

As the first big wave subsided in 2020, as it was doing before the lockdown was introduced, I could not discern any benefit other than to prevent a few people from hospitalisation. What it did do, however, was set the scene for a narrative of fear, spinning the tale that there was nothing that could possibly help with this virus, except a vaccine, which would be necessary to save us all!

The vaccine had been rushed through development and almost certainly appears to have been part of a pre-ordained plan. As life stopped, we waited for the vaccine to come to save us. It is now clear that agents such as hydroxychloroquine, some antibiotics and in particular Ivermectin were so effective in treating patients with severe early COVID that there was no need for a vaccine. I was given a slot in the Daily Telegraph to point out that the best vaccines for this type of disease are heat killed Mycobacteria. I was allowed to point out that all my patients on a heat killed mycobacterium product called IMM-101 that boosts the innate immune system, which was given as part of a trial in melanoma patients, induced such a good immune response that none of these at-risk, elderly patients developed COVID in 2020.

I pointed out to everyone that the secret was the T-cell response. It appears that the team that commissioned Astra Zeneca to go ahead with their vaccine were unaware of this until I pointed it out. Then they announced that they were very pleased to see the vaccine did induce a T-cell response.

Although I had great misgivings about the Astra Zeneca vaccine, when it was rolled out we were shown figures that demonstrated clear efficacy and no side effects in early trials. I was misled into recommending that such an agent would have a role in preventing widespread infection. However, courtesy of many good colleagues who shared their evidence, it became rapidly clear that the vaccine was not effective at all and that the evidence presented to the regulatory authorities could essentially be interpreted as two things:

1. The evidence was fraudulent, misleading and heavily edited.
2. The regulatory authorities were either completely incompetent or incentivised to look for no other solution.

It did not take long before I realised that the vaccine was causing more harm than good and that patients who were getting the vaccine did not seem to be protected from getting the next strain of COVID. I even asked the question whether the vaccine actually encouraged development of the next strain.

The next chapter of this global story concerns the Omicron virus, which was reported from South Africa as being very infectious and not nearly as dangerous, with the overall interpretation that there was no difference in health outcomes in vaccinated and unvaccinated patients. Indeed, this was tremendous news as it suggested the virus was going through the predicted arc of attenuation, increased infectivity and less virulent. This was received by the British authorities as evidence for more fear and more lockdown, etc. There was no scientific debate and the mantra 'follow the science' was used again and again. There was no science followed. In the future, proper scientific debate must be at the forefront of any policy decisions, not the draconian Orwellian policies imposed worldwide.

More and More Damage, Less and Less Evidence

When the vaccine clearly was not "working" due to waning antibody levels, someone, somewhere, decided we needed a booster vaccine. I have been working with vaccines for many years and any vaccine that needs a booster clearly is not working. My simple reason for this opinion is that if it had induced a good enough T-cell response, one would not need a booster as the T-cell would detect any new virus or variant and mount the necessary immune response.

Equally, my colleagues and I were horrified that the vaccine was subsequently rolled out to all age groups. Dr Ross Jones, Dr Claire Craig and I, with many others, pointed out that this was unjustified as the virus was only killing elderly people, with no significant death in young people, unless suffering multiple comorbidities. U.K. Chief Medical Officer, Chris Whitty gave the laughable explanation that children needed to be vaccinated to protect against their parents and grandparents. With this one sentence he proved that he was not fit for purpose or his office, as you do not vaccinate people to protect against others.

The Result of the Booster Programme

Basic science tells us that booster vaccines should not be given if there is a good immune response from primary doses. Especially not without testing for this first. I explained this all over the media. However, it slowly dawned on me that patients were being bullied, cajoled by GPs following orders, into accepting useless booster vaccines, creating more medical emergencies.

In my own clinic I began to see patients who had been stable for years with melanoma who started to relapse. This is not completely unusual. I have been prescribing experimental immunotherapy for nearly 30 years and I had noticed previously that patients who had become stable or disease free would relapse if put under a prolonged intense stress from life events such as death, divorce or bankruptcy. Initially, I noticed at least half a dozen patients, then more and more, relapsing. None of these patients had high stress events in their lives, but all had been coerced into having booster vaccines by their GPs.

There was clear evidence that this was a global phenomenon. I spoke to oncologists in Australia, New Zealand, Canada and America, all of whom were witness to the same patterns. They were told it was anecdotal and warned not to voice their concerns. Why on earth would you do this?

We now know that it was not just melanomas relapsing, but many other tumour types such as leukaemias, lymphomas, kidney cancer, colorectal, pancreatic and others, suddenly appearing after the booster shots. I was delighted to see that others were publishing on the effects of the vaccines on T-cell response, showing that the boosters, i.e., the third and fourth vaccine were causing T-cell suppression or, as one publication put it, T-cell exhaustion. The immune system was being overstimulated to exhaustion by the shots. Other groups showed that the immunoglobulin response (IgG) antibodies produced were switching from an antiviral neutralising destructive response, to a tolerising response, one more likely found in a successful transplant of a kidney or liver.

The stage was set by the booster vaccines to suppress the T-cell response and tolerise the antibody response. In other words, to remove the body's natural immune policemen from the system, allowing the tumours, normally successfully controlled by a healthy T-cell response, to start escalating.

For my pressure in making this medical catastrophe clear, I was hauled before my own hospital medical directors and the Royal College of Physicians. It promptly became clear that nobody on any of these boards had any understanding of the immune system, viruses or cancer. I made it very clear that the initial problem in pushing the boosters was medical incompetence. But after a full explanation, to persist in administering the vaccines would be medical negligence.

We, as doctors have been vilified, struck off, careers ruined, for asking sensible questions about the vaccine programme. The more we asked questions of the morons who pushed these vaccines from the Government, the Department of Health, the NHS, MHRA, the more we were met with silence. Unless we confront this failure now, the same thing will happen in the future, particularly if the WHO gets its way, controlling world health responses. They go out of their way to threaten new pandemics, such as bird 'flu, and have become hysterical and have induced fear over one case which has jumped to a human. They must not be allowed to control any future pandemic.

The Role of The Vaccines and Future Long term Health.

I have already addressed the way in which COVID vaccines can suppress T-cells and tolerise antibodies, allowing cancer to take off. I was told that there is no evidence that this is related to the COVID vaccines. However, there is now clear evidence from many countries, including Australia and Japan, that excess deaths correlate perfectly with the roll out of the vaccine programme. A large study from Japan published in Cureus shows a clear link with the booster vaccines and increase of death from many conditions, but particularly in cancer of all types.

A further reason that the vaccines promote cancer, is that they promote micro clots. These micro clots are associated with cancer dissemination. Indeed, clotting disorders associated with progressive disease in pancreas and prostate cancer have been recognised for decades. The ability of the spike protein to induce not only inflammation, but to bind receptors, enhancing this inflammation, is well documented.

Unfortunately, there are many other reasons that the messenger RNA vaccines in particular can cause cancer. First of all, they have been stabilised to last long enough for them to be recognised as a foreign antigen and make an immune response. Unfortunately, this science is far from established.

It's a fact that after over fifteen years of messenger RNA development, no product has been approved for cancer, indicating the seriousness of this problem. The pandemic was used as an excuse to allow mRNA vaccines to be rolled out to the general population. Now we see the consequences. First of all, the batch to batch variation is diabolical, as is the contamination, with DNA plasmid and known oncogenic sequences, such as SV40. Moreover, the early data suggesting that the mRNA binds to suppressor genes has been clearly confirmed by a number of studies. There is a serious concern that we are on the brink of a tsunami of new, unexpected cancers. My colleagues and I believe this has already started, particularly turbo or explosive cancers in young people.

There are many other potential reasons why mRNA could end up being oncogenic but I believe that beyond the scope of this chapter. Suffice to say that the use of mRNA vaccines of any kind is a clear and present danger for future health and they should be banned.

I am afraid to say that I have been a Canary with regards to the origin of the virus and its escape. I've also been a Canary who sang that the spike protein must not be used for a vaccine because it has far too many similarities to human epitopes. I was the Canary who chirped loudest about lockdown; that the benefits could not possibly outweigh the disastrous and obvious long term effects. Unfortunately, all these predictions have been proven correct. The vaccine programme was clearly the result of fraud, corruption and incompetence, at best. I have squawked long and loud that it should never have been given to children and young adults; that it should never have been given as a booster vaccine.

Unfortunately, we Canaries must now unite to sing our song at top volume. We must bring attention to the disaster of the COVID pandemic policies, the fallout from which will continue to cause catastrophic loss of life, to say nothing of a massive negative effect on the economy and democracy.

We say Never Again.

CHAPTER 16

The Rescue of John O'looney

By Dr. Sam Dubé

Mathematician, physician, strength coach, and broadcaster

Dr. Sam Dubé is a mathematician, retired award-winning university faculty, educator, academic physician, master strength coach, and broadcaster. He was one of the first Canadian physicians to attempt to expose the truth during the pandemic of fear, and continues to do so on his Rumble channel "The Fifth Doctor", and abroad.

"I'm not afraid of dying. I'm afraid of not doing the right thing while I'm alive."
– John O'Looney, U.K. Funeral Director & Whistleblower

It was late in 2021 and the "Pandemic of Fear" had truly come into its own. Fuelled by fear-mongering government propaganda and completely "in sync" mainstream media outlets, we went from "two weeks to flatten the curve" to a new normal including rotating lockdowns, social distancing, rampant "testing," mandatory yet nonsensical masking, and school closures. Despite extremely limited and dubious published data in support of the mainstream media and government universal claims that the vaccines were "safe and effective," vaccine mandates were implemented to force compliance. The unvaccinated were being vilified, with U.S. President Biden calling COVID-19 "a pandemic of the unvaccinated."

The public had been told simply to stay home and self-isolate and only to wait until becoming seriously ill before presenting to a hospital. No official recommendations for early treatment were made, despite strong evidence from frontline physicians like Dr. Pierre Kory and Dr. Paul Marik that well-known, safe, affordable, generic repurposed medications such as ivermectin and hydroxychloroquine could effectively treat COVID, especially in its early stages. Typically the most vulnerable populations for respiratory illnesses are the aged and those with serious co-morbidities, the published mortality figures for COVID were purposely not age-stratified. The authorized "emergency use" protocols had more to do with money and the urgings of Big Pharma than safety and effectiveness. Spurred by financial incentives for COVID diagnoses, the very ill were treated with expensive drugs that had been rapidly authorized despite questionable effectiveness and terrible safety records. One such drug, remdesivir, essentially a very expensive failed Ebola drug, had acquired the nickname "run-death-is-near" among nurses due to its reputation for killing patients through kidney failure. In the meantime, the known generic repurposed medications were suppressed and vilified by the legacy media, public health agencies and even scientific journals. Typically a last resort to assist breathing in patients, ventilators became a standard of care motivated by monetary impetus for their use. Hospitals had earned the reputation as the place people went to die. All of this served to escalate the fear campaign we experienced.

In Canada, there were additional government regulations that were bewildering in their inconsistency from province to province. For instance, did you know that the COVID virus could differentiate between a standing restaurant patron and a seated one? And the province of Quebec had curfews enforced by huge fines and arrest, while the directly adjacent province of Ontario did not. I vividly recall racing over the interprovincial bridges after work making it back to Ontario in the nick of time. In a power play of horrendous overreach, the Canadian government had also ordained travel restrictions for the unvaccinated. This violated the Charter of Rights and Freedoms as the requirement to "demonstrably justify" the new legislation was conveniently ignored. Many Canadians were prevented from travelling for work, to visit or care for friends and relatives, and even to attend funerals or a deathbed. There was an epidemic of job loss, financial ruin, mental health crises, drug addiction, and suicide. So many people succumbed to the pressure, threats, and fear of losing their job, their home, and even loved ones that they took the experimental gene therapy shots unwillingly, often with dire consequences. The Great

Canadian Freedom Convoy of early 2022, which brought attention to these draconian policies and their horrific consequences, as well as emboldened other major protests worldwide, had yet to happen.

While struggling to make ends meet and deal with the "policy-based science" of the aforementioned COVID regulations, the online world had grown in significance and become both a solace and a battleground. I founded my podcast The Fifth Doctor[1] on Rumble in the wake of the success of my "Exposed" videos in mid-2021. Having generated millions of views, along with an outpouring of public sympathy and outrage, they had given a collective voice to the brave and intrepid Canadian physicians who had openly resisted the public health pandemic narrative. I became very busy online, presenting, attending meetings, and moderating discussions.

The main online group I joined was Medical Doctors for COVID Ethics (MD4CE). The founder was Welsh radiologist Dr. Stephen Frost, a passionate and vocal opponent of the COVID injections and the near worldwide lockstep response to the pandemic. Initially, MD4CE brought together like-minded physicians and scientists, but the network quickly expanded to include professionals and experts from many fields, occupations, and positions. The heart and soul of the group was its online bi-weekly meetings, which at the time had rotating moderators - me among them - and discussions often went into the wee hours of the night. This initial incarnation of MD4CE featured a prohibition on recording, a vow of confidentiality, the freedom to speak one's mind and a focus on congregating and developing plans of action. The goal was to help expose corruption, publicize truth, and provide assistance where possible. It became a haven for the early movers and shakers of the medical freedom movement worldwide. MD4CE was where whistleblowers sang, corruption was revealed, and heroism was lauded. It gave the despondent hope, the persecuted support, and the enraged a constructive outlet. For some, it was even a lifeline.

I was blessed to have met so many dedicated and passionate freedom fighters through the MD4CE group. One of those was John O'Looney; the U.K. funeral director and whistleblower who publicly exposed the artificial inflation of COVID death numbers through the use of fake death certificates. This tactic was perpetrated by the British government, one of many, to scare the population into complying with COVID vaccination and the public health pandemic narrative in general. John was a leader in exposing the excessive use of the drug midazolam in "treating" COVID in U.K. nursing homes, resulting in thousands of unnecessary deaths which further inflated the COVID death toll. He presented his testimony to key medical freedom fighters as well as members of the U.K. parliament. John's public revelations eventually encouraged many others worldwide, including embalmers, emergency personnel, nurses, and physicians to expose the medical crimes they had witnessed. A humble, sincere, and endearing man of great conscience and fearless in his convictions, John was a great warrior for medical freedom and an enemy to government corruption everywhere.

I had conducted two long form interviews[2] [3] with John in October of 2021 where we had discussed all of these issues. I got to know John fairly well, and kept in touch with him and his latest efforts to expose what he'd witnessed. My buddy Maverick, an equally fearless ex-cop and former European secret service agent, met and befriended through MD4CE, became close friends with John. So it was with considerable confusion and concern that I picked up the phone one day to Maverick blurting out, "Sam! Are you aware that John O'Looney is in the hospital with what appears to be COVID?"

It was immediately before Christmas 2021, and I had just got off the phone with a Canadian physician who was seeking help. The doctor was being mandated to either take the COVID shots, or lose the position that was the pinnacle of a long and arduous academic career with many sacrifices and health challenges. The latter was a major reason for his reluctance to to take the injections. No exemption would be given regardless of provided medical records, conscientious objection, and pleading. The anguish and terror in his voice was absolutely heartbreaking, and I could only offer suggestions for personal and legal support. He was at his wits' end, and I felt powerless.... So I was determined to do everything I could to help John. Maverick, who had been monitoring John's fledgling Telegram channel at the time, had intercepted a truly pitiable message from him announcing that he was in hospital on 10 litres of oxygen, with no further information. We subsequently discovered that John had been in and out of consciousness, and was terrified.

How would John have ended up in hospital? Given his firsthand knowledge, he was very wary of them. Why had we not heard anything else? Were John's friends and colleagues in the U.K. freedom network aware? Then I also recalled the self-deprecating John telling me that if anybody were to die from a respiratory illness like COVID, given his large size, history of heavy smoking, and a lifestyle that admittedly could have been a lot healthier, it would be him. He was also painfully aware that given his whistleblower status, he could very well be a target for those he had implicated or exposed. "Try to find out what hospital he was admitted to", I said to Maverick. "I'll reach out to my contacts in the U.K. and see if they know what's going on."

Two of the world's most stalwart and resourceful freedom fighters, Dr. Dolores Cahill and Dr. Tess Lawrie, and a third, Croatian-born American physician Dr. Kat Lindley, were all as shocked as I had been when I told them of John's apparent hospitalization and life threatening condition. All had had recent contact with John, with Tess having spoken to his wife not three days prior, and everything had been fine. With what we had all heard and witnessed during the pandemic to that date, especially with regard to the treatment protocols used in hospitals, we decided that a team needed to be sent to rescue John O'Looney.

I can't describe everything that happened next because even to this day it would put some people in jeopardy. But those who feature here have given their blessing for this story to be told. The story of how John O'Looney escaped hospital alive. The entire operation hung by a thread more than once.

Teresa, another member of MD4CE, announced John's plight on one of our online forums, looking for volunteers to go to the hospital as soon as possible. With a background in physics, and a nature more stubborn than a mule, I knew she would not let John down. We spent nearly three hours on the telephone that night, pulling together a team and a plan of action. Throughout, I was bedside in another hospital, this one in Canada, acting as the advocate for the mother of a friend of mine, stuck in the U.K. due to his unvaccinated status, as she awaited cancer surgery.

U.K. lawyer Phil Hyland and former police officer Peter Huge joined the "Rescue John" team to handle legal issues. Teresa called MD4CE founder Dr. Stephen Frost to put out a call to find people to go to the hospital, among them Mark Sexton, a retired 15-year-veteran of the Birmingham police force, who volunteered for the rescue team.

We were very afraid of what might happen to John in hospital overnight. Stories about the new "COVID protocols" being implemented without mercy – sedation, ventilation, and remdesivir, followed by rapid decline then "death due to COVID", regardless of the ailment. Maverick's investigation had confirmed that John was in the COVID ward on oxygen, with a very grim prognosis from hospital staff. We knew that a physician on the team was of paramount importance. Teresa's call for medical help prompted a brave physician - for the purposes of this story and his anonymity called Dr. Heroic - to volunteer. The plan was to have John discharged from hospital into the professional care of Dr. Heroic where he would be treated using the protocols that included natural supplementation, oxygen if necessary and the known safe and effective generic repurposed medications that the public health narrative had suppressed and vilified. But Dr. Heroic was five hours drive from the hospital; time was of the essence.

A few days earlier, John had become increasingly short of breath at home. He had not smoked in over a decade. But when his oxygen saturation dropped to 78%, his wife called an ambulance. "I couldn't breathe, and I was absolutely terrified," John later confessed to me. In the ambulance, one of the attendants kept berating him for being unvaccinated while withholding the oxygen he needed. When he arrived at hospital, John was the only patient in the triage unit. He was told that he would have to be put on a ventilator or that he would die. He adamantly refused. He was admitted to a "COVID ward" with two guards stationed outside the doors. He was told that everyone in that ward was unvaccinated. When John declared that he did not want to be there and tried to leave, the guards physically prevented him from doing so, which wasn't difficult given his weakened state. They then threatened to have him arrested as a danger to the public. John was terrified of what they might do to him when unconscious. He surreptitiously managed to post the brief message on his Telegram channel that Maverick had intercepted.

John was given three lateral flow tests for COVID. Aware of its unreliability, he had repeatedly refused the PCR test, and had even defiantly spat on it when they had tried to administer it without his consent. All of the lateral flow tests came back negative. After the third, a nurse told him explicitly that he did NOT have COVID. John never received a COVID diagnosis during his hospital stay.

Two "consultants" visited John. The first claimed to be a representative from Oxford University. He told John that he was there to save his life from COVID, and wanted him to sign a waiver to be treated with the drug remdesivir. John refused treatment with "run-death-is-near", refuted the man's claim that he had COVID as he had not received the diagnosis, and confronted him concerning the serious side effects of the drug and its abysmal track record. The man walked out. Shortly afterwards, a woman appeared and sat on his bed, similarly claiming "I'm here to save your life" while brandishing waivers for the immunosuppressive drugs Baricitinib and Tocilizumab. She insisted that if John did not consent to the treatment, he would surely die. But John had done his research and once again confronted the consultant regarding how the drugs worked, their side effects and the dearth of evidence for their effectiveness. She left empty handed as well. "It was terrifying," said John. "It was clear to me that they KNEW the drugs would not work." He was told repeatedly that every single patient in his ward was unvaccinated and was shamed for his choice. He spoke to two other patients in the ward, both of whom had consented to the drug treatments the hospital claimed would save their lives. John never saw either of them again.

Meanwhile, John's wife called the hospital and reiterated John and his family's wish to be discharged directly into the care of Mark and Dr. Heroic. In a call with a hospital respiratory consultant, recorded by John's 11-year-old son, the doctor opposed the idea strongly. "The moment he goes out of the ward, he will just collapse and die," he said, ignoring the fact that he was to be discharged into the care of a doctor, equipped with oxygen for home use.

When Mark and Dr. Heroic arrived early in the morning, it took more than two hours on the telephone for them to be granted access to John's ward, with guards at the door. They were told by two doctors that everyone in the ward was unvaccinated against COVID including John, and that he would die within minutes if taken off his oxygen. An administrator cited the Coronavirus Act as justification to keep John locked up. Mark and Dr. Heroic made it very clear that John had never been diagnosed with COVID; that he was being released into the care of a physician; and he was not simply wandering out into the general public. It may have been implied that "forcible confinement" would be a legal concern for the hospital if John were held against his will. All of this took a further two hours before his release.

"This was not the John I knew", Mark recalled. "He was white as a ghost, gaunt and fearful." On the ride down in the elevator, a nurse turned desperately to Mark and pleaded, "I know who you are. Please help us. It's the vaccines that are killing people." When Mark asked her why she hadn't spoken up and gone public, she explained that she was a single mother and needed the job, and that she and her colleagues were very afraid. "She begged me for help," Mark recalled sadly. She also confirmed that every patient in the COVID ward had been vaccinated *except* for John. The doctor and consultant lied directly to perpetuate the charade of a "pandemic of the unvaccinated".

John was able to leave the hospital without the use of the supplemental oxygen brought for him. In the car, he gleefully announced on his Telegram channel the circumstances of his "rescue" to his followers. Dr. Heroic treated him at home with supplements and ivermectin. Within 24 hours of leaving hospital, John was up and about as normal. Under the care of Dr. Heroic, he was back to full time work four weeks after his discharge. A few weeks before his hospital experience, he was warned by a Communications Officer from British Intelligence, "they'll target you."

"I'm a soft target, Sam" John told me. John reached out to the hospital to discuss his "stay" in their care. They never responded. He often thinks about the two men he had spoken to, patients like himself. "I know they didn't survive. I feel survivor's guilt. I'll never live it down", John says with sorrow. "I'm not afraid of dying. I'm afraid of not doing the right thing while I'm alive."

John has continued to do the right thing. Flash forward to June of 2022; John O'Looney was among the first to publicly present evidence of the abnormal blood clots found in the bodies of the COVID vaccinated.

In an online meeting with some of the members of MD4CE, he showed us the abnormal long, stringy white clots in the bodies of the vaccinated. We published this on Odysee.com[4] and at the 18-minute mark John shows the world the isolated clots. In July 2024 he appeared on the Nova Scotia Free Speech Bulletin podcast[5] where polymer chemist Greg Harrison discussed the evidence for phospholipid-fibrinogen polymer formation and subsequent abnormal clotting, facilitated by the spike proteins, from the lipid nanoparticles (LNPs) of the shots.

My goal in telling John's story is to help bring attention to the vast number of people who were hospitalized in similar situations, but were not as lucky as John; victims of the Pandemic of Fear. People like my unvaccinated uncle, who died in a hospital in France having been sedated, ventilated, and given remdesivir. I also want to highlight the countless people who were frightened and coerced into taking the COVID shots. People like one of my best friends, threatened with non-payment and job loss. He died full of blood clots, comatose, and severely brain damaged in an ICU in British Columbia after I gave the consent to have him removed from life support.

There are so many who have suffered. Those of us still standing and healthy need to listen and seek accountability for them. There are so many for whom we must DO THE RIGHT THING.

[1] https://rumble.com/c/c-1060561/videos

[2] https://rumble.com/vo9tpl-the-5th-doctor-ep.-6-british-funeral-director-john-olooney-exposes-covid-de.html

[3] https://rumble.com/vo9w67-the-5th-doctor-ep.-7-british-funeral-director-john-olooney-exposes-covid-de.html

[4] https://odysee.com/@MAVERICK:8b/Interview-ICR:d

[5] https://rumble.com/v57fkwc-funeral-embalmers-directors-and-new-evidence-on-white-clots-presented-in-pr.html

CHAPTER 17

How The Deadliest Vaccine in History Targeted the Most Vulnerable

James A. Thorp MD

board-certified in Obstetrics and Gynaecology (OB/GYN) and also in Maternal-Fetal medicine

Dr. Thorp is a Board-Certified Obstetrician Gynecologist and Maternal Fetal Medicine Physician with almost 44 years of obstetrical experience. While serving as a very busy clinician his entire career he has also been very active in clinical research with almost 200 publications. Dr. Thorp has seen about 25,000 high risk pregnancies in the last 4 years. He has served as a reviewer for major medical journals and served on the Board of Directors for the Society of Maternal Fetal Medicine for four years, and served as an Examiner for the American Board of ObGyn. He served in the United States Air Force as an Obstetrician Gynecologist having been awarded a Health Professions Scholarship for his medical school education. Dr. Thorp testified in the US Senate under the Bush administration in 2003 for his expertise in treating the fetus as a patient with in-utero therapies. On December 7th 2022 he testified in the Senate with Senator Ron Johnson and others. Most recently Dr. Thorp has focused his research efforts on the COVID-19 pandemic and published over 15 peer-reviewed scientific publications and a book documenting the dangers of the vaccine in women of reproductive age and in pregnancy.

This chapter will focus on targeting the most vulnerable, pregnant women, pre-borns, and newborns, by the Covid-19 vaccines, by far and away the deadliest and most injurious vaccines in history. How did this happen? How could 60,000 ObGyn physicians and their three professional organizations, American College of Obstetricians and Gynecologists (ACOG), American Board of Obstetrics and Gynecology (ABOG), and Society for Maternal-Fetal Medicine (SMFM), simultaneously reject the "Golden Rule of Pregnancy" after the obstetrical disasters involving Diethylstilbestrol (DES) and thalidomide in the last half of the twentieth century? This Chapter will definitively answer that very question - with exacting proof, precision and clarity.

The Golden Rule of pregnancy was emblazoned on the collective consciousness of the global community after the thalidomide and diethylstilbestrol (DES) pregnancy disasters of the 20th century. Novel and untested medical interventions introduced during any stage of pregnancy are always avoided, due to their high potential to cause short and long-term multigenerational harms that may not be discoverable for years or even decades. The thalidomide and DES disasters demonstrate how easily delicate and intricate processes in the developing embryo/fetus can be catastrophically damaged when a novel teratogenic agent is given during pregnancy. During the vulnerable embryonic stage, the intricate blueprint for a new human life is created, including formation of all major systems and structures. During the fetal development stage, critical growth and development of all the major organ systems takes place. Because of the graphic nature of severe birth defects caused by thalidomide, it is perhaps better remembered than DES. Yet thalidomide (which we discuss in part II) caused far less morbidity and mortality in pregnancy than did DES.

1938 -1980 The Golden Rule of Pregnancy Devastatingly Violated with Diethylstilbestrol (DES) and Thalidomide with Consequences the World will Never Forget – That is Up Until the Roll Out of the COVID-19 Vaccines

The Golden Rule of Pregnancy was emblazoned in the collective consciousness of the global community after the catastrophic diethylstilbestrol (DES) and thalidomide pregnancy disasters. DES was prescribed to pregnant women for several decades with as many as 10 million exposed globally. [1] The carnage caused by DES was unprecedented up until the Covid-19 vaccines. All physicians, especially obstetricians, know that DES was associated with cervical malformations in the daughters exposed in-utero resulting in infertility, recurrent pregnancy loss, ectopic pregnancy, miscarriage, cervical insufficiency, preeclampsia, premature delivery, stillbirth, and neonatal death. [1] Ironically, the pharmaceutical industry marketed DES in pregnancy as a method to avoid pregnancy loss. DES also caused clear cell adenocarcinoma of the cervix, vagina, and breast cancer. [1] DES complications were multigenerational and were not limited to reproductive disasters in women. DES caused multiple complications in both sexes including autoimmune disease, neurodevelopmental alterations, psychosexual disorders, depression, immunologic complications, pancreatic disorders, early menopause, and cardiovascular problems. [2] [1] Epigenetic alterations have been detected, and generational effects are observed in both DES daughters/sons, and DES granddaughters/grandsons, possibly even great granddaughters/grandsons. [2] [1]

The German pharmaceutical company Chemie-Grünenthal launched thalidomide in the 1950's for morning sickness in pregnancy. [3] While DES was probably a far greater disaster, thalidomide is more well known because of the tragic visual images of the malformations known as phocomelia - some or all the newborn's limbs were missing. In addition to the limb deformities, survivors had other severe handicaps including early onset of age-related issues such as osteoarthritis, joint mobility issues, and coronary heart disease. A single 50 mg tablet of thalidomide during the time-sensitive window is sufficient to cause birth defects in up to 50% of pregnancies. [3] It is estimated that about 20,000 were injured and 80,000 died from thalidomide. Tragically, no individual, nor anyone from Grünenthal itself, was successfully prosecuted over the disaster. Reports suggest that Grünenthal entered into an agreement with the German Federal Prosecutors to withdraw criminal prosecution against them. [4]

February 28, 2021 - Pfizer's 5.3.6 Post-Market Analysis Completed and the Outcomes were Catastrophic

The Pfizer 5.3.6 legally mandated post-market analysis [5] documents Covid-19 vaccines to be the most injurious and lethal medical product ever rolled out to the public with 42,098 casualties (AE's) including 1,223 deaths in just 10-11 weeks (see page 7) thus documenting an "injure-to-kill" ratio of 33.4 (42,098-1,223/1,223). On page 12 of this report [5]there is also concerning pregnancy outcome data including the following:

- A miscarriage rate of 81% (26/32; 238/270 had no follow-up),
- A five-fold increase in stillbirth rates from an expected rate 5.8/1000 to 31/1000 (1/32 rate),
- An eight-fold increase in neonatal death rate from expected rate of 3.9/1000 to 31/1000 (1/32 rate),
- A 14% incidence of breast-feeding complications in those newborns whose mothers received the Covid-19 vaccines in pregnancy.

April 1, 2021 - Enlisting "Trojan Horses" to do the CDC's Ugly Bidding: HHS launches COVID-19 Community Corps

Pfizer and the FDA attempted to conceal the post-market analyses [5] of adverse events for 55-75 years [6] [7] while at the same time investing unprecedented amounts of US tax dollars to promote the safety, efficacy, and necessity of the Covid-19 vaccines [8] - even in the most vulnerable population, pregnant women, pre-borns, and newborns. Instead of hitting pause on rollout of the vaccines however, on April 1, 2021, the HHS launched COVID-19 Community Corps [9][1] – a colossal COVID-19 vaccine propaganda machine designed to exploit "trusted" private entities and individuals across the country, turning them into covert government agents to push the vaccines. As part of the strategy to get a shot in every arm, HHS used COVID-19 Community Corps to recruit private, non-government "trusted" sources to push the CDC's message that the novel mRNA genetic injections were safe (despite clear evidence to the contrary) – but without directly disclosing that these messages were from the government. [10]

Under the guise of COVID-19 Community Corps, HHS awarded billions of federal dollars to recruit what HHS referred to as "trusted community leaders" who could push the "vaccines" within our most private relationships. [10] Much like modern-day trojan horses, these "trusted messengers" would be unique in their ability to permeate all facets of private life. Essential to successfully deploying its strategy on the public, HHS sought to identify credible and influential community leaders, enlist them to join its COVID-19 Community Corps, and then exploit these "trusted sources" to convince those around them to take the COVID-19 vaccines. [10] The focus was on finding people with not just local, but also uniquely interpersonal influence. As Harvard public health professor Jay Winsten, [11] who has advised previous administrations, reportedly explained to CBS News in a December 2020 article about the HHS' monumental effort, "You want to go for the low hanging fruit, those that are easiest to pick and harvest." [11] Noting that the focus should be on finding locally influential people to push the vaccines, Winsten added, "People trust their own doctors, their own nurses, their own pastors, their own social networks. That's very, very different from a distant figure." [11] And indeed it was.

In the last 6 months of 2020 the reigning obstetrical narrative was that COVID-19 vaccination in pregnancy was experimental without safety data or long term follow up of newborns. The purposeful strategy to target pregnant women began to manifest itself on April 1, 2021 when HHS used the COVID-19 Community Corps to enlist the American College of Obstetricians and Gynecologists as a founding member, thus controlling 60,000 ObGyn physicians in several countries on two continents including the United States, Canada, and several countries in South America. The purpose of targeting women? Quite simple. Despite their shoddy medical research, their marketing research was beyond reproach. Mark Weber, then Deputy Secretary of HHS, collaborated with Winsten et. al. at Harvard

University pointing out that they could pick the "low hanging fruit" and capture women as they are known to make 90% or more of the medical decisions in all extended family members, regardless of race, ethnicity and country of origin. HHS/Harvard et all would blitz the media and trusted messengers with the false narratives that the COVID-19 vaccines were safe, effective and necessary in pregnant women to save their own lives and their pre-borns', and newborns' then 'game over with victory'. It logically follows that every human on the planet should be vaccinated since it is safe, effective and necessary in pregnant women - the most vulnerable patient population.

April 16, 2021 – New England Journal of Medicine (NEJM) Audio Interview: Covid-19 Vaccines and Pregnancy – A conversation with CDC Director Rochelle Walensky.

Time marks for Walensky's NEJM audio publication statements are detailed in this reference. [12] In the NEJM discussion, NEJM Editor-in-Chief Eric Rubin, NEJM Managing Editor Stephen Morrissey and Rochelle Walensky promoted fear tactics that were unsupported by research studies involving morbidity and mortality of unvaccinated pregnant women and their fetuses/newborns from COVID-19 infection. Walensky stated the following: "women who are pregnant have a 2-3 fold increase in risk of ICU [intensive care unit] stay, a 2 fold increased risk of mechanical ventilation as well as ECMO [extracorporeal membrane oxygenation], and the babies actually having somewhere between a 2-4 fold increased risk of adverse outcomes". In stark contrast Pineles and colleagues [13] published a study just 20 days later on May 11, 2021 reporting that pregnancy imposed a protective effect to COVID-19 infections. In a large cohort of 1,062 pregnant and 9,815 nonpregnant women all hospitalized with COVID-19 and viral pneumonia, Pineles found that pregnancy had a dramatic protective effect compared to non-pregnant women. Pregnancy was associated with a 75% reduction in maternal mortality rates compared to that of the non-pregnant women (0.8% vs 3.5%; OR 0.24, 95% CI 0.12-0.48, p < 0.0001). Pineles [13] states that rates found in their study "are consistent with results of multiple other studies" citing the studies of Knight [14] from June 8, 2020 and Metz [14] from February 8, 2021. Both the Knight [15] and Metz [14]studies were published prior to the statements published by Walensky/Rubin on April 21, 2021.

The two NEJM Editors Rubin and Morrissey hosting then Director of the CDC Walensky to push and promote an experimental COVID-19 vaccine in pregnancy is unprecedented. Worse, publishing it in the NEJM, a journal many perceive to be the most influential medical journal in the world, wreaks with danger signals, ethical concerns, and conflicts of interest [12]. One recent publication [16] documents flow of monies from the U.S. Department of Health and Human Services (HHS) including the CDC through the Massachusetts Department of Public Health to the owners of the NEJM, the Massachusetts Medical Society as outlined in the authors' Figure below.

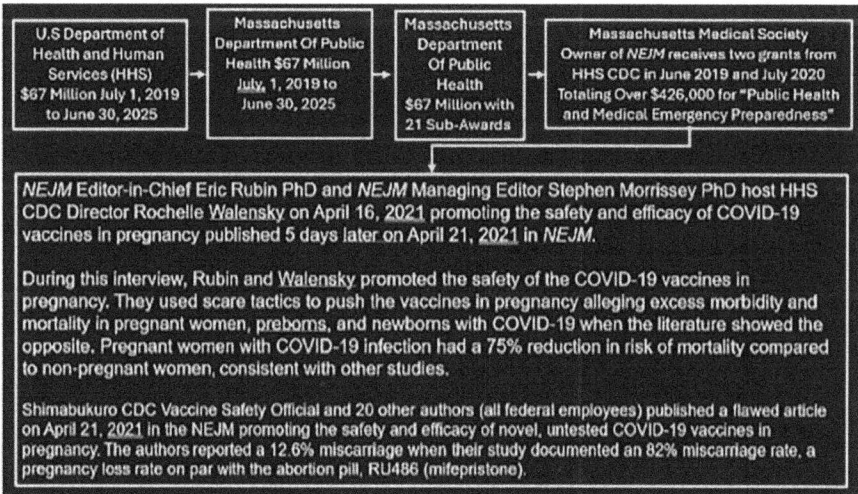

U.S Department of Health and Human Services (HHS) $67 Million July 1, 2019 to June 30, 2025	Massachusetts Department Of Public Health $67 Million July, 1, 2019 to June 30, 2025	Massachusetts Department Of Public Health $67 Million with 21 Sub-Awards	Massachusetts Medical Society Owner of NEJM receives two grants from HHS CDC in June 2019 and July 2020 Totaling Over $426,000 for "Public Health and Medical Emergency Preparedness"

NEJM Editor-in-Chief Eric Rubin PhD and NEJM Managing Editor Stephen Morrissey PhD host HHS CDC Director Rochelle Walensky on April 16, 2021 promoting the safety and efficacy of COVID-19 vaccines in pregnancy published 5 days later on April 21, 2021 in NEJM.

During this interview, Rubin and Walensky promoted the safety of the COVID-19 vaccines in pregnancy. They used scare tactics to push the vaccines in pregnancy alleging excess morbidity and mortality in pregnant women, preborns, and newborns with COVID-19 when the literature showed the opposite. Pregnant women with COVID-19 infection had a 75% reduction in risk of mortality compared to non-pregnant women, consistent with other studies.

Shimabukuro CDC Vaccine Safety Official and 20 other authors (all federal employees) published a flawed article on April 21, 2021 in the NEJM promoting the safety and efficacy of novel, untested COVID-19 vaccines in pregnancy. The authors reported a 12.6% miscarriage when their study documented an 82% miscarriage rate, a pregnancy loss rate on par with the abortion pill, RU486 (mifepristone).

The NEJM Editors Rubin and Morrissey failed to disclose this conflict of interest and by doing so they violated their own ethical standards published in their own journal: "to ensure that authors disclose all relevant financial associations and that such associations in no way influence the content NEJM publishes" [17].

Rubin and Walensky boasted about the validity of VAERS and that it demonstrated no safety concerns for pregnant women in their NEJM interview [12]. Yet CDC Director, Walensky and her colleagues at the FDA would have already received the damning Pfizer 5.3.6 post-marketing data completed February 28, 2021 already discussed above [5]. Moreover, Pfizer's post marketing report bears a Bates stamp [5] printed on each page indicating receipt by the FDA and its Center for Biologics and Evaluation Research (CBER). As CDC Director, it was Walensky's responsibility to have reported that document to the world and to have immediately halted the COVID-19 vaccinations. In early 2021 a whistleblower widely circulated this Pfizer document [5] on the internet available for everyone that did their own due diligence. Attorney Aaron Siri of Informed Consent Action Network (ICAN) obtained the official release of the Pfizer document [5] by a Freedom of Information Act request on April 1, 2022. As of their April 16, 2021, published "discussion" which shamelessly promoted the untested COVID-19 vaccines in pregnancy, Rubin, Walensky, and Morrissey certainly would have been aware that multiple pregnancy AEs had already breached VAERS safety signals set forth by the CDC/FDA.

April 21, 2021: NEJM Editor in Chief Eric Rubin then Promotes Safety, Efficacy and Pushing of the COVID-19 vaccines in "Pregnant Persons"

Lead author Shimabukuro along with 20 other authors, appearing to have colluded with the two aforementioned Editors of the NEJM, published an online article entitled "Preliminary Findings for mRNA Covid-19

Vaccine Safety in Pregnant Persons" by electronic publication on April 21, 2021, [18] and on in a print edition (PubMed) on June 17, 2021 [19]. Coincidentally the audio interview with the NEJM Editors and Walensky [12] was published on the exact same day as this Shimabukuro study [18] and once again Rubin, Morrissey, Walensky, and Shimabukuro all violated ethical standards of the NEJM by not disclosing their conflicts of interest [17]. Other major conflicts of interest in the Shimabukuro study [18]appear unprecedented with all 21 authors being federal employees. Even more egregious, the lead author Shimabukuro first came to the Immunization Safety Office (ISO) at the CDC in 2010 and served in multiple positions including senior medical officer, Vaccine Adverse Event Reporting System (VAERS), team lead, acting Vaccine Safety Datalink team lead, and vaccine safety team lead in the COVID-19 Vaccine Task Force, and deputy director. [20]

The mere appearance of Rubin, Walensky, Shimabukuro and their strongly pro-pregnancy COVID-19 vaccination hosted in their April 16th, 2021, audio interview published in the NEJM [12] wreaks of collusion, conflict of interest and potential criminal activity. Multiple studies have pointed out the major flaws of the Shimabukuro article including the use of the V-safe system that has subsequently been shown to have been corrupted and manipulated [21] [22], only an arbitrary 10 week study period of study when pregnancy lasts for 40 weeks, and finally a miscarriage rate of 82% that was falsely manipulated to appear in print as a 12.6% rate [23] [24]. These manipulations are documented in the Figure below.

The NEW ENGLAND
JOURNAL of MEDICINE

JUNE 17, 2021

Preliminary Findings of mRNA Covid-19 Vaccine Safety
in Pregnant Persons

Among 827 participants who had a completed pregnancy, the pregnancy resulted in a live birth in 712 (86.1%), in a spontaneous abortion in 104 (12.6%), in stillbirth in 1 (0.1%), and in other outcomes (induced abortion and ectopic pregnancy) in 10 (1.2%). A total of 96 of 104 spontaneous abortions (92.3%) occurred before 13 weeks of gestation (Table 4), and 700 of 712 pregnancies that resulted in a live birth (98.3%) were among persons who received their first eligible vaccine dose in the third trimester. Adverse out-

NEJM June 17, 2021 Vol 384 No 24, on page 2276: Shimabukuro et al shifted the denominators to dilute the spontaneous abortion rate of 82% (104/127) to 12.6% (104/827). 700 patients receiving the vaccine in the third trimester is gross misrepresentation because a spontaneous abortion is defined as a pregnancy loss before 20 weeks gestation. The 82% spontaneous abortion rate in this NEJM report is on par with the "abortion pill" RU486 (Mifepristone). Is this complete ignorance or willful deception?

American College of Obstetricians and Gynecologists (ACOG): A "Trusted Messenger"

Along with 275 other organizations, twenty-five of which were health and medical organizations, the American College of Obstetricians and Gynecologists (ACOG) jumped on board as a founding member of COVID-19 Community Corps [25], ultimately receiving millions in federal grant money [26]. Shortly thereafter, on July 30, 2021 ACOG began recklessly endorsing COVID-19 vaccination in pregnancy, even though the clinical trials failed to include pregnant women.

Perhaps no other medical organization had as much potential to persuade Americans into taking these experimental injections as did ACOG. A pregnant patient's relationship with her ob-gyn is arguably one of the most intimate and sacred physician-patient relationships in all of medicine. This is not without reason – as one patient and writer notes, "They're right next to you for the most momentous occasion of your life" [27]. Pregnant mothers trust their ob-gyn doctor with the most intimate and sensitive information about their own bodies, their sex lives, and, if pregnant, about the new life growing inside of them. Some individuals have even reported the development of a non-romantic affection for their ob-gyn that rivals that of the baby's father in some ways, due to the "complete vulnerability" many women reportedly experience with their gynecological and pregnancy specialists [27].

Government capture of ACOG would capitalize on this unique and sacred doctor-patient relationship, using ob-gyn doctors – with their unparalleled physician influence – as pro-vaccine "trusted messengers." Additionally, convincing pregnant women to take novel mRNA shots would yield an exponential harvest of "low hanging fruit." This is because women reportedly make a full 90% of all healthcare decisions about their household and have long been considered "A Brand's Powerhouse" by professional marketers. [28] Convincing pregnant women to take the COVID-19 shots was almost a guarantee that they would become pro-vaccine "trusted messengers" within their own families.

Moreover, the optics were exceptionally good for persuading other "vaccine" hesitant Americans to roll up their sleeve for the experimental shots – if the COVID-19 "vaccines" were considered safe enough to administer to pregnant patients (and thereby trans-placentally to their unborn babies) – certainly they were safe enough for everyone. If HHS and CDC could pull off government capture of ACOG and convince its ob-gyn members to push the shots on their patients, this would be a bonanza for reaching the "vaccine" hesitant – what HHS Deputy Assistant Sec. Mark Weber, referred to as the "moveable middle" [29].

As it would turn out, the HHS' grand marketing strategy worked. The methods utilized by HHS to push the COVID-19 "vaccines" – including the creation of COVID-19 Community Corps – were so vastly different from any other HHS effort that an academic article was published in Journal of Health Communication in April of the following year, detailing the process and commending its success [30]. Featuring now-retired HHS Deputy Assistant Sec. Mark Weber as lead author, the article confirms that HHS did, in fact, target interpersonal relationships [30]. Weber and his colleagues "vaccine" marketing efforts were so successful that, after retiring from HHS, Weber apparently formed his own private company aimed at "Achieving bold goals at the Federal Level" [31] – in revolving door fashion.

ACOG: A Revealing Case Study of Government Capture of Medical Non-Profit Organizations

On February 1, 2021, ACOG had been awarded the first of what would eventually be three HHS and CDC "Cooperative Agreement" grants made during the pandemic [32]. Under these three Cooperative Agreement grants, ACOG would receive over $11 million in federal money over coming years [32]. But there was a catch: Documents obtained in a Freedom of Information Act (FOIA) request made in connection with these three Cooperative Agreement grants have recently exposed that ACOG relinquished independent control over its COVID-19 recommendations for patients to the CDC when it accepted the federal grant money [32]. Receipt of grant money by ACOG was contingent on ACOG's full compliance with CDC guidance on COVID-19 infection and control [33]. Eerily similar to what former HHS Deputy Assistant Sec. Mark Weber writes that the FOIA documents reveal that HHS and CDC seemed to be using ACOG to "deliver messages without the Federal government being directly involved (even though the information may come from a Federal source)" [30].

Although they were heavily redacted, the FOIA documents revealed startling information about the extent of control CDC wielded (and still wields) over ACOG. For example, the FOIA documents show that CDC grants totaling $3,300,000 were awarded to ACOG on Sept. 2,

2021 for two separate programs, entitled "Engaging Women's Health Care Providers for Effective COVID-19 Vaccine Conversations" and "Improving Ob-Gyns' Ability to Support Covid-19 Vaccination, Mental Health, Social Support" [34]. As part of receiving funds under these awards, ACOG is required to "comply with existing and or future directives and guidance from the [HHS] Secretary regarding control of the spread of COVID-19" [34]. The award is also expressly contingent on ACOG's agreement "to comply with existing and future guidance from the HHS Secretary regarding the control and spread of COVID-19" [34]. In addition, ACOG must also "flow down" these terms to any person or entity who receives a "subaward" [34]. Moreover, the CDC is expressly authorized to terminate any award due to material failure to comply with "the terms and conditions of the federal award" [34].

Sub-awardees likely included the American Board of Obstetrics and Gynecology (ABOG) and the Society for Maternal-Fetal Medicine (SMFM) thus requiring them to also remain in lockstep with ACOG/HHS/CDC/ FDA's narratives. Evidence pointing to this would come just a few months later as ACOG/ABOG/SMFM announced their recommendation for the COVID-19 vaccination in pregnant women on July 30, 2021 [35]. On September 27, 2021 ABOG, the only one of the three organizations having punitive authority, issued a statement threatening 60,000 ObGyn physicians with removal of medical licenses and revocation of their board certifications if they did not comply [36]. If this sounds like government capture of ACOG – it is. Disturbingly, the FOIA documents show CDC working through ACOG, in essence exploiting ACOG's authority and sway to influence not only doctors and patients, but also a host of others, including public health entities and "partner organizations" [34]. The FOIA documents obtained make it difficult to tell where ACOG ends, and CDC begins [37].

January 12, 2022: Senior Ob/Gyn, Maternal-Fetal Medicine Physician Openly Challenges ABOG's Threat and the Unacceptable risks of COVID-19 Vaccination in Pregnancy

In response to the concerning threat from ABOG threatening punitive measures to 60,000 Ob/Gyn physicians,[36] a senior physician and former ABOG Board Examiner and former Board of Director of The Society for Maternal-Fetal Medicine (SMFM) compiled an open, public letter to ABOG published on January 12, 2022 [38]. This 98-page open letter to ABOG specifically reviewed the unacceptable breach in VAERS safety signals to the attention of ABOG's senior officers and examiners. Under a section entitled "The VAERS Data Has Signalled Warnings that Can No Longer be Ignored" on page 12, the letter specifically detailed unprecedented deaths, fetal malformations, and pregnancy losses in the VAERS database. The letter also warned ABOG of multiple other major concerns among others not listed here:

- Lipid nanoparticles (LNPs) were clearly designed to cross "all God-made barriers, including the blood brain barriers, the placental barrier, and the fetal blood brain barriers",

- LNPs were concentrated in ovaries,

- A female fetus has only about 1 million gametes (ova) and each is exposed to the potentially toxic substances in the LNP's including vaccine-mRNA,

- Any inflammatory substance such as the COVID-19 vaccine, is dangerous in the developing embryo/fetus and may cause permanent damage, malformation, death, placental insufficiency, and potentially lifelong chronic diseases,

- Disruption of the TOL7 and TOL8 receptors on cell may increase risk to infections and cancers,

- An unprecedented number of stillbirths in the US, Canada, Scotland, Europe and many other locations, and

- Scott Davison the CEO of OneAmerica insurance company has reported all-cause death rates up 40% in ages 18-64 years after the vaccine rollout and that a 10% uptick in all-cause mortality was catastrophic for the insurance industry.

The open letter to ABOG published January 12, 2022, also provided ABOG with references for 1,019 peer-reviewed medical journal publications in just 12 months after COVID-19 vaccines rolled out, documenting severe injuries and death [32]. As of June 2024, 42 months after the COVID-19 vaccine rollout, there are now 3,580 such studies [39]. ABOG never responded to the letter but continued to recertify this physician in 2022 and in 2023.

April 2023: VAERS Analysis of Adverse Events (AEs) in Pregnant and Menstruating Women

In a prior publication Thorp and colleagues [16] compared 18 AEs over 18 months after COVID-19 vaccination to AEs after influenza vaccines occurring over 282 months. This analysis used PRR based on three different variables: AE per time, AE per inoculation, and AE per individual vaccinated. There were 17 obstetrical AEs and 1 AE assessing abnormalities in menstrual function. All 18 AEs documented significant breaches in the CDC/FDA's safety signal of a PRR $\geq$ 2 including. The PRRs by time for menstrual abnormalities - 4257; miscarriage - 177; fetal malformation - 21; preeclampsia - 83; preterm delivery - 32.3; low amniotic fluid volume - 17; abnormal fetal surveillance - 83; and stillbirth - 135; all exceeded safety limits. All foregoing AEs had a p value of less than one in a million [16].

July 2023 Pfizer's: Randomized, Double-Blind, Placebo Controlled Clinical Trial in Pregnant Women, COVID-19 vaccine versus Placebo

Also consistent with the findings in this present study is Pfizer's "Randomized, Double-Blind, Placebo Controlled Clinical Trial in Pregnant Women, COVID-19 vaccine versus Placebo" released in July 2023. Pfizer's phase 2/3 clinical trial, allegedly a randomized, double-blinded, placebo-controlled trial, was grossly underpowered [40]. There were only 324 pregnant women, 161 randomized to COVID-19 vaccines and 163 to placebo, resulting in at least 8 newborn outcomes of grave concern. These included the following:

1) low Apgar Scores (depressed newborns) increased by 100%;

2) meconium aspiration syndrome substantially increased;

3) neonatal jaundice increased by 80%;

4) congenital malformations increased by 70%;

5) atrial septal defect increased by 220%;

6) fetal growth restriction substantially increased;

7) congenital nevus increased by 200%; and perhaps most concerningly,

8) congenital anomalies with developmental delays at 6 months of life, increased by 310%.

How many women would have ever considered taking COVID-19 vaccines in pregnancy if their Ob/Gyn physicians informed them of these 8 newborn outcomes from Pfizer's phase 2/3 clinical trial? It would seem unlikely that any women would have willingly taken the COVID-19 vaccines in pregnancy had they been given honest informed consent required by the Nuremberg Code of Ethics.

July 2024 Updated Analysis of the CDC/FDA's VAERS Adverse Events (AEs) in Pregnancy

In July, 2024 Part I [41] and Part II [42] of a three-part series was published entitled Are COVID-19 Vaccines in Pregnancy as Safe and Effective as the U.S. Government, Medical Organizations, and Pharmaceutical Industry Claim? Data were collected from the CDC/FDA from January 1, 1990, to April 26, 2024, for adverse events (AEs) involving pregnancy complications following COVID-19 vaccination. The time-period included 412 months for all vaccines except COVID-19 vaccines, having been used for only 40 of the 412 months (December 1, 2020, to April 26, 2024). Proportional reporting ratios (PRR) by time compared AEs after COVID-19 vaccination to those after influenza vaccination, and after all other vaccine products administered to pregnant women. The CDC/FDA's safety signals were breached for all 37 AEs following COVID-19 vaccination in pregnancy, 27 antepartum (before birth) and 10 postpartum (after birth) in newborns:

Miscarriage	fetal chromosomal abnormality
fetal malformation	cervical insufficiency
premature rupture of membranes	premature labor
premature delivery,	placental calcification
placental infarction	placental thrombosis
placenta accreta	placental abruption
placental insufficiency,	placental disorder,
fetal maternal hemorrhage,	fetal growth restriction,
reduced amniotic fluid volume,	preeclampsia,
fetal heart rate abnormality,	fetal cardiac disorder,
fetal vascular mal-perfusion,	fetal arrhythmia,
fetal distress,	fetal biophysical profile abnormal,
hemorrhage in pregnancy,	fetal cardiac arrest,
fetal death (stillbirth),	premature infant death,
neonatal asphyxia,	neonatal dyspnea,
neonatal infection,	neonatal hemorrhage,
insufficient breast milk,	neonatal pneumonia,
neonatal respiratory distress	neonatal respiratory distress syndrome
neonatal seizure	

Are Any of Pfizer's "Randomized, Placebo-Controlled, Double Blinded Clinicals Involving COVID-19 Vaccines Valid?

Turtles All The Way Down: Vaccine Science and Myth, a book of over 500 pages with more than 1200 references, states that there has never been a randomized, double-blind, placebo-controlled trial for any of the vaccines currently on the FDA schedule [43]. This book was originally published in early 2019 by two Israeli researcher-scientists who purposely remained anonymous so the world would focus on the content of the data rather than personally attacking them as has been done over the past century in vaccinology. No statement of fact in this book has ever been disproven. There has never been a randomized, double-blinded, placebo-controlled trial for any of the approximately 80 vaccines on the FDA schedule [43]. All alleged clinical trials conducted by Pfizer and other vaccine manufacturers are not compared with a true placebo group [43]. Legal claims challenging the integrity and veracity of Pfizer's clinical trials are pending in state and federal courts. Whistleblower Brook Jackson working for Ventavia Research Group observed gross breach of standard clinical practices in Pfizer's clinical trials stating that the company falsified data, unblinded patients, employed inadequately trained vaccinators, and was slow to follow up on adverse events reported in Pfizer's pivotal phase III trial. Jackson's testimony is detailed in the British Journal of Medicine [44]. Jackson stated that staff who conducted quality control checks were overwhelmed by the volume of problems they were finding. Jackson sued Pfizer in Federal court under the False Claims Act for fraud. Additionally, Pfizer is currently being sued by the Texas Attorney General for violation of the Texas Deceptive Trade Practices Act [45] and by the Kansas Attorney General [46] on multiple counts of misleading consumers. Five states are reported to be suing Pfizer [47].

Are Any of the Numerous Studies in the Peer-Reviewed Medical Journals Promoting the Safety and Efficacy of the COVID-19 Vaccines in Pregnancy Valid, Truthful and Without Major Conflicts of Interest?

The government and their co-opted private actors including the medical journals were deeply involved with driving the narratives promoting the masses to get inoculated with the COVID-19 shots. This should have been obvious from the beginning. The government's attempt to conceal the damning Pfizer 5.3.6 post marketing analysis for 75 years should send a powerful message to global citizens. The unethical promotion of two fatally flawed NEJM publications on April 21, 2021 pushing the most lethal-injurious "vaccines" in history in pregnant women is unparalleled and reviewed extensively above.

The tide appears to be turning in favor of truth and freedom. On June 25, 2024 Rousculp and colleagues studied the inflammatory symptoms in the first 2 days after different COVID-19 vaccines in 1,130 participants [48]. Symptoms occurred in 56.5% in the Novavax group, and 84.4% in the mRNA vaccine in just the first 48 hours after vaccination. Ten authors, five from NovaVax and another five, Rousculp and colleagues, published provocative studies proving that the vaccines were associated with significant symptoms within 48 hours:. These symptoms were moderate or severe in 27.8% in the Novavax and 49.3% in the mRNA vaccine. This NovaVax-authored study limited their analysis to 48 hours post injection, and concluded that this is an extremely inflammatory substance, likely the most inflammatory ever injected in humans. From the perspective of pregnancy outcomes, it is a proven assertion that inflammation in pregnancy is associated with a multitude of abnormal outcomes in the embryo/fetus/newborn.

Conclusions

This chapter focused on how 60,000 ObGyn physicians and their three professional organizations, the American College of Obstetricians and Gynecologists (ACOG), American Board of Obstetrics and Gynecology (ABOG), and Society for Maternal-Fetal Medicine (SMFM) simultaneously rejected the "Golden Rule of Pregnancy" in 2021 despite their knowledge of the obstetrical disasters involving diethylstilbestrol (DES) and thalidomide in the last half of the twentieth century. HHS/CDC/ACOG/ABOG/NEJM targeted the most vulnerable with the deadliest and most injurious vaccines in history. How did this happen? Simple. It happened because of the age-old flaw of humanity, corruption by power, greed, and money. The government didn't stop at just the medical organizations and medical journals, they co-opted every single thread of the fabric of our society to push these lies of the COVID-19 vaccines. They purposely mislead consumers by granting US tax dollars to promote COVID-19 vaccines in many private entities [51] including medical organizations [52], hospitals [53], faith leaders [54], and even retail pharmacies including CVS and Walgreens [55].

In this chapter we clearly outlined how the CDC Director Walensky and her vaccine safety officer Shimabukuro were deeply entangled with the NEJM with money transfers to NEJM's owners, the Massachusetts Medical Society. Two NEJM Editors Rubin and Morrissey while hosting Walensky in their published audio interview breached their own published ethical standards and targeted pregnant women globally by their two simultaneous publications on April 21, 2021. They had or should have had knowledge of the disastrous Pfizer 5.3.6 post market analyses. The HHS/CDC captured ACOG, ABOG and SMFM that controlled the 60,000 ObGyn physicians to promote the lethal and injurious COVID-19 vaccines in pregnant women under threat of punitive measures including license and board certification removal.

Every lie incurs a debt against the truth. The lie will ultimately be revealed and the debt against truth harming every person and entity will be paid back in full.

References

[1] Zamora-Leon P. Oct, "Are the Effects of DES Over? A Tragic Lesson from the Past.," Int J Environ Res Public Health , vol. 18, no. 19, October 2021 .

[2] N. N. C. Institute, "Diethylstilbestrol (DES) Exposure and Cancer.," [Online]. Available: https://www.cancer.gov/about-cancer/causes-prevention/risk/hormones/des-fact-sheet.

[3] V. N., "Thalidomide-induced teratogenesis: History and mechanisms.," Wiley Online Library. Birth Defects Research, Part C. Embryo Today: Reviews. , [Online]. Available: https://onlinelibrary.wiley.com/doi/full/10.1002/bdrc.21096.

[4] "Thalidomide: how men who blighted lives of thousands evaded justice.," The Guardian , November 14, 2014 2014 . [Online]. Available: https://www.theguardian.com/society/2014/nov/14/-sp-thalidomide-pill-how-evaded-justice.

[5] Celia Farber. Court-Ordered Pfizer Documents They Tried To Have Sealed For 55 years Show 1223 Deaths, "Court-Ordered Pfizer Documents They Tried To Have Sealed For 55 years Show 1223 Deaths, 158,000 Adverse Events in 90 Days Post EUA Release. The Most Shocking Document Release Of The Last 100 years," 5 December 2021. [Online]. Available: https://celiafarber.substack.com/p/court-ordered-pfizer-documents-they . [Accessed 7 July 2024].

[6] CTV News, Windsor. "Michelle Maluske. CTV News. 'Data is power': Experts weigh-in on court-ordered release of Pfizer vaccine documents. March 11, 2022. https://windsor.ctvnews.ca/data-is-power-experts-weigh-in-on-court-ordered-release-of-pfizer-vaccine-documents-1.5816089," 11 March 2022 . [Online]. Available: https://windsor.ctvnews.ca/data-is-power-experts-weigh-in-on-court-ordered-release-of-pfizer-vaccine-documents-1.5816089. [Accessed 7 July 2024].

[7] Maggie Thorp JD and Jim Thorp MD. America Out Loud. Tentacles of a Covert and Exploitative Propaganda Machine Compliments of the US Government," 28 October 2022. [Online]. Available: . https://www.americaoutloud.news/tentacles-of-a-covert-and-exploitative-propaganda-machine-compliments-of-the-us-government/.

[8] Maggie Thorp JD and Jim Thorp MD. America Out Loud. Tentacles of a Covert and Exploitative Propaganda Machine Compliments of the US Government.," 28 Octobe 2022. [Online]. Available: . https://www.americaoutloud.news/tentacles-of-a-covert-and-exploitative-propaganda-machine-compliments-of-the-us-government/.

[9] U.S. Department of Health and Human Services Launches Nationwide Network of Trusted Voices to Encourage Vaccination in Next Phase of COVID-19 Public Education Campaign. (Screen Snapshot captured on April 1, 2021, at 22:51:02, by Internet Archive Wayback," 1 April 2021. [Online]. Available: https://web.archive.org/web/20210401225102/https://www.hhs.

gov/about/news/2021/04/01/hhs-launches-nationwide-network-trusted-voices-encourage-vaccination-next-phase-covid-19-public-education-campaign.html.. [Accessed 2024 July 2024].

[10] P. Harvard T.H. Chan: School of Public Health. 2023. "Jay A. Winsten, "Harvard T.H. Chan: School of Public Health. 2023. "Jay A. Winsten, Ph.D." Accessed May 6, 2023. https://www.hsph.harvard.edu/jay-winsten/," 2023. [Online]. Available: https://www.hsph.harvard.edu/jay-winsten/. [Accessed 7 July 2024].

[11] Rubin EJ, "Audio Interview [April 16, 2021]: Covid-19 Vaccines and pregnancy – A Conversation with CDC Director Rochelle Wallensky. April 21, 2021. N Engl J Med 2021;384:e73. DOI:1056/NEJMe2106836.," New England Journal of Medicine, vol. 384, no. e73, 21 April 2021. https://www.nejm.org/doi/full/10.1056/NEJMe2106836

[12] Pineles BL, Goodman KE, Pineles L, O'Hara M, Nadimpalli G, Magder LS, Baghdadi JD, Parchem JG, Harris AD. "In-Hospital Mortality in a Cohort of Hospitalized Pregnant and Nonpregnant Patients With COVID-19," Ann Intern Med, vol. 174, no. 8, pp. 1186-1188, 17 August 2021.

[13] Knight M, Ramakrishnan R, Bunch K, Vousden N, Kurinczuk JJ, Dunn S, Norman L, Barry A, Harrison E, Docherty A, Semple Calum. "Females in hospital with SARS-CoV-2 infection, the association with pregnancy and pregnancy outcomes: a UKOSS/ISARIC/CO-CIN investigation," BMJ . https://pubmed.ncbi.nlm.n, vol. 8, no. Scientific Advisory Group for Emergencies:m2107, p. 369, 2021.

[14] Metz TD, Clifton RG, Hughes L, et al. Disease severity and perinatal outcomes of pregnant patients with coronavirus disease 2019 (COVID-19)," Obstet Gynecol, vol. 137, pp. 571-580, 2021.

[15] Public Health and Medical Professionals for Transparency (PHMPT). "BNT162b2 5.3.6 Cumulative Analysis of Post-authorization Adverse Event Reports," Pfizer, 1 April 2021. [Online]. Available: https://phmpt.org/wp-content/uploads/2022/04/reissue_5.3.6-postmarketing-experience.pdf. [Accessed 6 July 2024].

[16] Shimabukuro TT, Kim SY, Myers TR, et al. Preliminary Findings of mRNA Covid-19 Vaccine Safety in Pregnant Persons," N Engl J Med, vol. 384, no. 24, pp. 2273-2282, 21 April 2021. https://www.nejm.org/doi/full/10.1056/NEJMoa2104983

[17] Shimabukuro TT, Kim SY, Myers TR, et al. Preliminary Findings of mRNA Covid-19 Vaccine Safety in Pregnant Persons, N Engl J Med, vol. 384, no. 24, pp. 2273-2282, 17 June 2021. https://www.nejm.org/doi/full/10.1056/NEJMoa2104983

[18] CDC Centers for Disease Control and Prevention. Tom Shimabukuro, "Safe Healthcare Blog: Tom Shimabukuro, MD," [Online]. Available: https://blogs.cdc.gov/safehealthcare/bios/tom-shimabukuro/. [Accessed 7 July 2024].

[19] HHS "U.S. Department of Health and Human Services Launches Nationwide Network of Trusted Voices to Encourage Vaccination in Next Phase of COVID-19 Public Education Campaign," 1 April 2021. [Online]. Available: https://www.hhs.gov/about/news/2021/04/01/

hhs-launches-nationwide-network-trusted-voices-encourage-vaccination-next-phase-covid-19-public-education-campaign.html. [Accessed 7 July 2024].

[20] USASPENDING.gov, "An official website of the United States government.," [Online]. Available: https://www.usaspending.gov/search/?hash=2b9bbf7349e6c520a55164cbe34c6321. [Accessed 7 July 2024].

[21] C. Pickworth, ""I'm in Love with my Obstetrician, and I'm not Alone."," News.com.au. KidSpot, 2 May 2023. [Online]. Available: https://www.kidspot.com.au/pregnancy/labour/im-in-love-with-my-obstetrician-and-im-not-alone/news-story/1fc5007077f517444c29fe53acecce56. [Accessed 7 July 2024].

[22] T. F. Powerhouse, "Statistics on Women''s Influence... and the power of the Women's Choice Award"," 2018. [Online]. Available: https://womenschoiceaward.com/wp-content/uploads/2018/01/WCA_FemalePowerhouse_Infographic_2018.pdf.. [Accessed 7 July 2024].

[23] Graham Kates CBS NEWS. "Inside the $250 Million Effort to Convince Americans the Coronavirus Vaccines are Safe," 23 December 2020. [Online]. Available: Kates, Graham. "Inside the $250 Million Effort to Convince Americans the Coronavirus Vaccines are Safe." CBS News, December 23, 2020. Accessed May 2, 2023. https://www.cbsnews.com/news/covid-vaccine-safety-250-million-dollar-marketing-campaign/.. [Accessed 7 July 2024].

[24] B. T. B. A. Weber MA, "Public Education Media Campaign: Applying Systems Change Learnings.," Journal of Health Communication, vol. 27, no. 3, pp. 201-207, 25 April 2022.

[25] W. MA, "Your success is my success!," LinkedIn , 2023. [Online]. Available: https://www.linkedin.com/in/mark-weber-595918a/. [Accessed 7 July 2024].

[26] USASPENDING.gov.2023., "Spending by Prime Award," [Online]. Available: USASPENDING.gov. 2023. "Spending byhttps://www.usaspending.gov/search/?hash=2b9bbf7349e6c520a55164cbe34c6321.. [Accessed 7 July 2024].

[27] CDC: Documents responsive to FOIA Request can be accessed at https://centersfordiseasecontrol.sharefile.com/d-sa6cdb04fbfef4f579490cc942fe74945. (See, e.g., Page 440.). [Accessed 7 July 2024].

[28] Centers for Disease Control and Prevention (CDC). 2023. Accessed May 3, CDC, 2023. [Online]. Available: https://centersfordiseasecontrol.sharefile.com/d-sa6cdb04fbfef4f579490cc942fe74945. [Accessed 7 July 2024].

[29] American Board of Obstetrics & Gynecology (ABOG). American Board of Obstetrics and Gynecology Statement Regarding Dissemination of COVID-19 Misinformation. September 27, 2021.," 27 September 2021. [Online]. Available: https://www.abog.org/about-abog/news-announcements/2021/09/27/statement-regarding-dissemination-of-covid-19-misinf. [Accessed 7 July 2024].

[30] Maggie Thorp JD and Jim Thorp MD. "FOIA Reveals Troubling Relationship between HHS/CDC & the American College of Obstetricians and Gynecologists," America Out Loud News, 7 May 2023. [Online]. Available: https://www.americaoutloud.news/tentacles-of-a-

covert-and-exploitative-propaganda-machine-compliments-of-the-us-government/. [Accessed 7 July 2024].

[31] The American College of Obstetricians and Gynecologists (ACOG), "ACOG and SMFM Recommend COVID-19 Vaccination for Pregnant Individuals," 30 July 2021. [Online]. Available: https://www.acog.org/news/news-releases/2021/07/acog-smfm-recommend-covid-19-vaccination-for-pregnant-individuals. [Accessed 7 July 2024].

[32] James A Thorp MD. Open Letter Sent to All American Board of Obstetrics & Gynecology Officers and Examiners. Dr. James Thorp's Letter to the American Board of Obstetrics and Gynecology on the Risks of the Covid-19 Vaccine in Pregnancy. Rodef Shalom 613, 12 January 2022. [Online]. Available: https://www.rodefshalom613.org/2022/01/dr-james-thorp-letter-to-american-board-obstetrics-gynecology-risk-covid19-vaccine-pregnancy/. [Accessed 7 July 2024].

[33] REACT19, "Science-based support for people suffering from long-term COVID-19 vaccine effects," React19.org, [Online]. Available: https://react19.org/. [Accessed 7 July 2024].

[34] Thorp JA, Rogers C; Deskevich, MP, Tankersley S, Benavides A, Redshaw, M.D.; McCullough, P.A. "Covid-19 Vaccines: The Impact on pregnancy Outcomes and Menstrual Function," Journal of American physicians and Surgeons, vol. 28, no. 1, pp. 28-34, Spring 2023.

[35] ClinicalTrials.gov, "A PHASE 2/3, PLACEBO-CONTROLLED, RANDOMIZED, OBSERVER-BLIND STUDY TO EVALUATE THE SAFETY, TOLERABILITY, AND IMMUNOGENICITY OF A SARS-COV-2 RNA VACCINE CANDIDATE (BNT162b2) AGAINST COVID-19 IN HEALTHY PREGNANT WOMEN 18 YEARS OF AGE AND OLDER," NIH Natioinal Library of Medicine, 7 July 2023. [Online]. Available: https://clinicaltrials.gov/study/NCT04754594?tab=history&a=21. [Accessed 7 July 2024].

[36] Thorp JA, Benavides A, Thorp MM, McDyer DC, Biss KO, Threet JA, McCullough PA. PART I. Are COVID-19 Vaccines in Pregnancy as Safe and Effective as the U.S. Government, Medical Organizations, and Pharmaceutical Industry Claim? Part I," Preprints.org, June 29, 2024. DOI 10.20944/preprints202406.2062.v1https://www.preprints.org/manuscript/202406.2062/v1

[37] Thorp JA, Benavides A, Thorp MM, McDyer DC, Biss KO, Threet JA, McCullough PA. PART II. Are COVID-19 Vaccines in Pregnancy as Safe and Effective as the U.S. Government, Medical Organizations, and Pharmaceutical Industry Claim? Part II," Preprints.org, 29 June 2024. DOI https://doi.org/10.20944/preprints202407.0069.v1https://www.preprints.org/manuscript/202407.0069/v1

[38] The NEW ENGLAND JOURNAL of MEDICINE. About NEJM: Policies and Practices.," [Online]. Available: https://www.nejm.org/about-nejm/about-nejm#:~:text=Our%20mission%20is%20to%20publish,practice%20and%20improve%20patient%20outcomes. [Accessed 8 July 2024].

[40] Aaron Siri JD. "V-Safe part 1: After 464 Days, CDC Finally Coughed up Covid-19 Vaccine Safety Data Showing 7.7% of people Reported Needing Medical Care. First part of an incredible

story that shows just how broken our public "health" apparatus is: very, very broken.," 23 November 2022. [Online]. Available: https://aaronsiri.substack.com/p/v-safe-part-1-after-464-days-cdc?utm_source=profile&utm_medium=reader2. [Accessed 8 July 2024].

[41] Aaron Siri JD. "V-Safe part 10: Federal Judge Orders CDC to Make public 7.8 Million V-safe Free-Text Entries within 12 Months. Tenth part of an incredible story that shows just how broken our public "health" apparatus is: very, very broken," 11 January 2024. [Online]. Available: https://aaronsiri.substack.com/p/v-safe-part-10-federal-judge-orders. [Accessed 8 July 2024].

[42] Thorp KE, Thorp MM, Thorp EM, Thorp JA. "COVID-19 & Disaster Capitalism – Part I. See pages 170-171 documenting the data manipulation revealing 82% miscarriage rate in the Shimabukuro article. https://www.doi.org/10.46766," The Gazette of Medical Sciences, vol. 3, no. 1, pp. 159-178, 27 July 2022. https://www.thegms.co/medical-ethics/medethics-rw-22071901.pdf

[43] Maggie Thorp JD and Jim Thorp MD. "Pushing COVID-10 Shots in Pregnancy: The Greatest Ethical Breach in the History of Medicine," America Out Loud News, 12 February 2023. [Online]. Available: https://www.americaoutloud.news/pushing-covid-19-shots-in-pregnancy-the-greatest-ethical-breach-in-the-history-of-medicine/. [Accessed 8 July 2024].

[44] Thorp JA, Benavides A, Thorp MM, McDyer DC, Biss KO, Threet JA, McCullough PA. PART I. Are COVID-19 Vaccines in Pregnancy as Safe and Effective as the U.S. Government, Medical Organizations, and Pharmaceutical Industry Claim? Part I," Preprints. org, June 29, 2024. DOI 10.20944/preprints202406.2062.v1https://www.preprints.org/manuscript/202406.2062/v1

[45] Anonymous Authors - Israeli Scientists/Researchers, "Chapter 1. Turtles All The Way Down: Vaccine Clinical Trials," in Turtles All The Way Down: Vaccine Science and Myth, Forward by Mary Holland JD. Edited by Zoey O'Toole and Mary Holland JD. 1 ed., Z. O. a. M. Holland, Ed., NYC, NY: Republished in English by Childrens Health Defense, 2022, pp. 35-83.

[46] Paul D Thacker. Covid-19: Researcher blows the whistle on data integrity issues in Pfizer's vaccine trial. The British Medical Journal (thebmj), vol. 375, p. n2635, 2021. doi: HYPERLINK "https://doi.org/10.1136/bmj.n2635" https://doi.org/10.1136/bmj.n2635 https://www.bmj.com/content/375/bmj.n2635

[47] J. F. Substack, "Kansas Attorney General Sues Pfizer for 'Misleading Claims It Made Related to the COVID Vaccine' (Video).," 17 June 2024. [Online]. [Accessed 9 July 2024].

[48] https://www.medrxiv.org/content/10.1101/2024.06.25.24309259v1.full

[49] Jon Fleetwood, "Kansas Attorney General Sues Pfizer for 'Misleading Claims It Made Related to the COVID Vaccine' (Video)," 17 June 2024. [Online]. Available: https://jonfleetwood.substack.com/p/kansas-attorney-general-sues-pfizer. [Accessed 9 July 2024].

[50] Peter Imanuelsen. HUGE: Five states will be SUING Pfizer. Kansas and Idaho among the states to be suing Pfizer over misleading claims about their covid injections," Peter Imanuelsen. The Freedom Corner with PeterSweden, 24 June 2024. [Online]. Available: https://petersweden.

substack.com/p/huge-five-states-will-be-suing-pfizer. [Accessed 2024 July 2024].

[51] Maggie Thorp JD and Jim Thorp MD. "The war on free speech! Medical boards accused of collusion with feds as 'State Actor' status looms," America Out Loud News, 12 June 2024. [Online]. Available: https://www.americaoutloud.news/the-war-on-free-speech-medical-boards-accused-of-collusion-with-feds-as-state-actor-status-looms/. [Accessed 9 July 2024].

[52] Interest of Justice, "Ninth Circuit Court Rules Correctly COVID-19 mRNA Injections Are Not Legitimate State Interest Due To Being A Treatment, Not A Preventative," Interest of Justice., 8 June 2024. [Online]. Available: https://interestofjustice.substack.com/p/ninth-circuit-court-rules-correctly. [Accessed 13 July 2024].

[53] Maggie Thorp JD and Jim Thorp MD. Tentacles of a Covert and Exploitative Propaganda Machine Compliments of the US Government. America Out Loud News , 28 October 2022 . [Online]. Available: https://www.americaoutloud.news/tentacles-of-a-covert-and-exploitative-propaganda-machine-compliments-of-the-us-government/. [Accessed 9 July 2024].

[54] Maggie Thorp JD and Jim Thorp MD. FOIA Reveals Troubling Relationship between HHS/CDC & the American College of Obstetricians and Gynecologists," America Out Loud News, 7 May 2023. [Online]. Available: https://www.americaoutloud.news/foia-reveals-troubling-relationship-between-hhs-cdc-the-american-college-of-obstetricians-and-gynecologists/. [Accessed 9 July 2024].

[55] Maggie Thorp JD and Jim Thorp MD. "COVID-19 Government Relief Funds Turned the Healthcare Industry on Its Head," America Out Loud News , 10 December 2023. [Online]. Available: https://www.americaoutloud.news/covid-19-government-relief-funds-turned-the-healthcare-industry-on-its-head/. [Accessed 9 July 2024].

[56] Maggie Thorp JD and Jim Thorp MD."US Government coerced leaders of faith to push COVID-19 vaccines on Americans," America Out Loud News, 14 January 2024 . [Online]. Available: https://www.americaoutloud.news/us-government-coerced-leaders-of-faith-to-push-covid-19-vaccines-on-americans/. [Accessed 9 July 2024].

[57] Maggie Thorp JD and Jim Thorp MD."Thorp MM, Thorp JA. The Government Cartel paid billions to Walgreens and CVS not to fill Ivermectin – the question is why," America Out Loud News, 20 May 2024. [Online]. Available: https://www.americaoutloud.news/the-government-cartel-paid-billions-to-walgreens-and-cvs-not-to-fill-ivermectin-the-question-is-why/. [Accessed 9 July 2024].

[58] Rousculp MD, Hollis K, Ziemiecki R, et al. Reactogenicity differences between COVID-19 vaccines: A prospective observational study in the United States and Canada.," medRxiv.org, 2024. doi: https://doi.org/10.1101/2024.06.25.24309259

[59] Maggie Thorp JD and Jim Thorp MD. "The war on Free speech! Medical boards accused of collusion with feds as 'State Actor' status looms," America Out Loud News, 12 June 2024. [Online]. Available: https://www.americaoutloud.news/the-war-on-free-speech-medical-boards-accused-of-collusion-with-feds-as-state-actor-status-looms/. [Accessed 11 July 2024].

[60] I. O. JUSTICE, "Ninth Circuit Court Rules Correctly COVID-19 mRNA Injections Are Not Legitimate State Interest Due To Being A Treatment, Not A Preventative," Interest of Justice, 12 June 2024. [Online]. Available: https://interestofjustice.substack.com/p/ninth-circuit-court-rules-correctly. [Accessed 12 July 2024].

[61] U.S. Department of Health and Human Services (HHS). 2021. "U.S. Department of Health and Human Services Launches Nationwide Network of Trusted Voices to Encourage Vaccination in Next Phase of COVID-19 Public Education Campaign." (Screen Snapshot captured on April 1, 2021, at 22:51:02, by Internet Archive Wayback Machine. Accessed May 1, 2023). https://web.archive.org/web/20210401225102/https://www.hhs.gov/about/news/2021/04/01/hhs-launches-nationwide-network-trusted-voices-encourage-vaccination-next-phase-covid-19-public-education-campaign.html.

CHAPTER 18

Death by Silence

Dr. Roger Hodkinson

Pathologist

Dr. Hodkinson received his general medical degrees from Cambridge University in the UK (M.A., M.B., B. Chir.) where he was a scholar at Corpus Christi College. Following a residency at the University of British Columbia he became a Royal College certified general pathologist (FRCPC). He was previously in good standing as a Fellow of the College of American Pathologists (FCAP) for forty years and is a Fellow of the Royal College of Physicians and Surgeons of Canada, Ottawa. Previously Chairman of General Pathology Examination Committee for the Royal College of Physicians and Surgeons of Canada, Ottawa

Dr. Roger Hodkinson has first hand experience in his fight with big-tobacco decades prior and how the current conditions of every aspect of the medical, pharmaceutical and health regulatory industries are in critical condition due to corruption and regulatory capture.

At its most basic, pathology is the study of how disease and illness progresses. Pathologists are known as the doctor's doctors. They're not just the people that do autopsies. They look at biopsies. They tell the doctors what is going on so that they can treat their patients. Pathologists are the backroom guys; we give other physicians the answers and they take all the credit!

In general pathology, it's important for everyone to realize that the word *general* is used because we simultaneously run the big labs with all the instruments that produce the hematology, chemistry, microbiology results, including virology investigations, while at the same time having a very different role. We look down a microscope at tissue biopsies and we perform autopsies. Those are very different roles. What that gives me as a general pathologist, is a very broad scope of practice that allows me to condense various facts and theories.

I was the first physician in Western Canada, and one of only two in Canada, to stand up against Big Tobacco in the late 1970s and 80s. In other words, I've been steeped in public health for decades. I would consider that I'd saved more lives trying to control Big Tobacco than I ever have as a pathologist. That experience with Big Tobacco was a huge education for me, because Big Pharma is operating in exactly the same way, using the same predatory marketing characteristics.

I would say that I understand real public health, not from an academic ivory tower perspective, which is what got us into all this trouble, but from a real practical, down to earth, street level; a level-headed, common sense approach, which of course is something that has been severely lacking.

My essay is about the most grave injustice Western society has ever experienced. I'm writing this because this is the most important moment in my medical career; indeed my entire life. It's the fight for freedom and the very preservation of democracy. The tyranny must be exposed and stopped dead in its tracks.

As you have heard, I'm an old school, traditionally trained medical specialist who has been a soldier for organized medicine and public health for over 50 years. But no more. I am ashamed of what medicine has become. I intend to paint a very big canvas of the terrible things that happened during COVID. It was never about public health, but all about control. The Alberta truckers were the first to battle against the despots. Not doctors. Not the church, not the media. Truckers. I was there with them on the hustings in Ottawa. Although they failed in their primary objective, they achieved two much bigger victories. They forced the hand of government to take extreme, unwarranted measures to suppress the democratic process using the Emergencies Act, and the truckers also started an international movement to push back on wokeism in all its dystopian guises, including climate change. Let me summarize what has happened to date. I call it the Big Kill of people, economies, and trust in all our previously cherished institutions.

Nothing was needed to manage COVID-19 except common sense and chicken noodle soup; vitamin D and reliance on our miraculous natural immunity. If we had done nothing more than for previous 'flu epidemics, no one would have noticed. It was never close to a viral pandemic, an epidemic at most. What it was a virulent Pandemic of Fear, largely based upon the monumentally flawed PCR test. I speak somewhat knowledgeably of that as a pathologist. We seem to have forgotten what Voltaire presciently said a long time ago; "the art of medicine consists of amusing the patient while nature cures the disease." Everything we were forced to endure predictably failed, with the singular exception of the orchestrated campaign of lies and deceit, which succeeded brilliantly. Yes, the virus is real, but the reaction was a hoax that raped our very soul. I define a hoax as a widely publicized fraud intended to invite unthinking acceptance. I steadfastly refuse to retract my use of the word. It is unquestionably correct. None of the many mandates had any evidence of effectiveness in the medical literature. Masks, social distancing, business closures, travel bans, contact tracing, asymptomatic testing, prohibited gatherings, etc., etc. etc. it was all lies. Nothing could work, nothing did work and therefore nothing will work now. Period.

The so-called modified mRNA vaccines were actually the first ever large-scale experimentation of gene therapy in humans. The majority of the world's population trusted the fraudulent propaganda and got willingly poisoned. It was not needed. It was not tested, didn't work, and has now been shown to have had calamitous consequences.

We know from the incredible work of Denis Rancourt (Canary Vol 1), Jessica Rose and Peter Halligan that it has killed approximately 1 in 1000 injected and about 20 million worldwide. Let that sink in. Ed Dowd has shown that the statistics on permanent disability are many times worse. Humanity essentially became lab rats for experimentation by Big Pharma and our bodies simply toxin factories. The cure was far worse than the disease and is now documented as the most catastrophic event in medical history.

It is also worth emphasizing how vital it would have been to perform autopsies and acurate diagnostic tests in the middle of the muddle created by the idiocrats in charge, in order to be certain of the actual cause of death, instead of relying on the notoriously inaccurate PCR-based test. Autopsies were actively discouraged by the 'authorities' during the alleged pandemic for fear of the outcome being counter narrative.

Certain specialized stains on tissue taken at autopsy that clearly differentiate COVID-19 infection vs COVID 'vaccine' injury have been well described by two prominent pathologists: Professor Arne Burkhardt (now deceased) in Germany and Dr Ryan Cole from the USA. Without getting too technical, they work like this:

> · Specific antibodies are raised in rabbits against two different proteins: the protein on the surface of the COVID-19 virus called the nucleocapsid protein, and the spike protein itself. When these antibodies react with tissue sections seen under a microscope to produce a specific colour it is called a positive reaction. No colour reaction is called negative.
>
> · The results are interpreted as follows:

- **Spike** Positive **Nucleocapsid** Negative = **'vaccine' effect**
  Rationale: The mRNA <vaccine> only codes for the spike protein, not the nucleocapsid protein of the intact virus
- **Spike** Positive **Nucleocapsid** Positive = **virus infection effect**

These tests should have been mandated (a word I have come to loathe in other illegitimate contexts) on autopsies of so-called SADS cases (Sudden Adult Death Syndrome), which was the commonest cause of death listed on death certificates in Alberta, Canada for a significant period. But they were not, perpetuating the lack of accurate information to better inform population health decisions.

Hulscher et al recently published in the *European Society of Cardiology Heart Failure*, a report on the largest series of autopsies of COVID-19 vaccine-induced myocarditis. They concluded, based upon the pathologic findings, that death was caused by the injection. Without vaccination, these 28 patients in the study with an average age of 44, would have been alive today. They also concluded, using the Bradford-Hill criteria, that cardiac death after vaccination can be inferred using epidemiological criteria; in other words, unexplained cardiovascular deaths in the vaccinated with no prior antecedent disease are likely caused by vaccination.

Professor Burkhardt performed the first series of 15 autopsies of people who died from seven days to six months following vaccination (ages 28 to 95), after the coroner or the public prosecutor found no association with the vaccine as the cause of death in any of the cases. However, further examination revealed that the vaccine was indeed implicated in the deaths of 14 of the 15 cases based upon significant infiltration of the heart and other organs with inflammatory cells called lymphocytes. To continue his research Professor Burkhardt contacted other pathologists to help with the findings but most refused to help for fear of repercussions. Luckily he had a second experienced pathologist join him, Professor Lang from Hannover. Professor Lang helped confirm the results, as well as many others who did not want their names published. In total they went on to perform 75 autopsies and concluded that in 78 percent of the cases, the death process was in some way influenced by vaccination.

The most sinister use of gene therapy shots with children has stopped in many international jurisdictions, but in Canada (and the US) it is still being advocated for from six months of age. This can only be called child sacrifice on the altar of the New Gods. No child in good health has died of COVID anywhere, and this gene therapy in children has resulted in untold numbers of senseless deaths. This is murder, plain and simple, and must be prosecuted to the fullest extent of the law.

With the total disinterest in investigating *any* unusual and unexplained death - be that of a child, an athlete, a healthy adult (SADS) - it is disgusting, willful blindness. We don't know what we don't know until we look.

Looking to the future, I believe we are going to see a delayed epidemic of premature heart failure and dementia due to silent, diffuse capillary thrombosis that kills random cells in those organs, only to be diagnosed later as a major organ dysfunction. Conveniently, when the perpetrators are themselves dead and buried. Even worse is the probability of the gene therapy causing permanent changes in the human genome due to a process called reverse transcription. That means the permanent incorporation of genetic information from the gene therapy into the DNA of rapidly dividing human cells in the bone marrow, gut, and testes. We have absolutely no idea what the consequences will be, but the human genome may have been changed. Transgenerationally for evermore. Reverse transcription into spermatozoa is currently being studied by Canadian molecular biologist Dr. David Speicher and others. If he shows this is happening, it will be a Nobel worthy discovery.

We must then ask the obvious question; how could this have possibly happened? In my opinion, this was not intentional genocide. It was the law of unintended consequences resulting from a program operated by the US Department of Defense, called Dual Purpose Research. That is the synergistic combination of gain of function research with preparation for mass vaccination with mRNA in response to actual biowarfare.

Gain of function, of course, is the supremely ridiculous concept that by making a virus more infectious and lethal, one can devise methods to control and treat it. The idiocy of that concept is that viruses, especially RNA viruses like COVID-19, mutate randomly all the time and their mutations are impossible to predict. But more than that, if a lethal virus were to be created with high transmissibility, gain of function research is clearly an existential threat to humanity. It must be stopped by international convention.

Gain of function work was quietly offshored to Wuhan in lock step, with the DoD funding aggressive research into mRNA gene therapy to rapidly counter a potential bioterrorism attack with an unrelated novel virus. When COVID-19 escaped from the Wuhan lab, the secrecy of that project was blown and the DoD went into immediate crisis mode with full bore production of a modified mRNA gene therapy shot to justify the existence of gain of function research. They were lusting to trial run a response to a potential future bio threat. It was a purely military operation from start to finish, tightly managed in every detail by the ex-military Dr. Birx. Fauci was just a front end stooge, acting as spokesperson. The response to the escape should have been based upon the founding principles of public health, namely, the duty to protect the public from risks they cannot manage themselves.

Carefully managing risks versus the benefits of intervention. That principle was rapidly dumped and replaced by four repulsive processes that have operated 24 / 7 for four unbelievable years, namely gargantuan greed by Big Pharma, stupendous stupidity by the idiocrats, Machiavellian manipulation by the mainstream media and intimidation of MD's, and information suppression by colleges of physicians.

Every jurisdiction simply copied the lead of China and the USA. The general operating principle was, 'don't trouble me with due diligence. It takes expertise, time and money that I don't have.'

But oddly, I can also say thank God for COVID as this unforgivable series of events has had two positive outcomes. Massive institutional corruption has been revealed for the first time involving Big Pharma. The courts, mainstream media, the alphabet agencies, by which I mean W.H.O., WEF, CDC, FDA and NIH, as well as organized medicine - colleges of medicine internationally - have been shown to be co-conspirators with the state in murder by intimidating physicians into compliance with the mandates and gene therapy. They have essentially told physicians to swear that the Earth is flat or risk losing their livelihood.

Those colleges are there principally to ensure that there is informed consent for treatment, and that treatment should do no harm. But they bowed to governments diktats and blatantly contravened their own ethical standards by persecuting physicians like me, and others who dared to uphold those time-honored principles.

One could summarize this by saying, the government is now your new doctor. Be worried. Be very worried. Politics playing medicine is a very dangerous game.

The other positive outcome is that the ultimate cause of all this evil has been revealed. Wokeism. The enemy is now revealed and has no clothes. One cannot fight an invisible enemy that wants to abolish religion, travel, money, cars, food, work, parents and family. Wokeism started insidiously in universities decades ago by an arrogant, self-perpetuating, intellectual elite that has been slowly eating away at traditional democratic freedoms. We are stupidly paying them to destroy us.

But then the bad. The very degree of corruption has resulted in the worst outcome of all; the loss of trust in all our previously cherished institutions. Trust is the cement that holds society together. Distrust leaves people feeling isolated. That makes them fair game for government control. The successful recipe has now been baked in. And is ready to be applied to the next hoax... climate change.

The unholy alliance of the WEF, unelected billionaires and multinational corporations otherwise known as fascism has furthered this dystopian nightmare.

To fight for a free future: get educated and get involved. Take your vitamin D and use cash, not credit. Here's to freedom, justice, and democracy now!

CHAPTER 19

Principle-less, Panicked and Power-Hungry: The Three 'P's of Society's Elites During COVID

Professor James Allan

Professor of Law at the University of Queensland, Australia

James Allan is a Canadian-born Garrick Professor of Law at the University of Queensland, Australia. He has lived in Australia for twenty years after practising law in Toronto and London, and teaching it in Hong Kong and New Zealand. He has had sabbaticals as far afield as the Cornell Hall Law School and the University of San Diego law school in the US, the Dalhousie Law School in Canada, and King's College Law School in London. He is a prolific book author and contributor to periodicals.

It is important to admit when one has been wrong, and even more so when one has been badly wrong. So let me start with myself. I go back to the years before the Covid pandemic. For a long time part of my work-related, peer-reviewed legal writings had focused on the failings around the English-speaking world of bills of rights and of the judges – committees of unelected ex-lawyers if we wish to be precise – and, indeed, of the lawyerly caste itself. And I believed that things were only going to get worse. That was in part due to what was happening in the law schools around the anglosphere. Let's just say that the law schools, and universities more generally, were incontestably getting more woke while viewpoint diversity was collapsing – just look at last year's Australian Voice referendum and the fact that Australia has some three dozen law schools yet the number of law professors across the whole country who came out openly against the proposal could be counted on one hand, one machine operator's hand in fact. But the country as a whole voted nearly 61 percent 'No'. In short, I was a fully signed-up member to the well-known sentiment that William Buckley had conveyed some years back when he said that he would rather be governed by the first 2,000 people in the Boston telephone directory than by the Harvard University faculty. For me, make that also the lawyerly caste that gives us our top judges. I was no great fan of juristocracy or of kritarchy or of lawyers as a group when it comes to driving public policy.

But before 2020 I had been quite a big fan of the doctorly caste. During my seven or eight years on New Zealand's University of Otago ethics committee, and from interactions more generally, I believed as a general proposition that doctors tended to focus on the evidence. That they did not tend to over-moralise and then attempt to impose their own moral worldviews on others. That they were better at standing up to groupthink and panic, and certainly better than the lawyerly caste. They put a hefty weight on individual autonomy, sometimes through the prism of the doctrine of 'informed consent' (about which I have grave doubts, as it happens, since ten plus years of education is really not able to be summed up in a ten minute little overview so the patient can give 'informed' consent – the proper question to the doctor is 'what would you do if this were your son?') but nevertheless I reckoned doctors valued individual autonomy and a large degree of patient choice. They also, as an aside of sorts, seemed to me to take a real interest in the arts and literature in a way that is dying out in the universities – including in those parts of our universities supposedly devoted to them such as history, literature, classics, even philosophy and which are dying out, in some measure, because the academics who staff them want to deconstruct and woke-ify even their own fields of expertise. Still, and in summary, I was a big fan of doctors and the doctorly caste. I certainly thought that as a group they were better than the lawyers.

And here's where we come back to my starting claim, the importance of admitting when one has been wrong. Because let's face it. Boy, was I wrong about doctors! The pandemic and Covid plainly showed the preponderance of them, as a class, to have been as pusillanimous, panicked and even principleless as the rest of our elites. Let's take the risk of having all of our blood pressure readings go through the roof and recall the nearly three years of governmental thuggery, heavy-handedness, imposition of idiotic and often irrational rules and resort to lockdown lunacy – not to mention that those imposing these sometimes inane and often unprece-dented public health measures virtually never paid the costs of what they were imposing. The police heavy-handedness verging on thuggery did not affect them. The school closures that shut down schools in a way that will see many children, especially the poor ones, disadvantaged for life did not much affect them – and under a fortnight ago, in late March 2024, a new study out of Stanford University's Hoover Institute came out and found that the total cost to the US economy of the educational loss from Covid school closures will be US$31 trillion, leave aside that the closures were completely needless and ineffective at preventing Covid transmission. There will be a proportionally enormous cost here in this country. And don't forget that Australia's educational results pre-Covid were already woeful – we scored below Kazakhstan – so it's not as though we could af-ford any drops in scores and attainment, let alone precipitous ones. In ad-dition to the police thuggery and school closures the people who brought us lockdowns did not pay the costs of devastating the small business sec-tor. Somehow that seems worse when it is a supposedly right-of-centre po-litical party doing the devastating of its core constituency in favour of the public service and while fostering an ongoing 'work from home' mind-set across society that has gutted productivity – no serious person really believes that working from home, in general terms, produces as much as working from the office – and that led to last year's biggest drop in living standards in this country in decades. Nor did a single public health type or politician or top bureaucrat take a big pay cut, or even a small one, all while seemingly flipping coins to decide which were, and which were not, essential businesses. Oh, and let's not forget that while doing all this they were mouthing the inane, false (but rhetorically effective) phrase 'we're all in this together', a phrase that was factually wrong on all sorts of levels including poor v. rich, young v. old, and private sector v public sector. Ba-sically, the lockdown imposers had no skin in the game, to borrow a phrase from Nassim Taleb. They didn't bear the costs of their decision-making. If they had, we would have had different, more liberal decisions.

Or what about the sort of massive government spending and increased debt and all the money printing during the lockdown lunacy? These measures effectively – in part via asset inflation – transferred huge wealth from the young to the old and from the poor to the rich. The pandemic years were the best years ever to be a billionaire. Again, the decision-makers had no skin in the game. Or what about, in a comparative blink of the eye, throwing away everything I had ever heard about the importance of informed consent during my years on a university ethics committee, in order to push vaccine mandates? All in all, these years amounted to 'the biggest inroads on our civil liberties in at least two hundred years' to paraphrase the retired UK Supreme Court judge Jonathan Sumption.

Which takes us back to doctors. The pandemic response was largely brought to you by public health types and by modellers. Imperial College's Neil Ferguson was the modeller who years earlier had given us modelled predictions on the threat of BSE ('mad cow disease') and foot-and-mouth disease that massively overestimated everything – by orders of magnitude. This was well-known at the start of the Covid pandemic. Yet it made no difference at all to the British and American governments' willingness to treat Professor Ferguson's forecasts wholly unsceptically and almost as holy writ. Apparently hugely over-estimating what the actual deaths will turn out to be, however repeatedly, does not affect one's career as a feted epidemiological modeller one iota; it seems, in fact, to bolster one's position and burnish one's credentials. Perhaps, though, if instead of over-estimating actual outcomes by orders of magnitude you were to under-estimate by just one death, well then we'd see some ramifications.

I need also to mention the incredible inroads into free speech and the marketplace of ideas during the pandemic. Censorship, shadow bans, social media blackouts, the legacy press operating more as a latter-day *Pravda* running the lockdownista line on everything and without even a hint of a trace of a soupcon of an echo of scepticism and questioning regarding that day's offerings from the public health cadre and government ministers. Heck, I even had a couple of published, peer-reviewed law articles offering a sceptical view of the pandemic response rejected for listing by SSRN (Social Science Research Network), presumably because only public health types were then deemed suitable to comment on this fiasco, and only lockdown cheerleader ones at that. Or consider the vitriolic response to anyone who suggested that the virus that was found a few hundred yards from the front door of a lab doing research on just this sort of virus – the only known one in that country – might, just might, have actually escaped from that lab. Mirabile dictu! Instead, charges of 'racism', were the accepted line of response from our elites, along with mocking anyone who suggested this as the source. Even a former head of MI5 who asserted the lab leak theory was censored and banned on social media. Or remember how the three authors of the Great Barrington Declaration were treated by their university colleagues, by the press, by social media. Mr. Fauci called these three 'fringe epidemiologists', although one day before the pandemic started, Professor Sunetra Gupta of Oxford University would have been widely picked as the world's most eminent epidemiologist. And the other two would have made the top ten list, those two being Professor Jay Bhattacharya of Stanford University and Professor Martin Kulldorff of Harvard University (then, not now, as Harvard recently fired him for being right about everything). During the frenzied panic and demand for conformity of the lockdown mania years, even the most credentialled experts in the world were censored, shadow banned and threatened with losing their jobs if they proffered an opinion outside the government and public health line. So much for any concern about free speech! Gosh, it was even a political party with the name 'Liberal' and Prime Minister Morrison, that to their eternal shame, offered up the first iteration of the free speech suppressing and truly woeful ACMA Bill, the one that uses the bogus notions of misinformation and disinformation to try to set up a privileged set of people who will tell us what is and is not true. And this, despite the fact that Professor Bhattacharya maintains to this day that the biggest source of disinformation throughout the pandemic was government. These are bleak times for freedom of expression.

And so if you are all sufficiently depressed, we are nearly ready to turn to the occupations and castes who in general terms were without principle, panicked and power-hungry. These were the various types of elites who let us all down so badly during the pandemic in this country and across the democratic world, outside of Sweden, Florida, South Dakota and a tiny few other jurisdictions. First, though, let me preemptively deal with a response one hears regularly. This is the line that goes something like: 'well, yes, in retrospect we made a fair few errors but at the time, in conditions of uncertainty, we made the safe, responsible choices that uncertainty demanded.' This is simply wrong. It is public policy nonsense in fact. Indeed, right from the start it seemed silly to me, verging on crazy, to think that in conditions of great uncertainty what you ought to do is to proceed directly to some version of an inverted precautionary principle on steroids, thereby mimicking the authoritarian response of the Chinese politburo – and in the process throw away a hundred years of data that informed the then pandemic plans of the British government (and the WHO for that matter) and that unambiguously rejected lockdowns. The smart response in an information vacuum is to carry on as you are making changes at the margins to protect those most at risk as you wait for more information. This is how virtually all of us behave all the time in general life. Nor do we focus obsessively on just one cause of death – let's say from car accidents – and so impose 5 kph speed limits that would undoubtedly save a decent number of lives currently lost in car crashes, but at the same time cause markedly more deaths (rising to myriad more) due to returning us all to the middle ages in terms of being able to move goods and people around efficiently. From very early on it was known that this virus was over a thousand times more deadly to the very old than to the under thirties. In most countries, for most of the pandemic, the average age of death from Covid was over the country's life expectancy. For governments to proclaim that 'we are all in this together' was not true in any sense, certainly not so that it that could lead to the sort of policy response we saw everywhere in the democratic world except for the few other outliers mentioned above that got their responses more or less correct (a fact that today's cumulative excess deaths data, from start of the pandemic to today, brings home in the bluntest fashion going). Not one thing that we knew in March 2020 justified going down the incredibly authoritarian, 'let's run government on the Chinese Politburo model' path that our elites opted to take. It wasn't caution. It was stupidity, a complete lack of commitment to both the liberal and the democratic components of 'liberal democracy', an incredible naivete about how handing huge, unfettered power to government and public health cadres affects the likelihood of their ever confining lockdowns to just a fortnight, and – let's be honest – an awful lot of cowardice on the part of an awful lot of people.

And lest anyone thinks this is all pure hindsight on Allan's part, I will remind doubters that from virtually day one this native born Canadian, who has lived in Australia for two decades, was an open sceptic of the lockdowns in the pages of the *Spectator Australia*, the British *Lockdown Sceptic* website (now *Daily Sceptic*) and once or twice in *Law & Liberty* in the US and in *The Australian* here. In fact, it was that early scepticism that led me to meet the incredibly insightful Ramesh Thakur, as we were fellow travellers right from the start. I think we got just about everything right!

In my opinion, the various castes the most responsible for the panicked, power-hungry, pusillanimous and principleless (four 'P's, not three!) response to Covid in Australia and around the non-Swedish, non-Florida democratic world are as follows:

5th: Lawyers, Judges and the Lawyerly Caste. Yes, there was next to no chance litigants anywhere in the democratic world were going to be able to use a bill of rights to roll back thuggish, heavy-handed governmental Covid regulations through the courts. I said so in print at the start of the crisis and I believe events have proved that true. My take was that we would have to wait until everyone calmed down and the panic subsided and then you would see the judges discover a tiny bit of a willingness to overturn some of these rules and regulations. But as far as the Covid years were concerned the entire edifice of human rights law, and all its accoutrements, was totally useless. Worse than useless in fact, thereby going a long way to proving the enervated, emasculated worth of bills of rights. You buy one and you are simply buying the views of the unelected judges. And they panicked as much as the rest of our elites. But the lawyers and judges come least bad in my list because I do not think we really should even want to live in a world where the lawyerly caste could decide these sort of issues through the courts. And that is true even when we strongly, even vociferously, disagree with what the government is doing, as I did throughout the pandemic. The remedy here had to be political. Elect a Ron DeSantis or the Social Democratic government of Sweden and let them stand up to the panic and show what should be done. There would be nothing left for democracy if a handful of unelected judges could dictate policy here. So only fifth worst.

4th: Here I'm putting the university caste, including the modellers at Imperial College. Yes, many of them disgracefully imposed vaccine mandates (explicitly or implicitly). Yes, the treatment of your Bhattacharyas and Guptas at the world's top universities was shameful. But the competition here is fierce so I'm scoring them just outside a podium finish.

3rd: Doctors get the bronze medal for the four 'P's of being panicked, pusillanimous, principleless and power-hungry. Sure, the public health wing of the doctorly caste carried more than its fair share of the load here.

And maybe this scoring was a tad affected by our disappointment with an occupation that had looked so good before Covid. But it's more likely that the gold and silver positions were denied the doctors because at least a noticeable chunk of them were dissidents and sceptics, including the terrific Anders Tegnell. Many even lost their practising certificates because of their bravery. And that would influence anyone's scorecard.

2nd: This was a tough call. But in the end I gave the silver medal for most pusillanimously panicked and power-hungry to the politicians. A good few who had come into politics preaching their commitment to freedom and to the individual showed that these protestations weren't worth the paper they hadn't been written on. They were too lazy and too fearful to do their jobs the way Governor DeSantis of Florida did. Or the way the Swedish government did. In fact, they shamed themselves while pretending they'd implemented good policies. They deserve to be voted out everywhere.

Absolute worst: The Jimbo gold medal goes to the journalistic caste. Here is a profession or occupation supposedly dedicated to questioning power and to bringing a sceptical mind to all assertions but especially those by government. It is a job that values an open-mind and not taking on trust what the elites are telling them. It is an occupation that is meant to be fearless, not cravenly fearful. So in a close finish, the journalists get the gold medal for being pusillanimous, panicked and without principle.

CHAPTER 20

From Pandemic to Control: How Vaccines Became Tools of Tyranny

Dr. Mike Yeadon

Former VP & Chief Scientific Officer of
Allergy & Respiratory at Pfizer Global R&D

Dr. Michael Yeadon, PhD, is a distinguished scientist and former Vice President & Chief Scientific Officer of Allergy & Respiratory at Pfizer Global R&D. Holding joint honors in Biochemistry and Toxicology along with a PhD in Pharmacology, Dr. Yeadon has spent decades at the forefront of pharmaceutical research. In 2011, after achieving the role of Vice President, he left Pfizer when the company decided to close its R&D operations in Kent, England.

Following his departure, Dr. Yeadon leveraged his expertise to negotiate access to a portfolio of early-stage exploratory compounds from Pfizer, which would have otherwise been discontinued. With these assets, he co-founded Ziarco Pharma Ltd., a biotech company dedicated to innovative drug development. Ziarco attracted significant backing from Pfizer Venture Investments and several other venture capital firms. In 2017, Ziarco was acquired by Novartis Pharmaceuticals for a reported $1 billion, underscoring Dr. Yeadon's impact on the field. Today, he continues his work as an Independent Consultant, contributing his deep knowledge of pharmacology and drug development to new ventures.

I hope to explain to you that the development of vaccines against this alleged pandemic virus was not an appropriate thing to do. And I think, more importantly, that the design choices about the so-called vaccines, in every case, had the consequence of producing toxicity and harm in human beings.

I was doing a limited amount of consulting when the alleged pandemic started in 2020 and I had plenty of time to pay attention to what was being said to me on television. And I quickly deduced and calculated that we were not being told the truth about whatever was going on.

Let me just jump past all of the lies, deceptions and hurts over the last few years and just say why, I am sure that the development of vaccines, the decision to develop vaccines was an obviously inappropriate, impractical, improper strategy, even if what you were being told was true, which it was not. Why am I saying that? Well, if I look through the history of the development of vaccines, I don't think you're going to find very many that were developed in less than about six years. Now, that's because it involves first discovering, or inventing the material you hope to make into a vaccine and conducting preclinical toxicology in test tubes and in animals and then a staged series of tests in human beings to see if it works and if it's safe. But it's much more than that. You have to manufacture on scale a complicated biological material and the processes required to make sure you have control of this complex biological manufacturing process itself takes no less than several years. It cannot be done faster. It doesn't matter that you want it done faster. It doesn't matter how much money you spend or how many people you apply to it. Some of the processes can't start until the results of the process ahead of it is known.

And the long and short of it is that it's absolutely impossible. Laughable to someone like me to pretend that a vaccine was conceived, created, tested, manufactured, and authorized in under a year. I'm absolutely certain, after 30 years in this industry, that is not what happened. Something else happened. There are other reasons why you wouldn't make a vaccine. In this particular case, a very important one is that there has not been a pandemic. You look at the work of Denis Rancourt in Canada, you will find there's no evidence whatsoever of increase in all cause mortality until the W.H.O., in my view, fraudulently declared a pandemic.

There were increases in deaths, of course, but what you probably don't know is that these only started to increase after W.H.O. fraudulently called a pandemic. They flowed from three major changes to medical management in Britain and every other country I've been able to find out.

First, in hospitals, many people who arrived and were declared COVID positive, were put on ventilators. I can assure you, my PhD, being in the field of respiratory control, I know quite a bit about this and it's not appropriate if someone is breathing and doesn't have chest wall damage; you don't sedate, intubate, and ventilate. If you do that, especially if the person's frail, you're really quite likely to kill them. In my view, large numbers of people were killed as a consequence of being wrongly treated in hospital. It wasn't an accident. That protocol was imposed upon them, upon every country from guidance given from a higher up authority that trickled down. It wasn't worked out by your local doctors in the hospital and other doctors who worked out alternative treatments were censored.

The second way in which large numbers of people died was in old people's care homes. Very many people were given sedative drugs that slowed their respiration. Midazolam and morphine were two common drugs and they were used at doses that caused people to literally fade away. They were given effectively lethal injections even though they weren't about to die. So those two things I think can be described as medical murder.

The third category of increased deaths that resulted from changes in medical procedures were people in the community, you and me. You might have got a cold or a flu, and then it went to your chest and you had a persistent cough. Maybe it became bronchial or bacterial pneumonia. Now, the normal course of treatment was seven days of antibiotics but in many, many cases these patients were denied treatment, access to doctors and hospitals because of lockdowns and fear, and they died of treatable bacterial pneumonia.

All of those deaths in hospitals, care homes and in the community were ascribed to COVID. There's your artificial pandemic.

I've given you one reason why you wouldn't develop a vaccine. It cannot be done in 12 months. It would take years and years and years. If you do it faster, you've done it badly or incompletely, or you have not obtained the data to say that it works or is safe. I don't know what they did exactly, but it was not a vaccine.

Few people are able to understand and tell you that the design of these molecular structures in the vaccines have been done intentionally or at the very least recklessly; the vaccines, not COVID, are killing and injuring millions of people. It's a huge claim but the data is unequivocal. All over the world we are seeing a rise in excess mortality through government databases. We are seeing huge reports of injury and death through the VAERS system in the U.S. and the Yellow Card system in the UK and similar tracking systems across Europe and worldwide. The CDC's VSafe app, which tracked 10 million injected persons in the U.S. reported that 7% (check percentage) of vaccine recipients experienced a severe adverse reaction which required medical intervention. We are seeing athletes collapsing on the sports field, we are seeing young people die suddenly.

The world is not connecting the dots. No government is going to admit they were wrong after scaring and mandating populations to get the COVID vaccine, it's political suicide, it's complete denial. It's up to us to talk up, educate and warn others. Pfizer knew there were problems, which is why ICAN through lawyer Aaron Siri sued the FDA and won the release of the trial data, which the FDA wanted hidden for 75 years. I wonder why?

I've worked over 30 years with colleagues in rational drug design. That is every synthetic medicine that is made from something not purified from nature. It consists of a series of atoms and molecules and formulations. Every single component in that vial, as it turns out, has to be chosen by a person. They're not there randomly. They're not there as a natural product. Someone decided to put them in there, and you put them in there because you have particular objectives for the drugs to be absorbed quickly or slowly, for it to last a long time or not, for it to go everywhere versus remaining in a certain area of the body, and so on.

So when I look at the design of these molecules, I do it with the mind of a drug hunter, someone involved in rational drug design. I will be able to tell you three or four things about these vaccines that are not accidental and undoubtedly, would have, as a consequence, toxicity that was predictable and indeed predicted.

Wolfgang Wodarg and I, in early December 2020, wrote a technical letter, an open letter to the European Medicines Agency. In that letter we expressed great concerns about the safety profile of these materials and begged that they not be developed further. Our objective was to reach many people. We did not succeed because of censorship. I can tell you that these are toxic by design; I knew that three years ago and unfortunately, I've been correct. This arises out of my experience of over 30 years of teamwork in designing molecules and then working out what happens.

The first obviously harmful decision made is the fact that these are gene based materials. I will focus on mRNA, but the principles are pretty much the same as the others. The mRNA vaccines encode a protein sequence. The key thing for me is that they're not your protein. They don't belong in your body. The reason is that your immune system is able to play nice with itself most of the time, but if you're infected, it will go to war. Your immune system is exquisitely aware of self, what's meant to be in your body and non self, or foreign things that are not meant to be inside you, such as when you are injected with mRNA encoding something that's not human. We were told it was a virus spike protein, but whatever it was, it's not human. Your body takes up that genetic instruction and starts to manufacture something that does not belong in your body. Your immune system goes to war and kills every single cell that has taken up that material and made the foreign protein, which is by design. It's what those particular formulae do.

I first encountered these products at least ten years ago at Pfizer. Like other companies in the industry, Pfizer was considering this technology for potential anti-cancer treatments. We figured if we could direct them to a rogue cell, a cancer cell, your immune system would recognize it now as foreign and kill it. It's quite a clever idea. It's called immuno oncology. So the technology does exist for a good reason.

But I knew four years ago that giving it to healthy people, in a mass market application, would induce a lethal autoimmune attack on every cell and tissue in your body to which that material went, which is why we are seeing continued dangerous and lethal side effects. Every person from the industry involved in the manufacture of these materials knew it as well, I would call it immunology 101. It's the first thing you would be taught about immunology, the difference between self and non-self. Now that's a devastating piece of information, but it's not the only one.

The second one I will point to is the protein that was coded by the mRNA, the so-called spike protein. The bits illustrated on the television as sticking out from the outside of the sphere. That is allegedly this virus. Spike proteins are not inert. They're biologically active in their own right and they are biological toxins. If you add spike protein to human blood cells, the blood begins to coagulate. This is what embalmers are reporting and pathologists are seeing when autopsies are performed, reported by Dr. Ryan Cole and others. These instructions cause your body not only to make something that was alien to you, not human, but also to manufacture something that was directly toxic to your body and would induce blood clots in the blood, and neurological harms if near any neuro nervous tissue. So that's the second one, the design choice was to manufacture something that's dangerous.

That design choice wasn't necessary. They could have chosen anything else about this alleged virus, but they chose the thing that was toxic. But there's worse even than that. The spike protein was supposedly the site of the highest rates of mutation. That means the vaccine would stop working very quickly as the spike protein changed. Then finally, the sequence of the spike protein is somewhat similar to some proteins in the human body. For females, it's somewhat similar to vital proteins of pregnancy. They're called syncytins. So, if you manufacture a situation where your body makes a powerful immune response to this foreign protein, it wouldn't be surprising if there was a little bleed over and your immune system starts attacking your own pregnant uterus. This was one of the specific things that concerned Dr. Wodarg and I in 2020. I'm afraid that's come true.

The final design choice I'm going to focus on is devastating. Drugs are normally formulated in a capsule or a tablet or a spray. In this case, they're liquids and they're formulated in essentially little fatty globule molecules called lipid nanoparticles. The lipids themselves are novel. Some of them are novel and are known to be toxic, so it was a bad idea to inject people with novel, and known-to-be-toxic lipids.

But putting that aside, the worst thing is that the lipid nanoparticles surround and protect this foreign genetic sequence. Why is that important? Well, if you just inject foreign DNA into your body, you will not be surprised to learn that your body doesn't like foreign DNA. Your body things it's very good idea to get rid of it so you preserve your own genetic instructions. But covered in lipids, it allowed the so-called vaccine to glide around the body and be distributed into your heart, your brain, your uterus, all over. That was the purpose of the formulation, to allow vulnerable compounds that otherwise wouldn't spread around the body to do so in a protected manner. They didn't stay in the shoulder, as was reported by Pfizer. They distributed swiftly all around the body. Byram Bridle in Canada originally confirmed this, thanks to a FOIA request of Pfizer's data submission to the Japanese authorities.

Particularly shocking is that 10 years ago, lipid nanoparticles were known to accumulate in the ovaries, which is simply dangerous. This is not news to vaccine developers or molecular biologists. I could come up with many more examples. There are clever molecular biologists who've looked at the sequences and believe that there are at least two or three other features of these injections that increase the propensity to harm.

I declare these products toxic by design. They are intentionally harmful. I think that fits perfectly with the lie you've been told about a pandemic. There isn't one. The purpose of the pandemic, I think, was to damage the economy, to get us used to doing what we're told under a mock emergency, and to roll up our sleeves to receive these dangerous materials.

Where are we now after almost four years? I think we're still being given fear-based messages almost every day. And here's where I think we're heading; it's not going to be over. It will just continue and morph into a more and more aggressive form of totalitarian dictatorship. I think it's malevolence and intentionally harmful and it will continue. I believe in short, if you do nothing, you don't speak up, you do what you're told, you will lose your freedom and then your life. I think some self-appointed group of very rich people have decided they don't like 8 billion people on the planet, and they want to reduce our numbers.

If we do not protest, if we do not refuse and fight back, we will lose freedom first and then our lives. I think it will be as simple as this; that unnecessary mandatory digital ID will be imposed. That's what they need in order to control us. Then, I think we'll lose cash and only have digital money. The combination of digital ID and digital money means control of every single thing you do, every movement, every purchase will be in the hands of a computer program and you'll never escape it. There's no way to turn it off. Don't sign up for it. If you ignore what I've said and I'm right, it will be the end. If, on the other hand, you think there's something in what I've said and you do something about it, the very worst that will happen to you is you'll be laughed at. I urge you to do something with this information.

Your Voice Matters

We hope this book has sparked thought and encouraged deeper reflection. If you feel the same, we'd appreciate it if you could take a moment to rate and review the book on Amazon. Your review helps others discover this work, and it's our most effective way of reaching new readers. Thank you for helping us spread the message!

CHAPTER 21

Pandemic Preparedness: The New Parasite

David Bell

Former medical Officer and scientist at
the World Health Organization (WHO)

David Bell is a clinical and public health physician with a PhD in population health and background in internal medicine, modelling and epidemiology of infectious disease. He has worked in global health and biotech for the past 25 years. Previously, he was Director of the Global Health Technologies at Intellectual Ventures Global Good Fund in the USA, Programme Head for Malaria and Acute Febrile Disease at FIND in Geneva, and worked in infectious diseases and coordinated malaria diagnostics strategy at the World Health Organization. He currently consults in biotech and international public health, co-leads the REPPPARE project on pandemics at the University of Leeds, and is a senior scholar of the Brownstone Institute.

"Epidemics and pandemics of infectious diseases are occurring more often, and spreading faster and further than ever..." (WHO)
"Since the beginning of the 21st century, the world has experienced major epidemics and pandemics every four to five years" (WHO)

So begin two 2022 publications from the World Health Organization (WHO). The reader may wonder whether they missed something, but this is the perception of the world that major international health agencies would like us to adopt. As the G20 Nations High Level Panel concluded the same year, advocating for over $10 billion in new money annually to support a response to this sudden crisis:

"...countering the existential threat of deadly and costly pandemics must be the human security issue of our times"

These claims, and others like them, are intended to encourage the diversion of over $10 billion in new international development assistance funding to the burgeoning pandemic preparedness and response (PPR) industry. Adding to another $20 billion to be found within country health budgets, this aims to set up a massive surveillance effort to find variants of viruses, proclaim them theoretical threats to health, and (with further funding) develop rapid mass-vaccine responses based on the model trialled for COVID-19. The World Bank is adding further funds to this, and advocating for $10 billion more annually.

In a world in which the total current budget of WHO is under $4 billion, and the entire world spends a little over $3 billion to address well over half a million children dying annually from malaria, these new sums would suggest something truly existential is brewing. Yet few are reporting bodies in the streets. Something very strange, but very human, is happening, but on a scale we have never before seen.

In the century prior to the COVID event pandemics were, in reality, not increasing. Their impact in terms of lives lost was steadily diminishing. WHO noted this in its 2019 pandemic guidelines. But a revolution in diagnostic and communications technologies from the 1960s had provided us with a new and remarkable ability to detect and distinguish pathogens we had never been aware of, and minor genetic variants of these. A background of indistinguishable disease syndromes had become a plethora of outbreak opportunities. Businesses are there to jump on such opportunities - it is their responsibility to their shareholders. The age of international health public-private partnerships had arrived, enabling the Global Health industry to move from its niche tropical health routes to a multi-billion-dollar industry, with potential for controlling a market in a way other industries could only dream.

So, the quotes above are not intended to reflect reality; rather, they are intended to push a product. A form of advertising - like showing stains on a shirt to sell soap powder or new laundry services. It is intended to paint a picture through which the public will perceive a false reality, made possible through advances in technology. Not unlike the virtual reality industry - and so perhaps it is not surprising it is backed by some of the same individuals and corporations.

By triggering fear and deference to expertise in an area with which most are unfamiliar, the wealth-concentrating response used so successfully through the COVID-19 response can be normalized and repeated. False assertions stated as accepted fact have proven very effective in increasing the industry's share of the global financial cake. International agencies have no advertising standards to comply with.

When an industry absorbs material value to produce mostly unquantifiable products, perceptions are vital. Growth in the public health industry can only occur in two ways. Firstly, the industry and the public can jointly identify mutually beneficent areas of work that the public considers worth funding. Secondly, the industry can mislead, coerce or force the public, with the assistance of cooperative governments, to provide support that is not in the public's interest. The latter is what parasites do.

As a disclaimer, I have spent the bulk of my working life employed by governments or on aid budgets, living off money taken from taxpayers so that I could have it. It can be a great lifestyle, as global health salaries and benefits are generally very attractive, offer travel to exotic locations, and commonly offer generous health and education benefits. It can still work for the public if the relationship is symbiotic, increasing their general health and well-being and improving the functioning of a moral, decent society. Sometimes that outcome can occur.

For public health to work for the public, the public must remain in control of this relationship. Oxpeckers, the birds that hitch a ride on rhinoceroses, have a useful symbiotic relationship with their host. They remove skin parasites from awkward crevices, providing the rhinoceros with a healthier skin and fewer irritating itches. If they pecked out the eyes of the host, they would cease to be of benefit, and become a marauding parasite. For a while, the oxpecker may gain more for themselves, feasting on the rhino's softer parts. Eventually their host will succumb as a blind rhinoceros, unless confined to a zoo, cannot sustain its being. But the oxpecker, if overcome by greed, may not have thought that far ahead.

To remain in charge and manage public health for mutual benefit, the public must be told the truth. But in a problem-solving industry where solved problems no longer require work, truth-telling risks job security. This is where the symbiotic relationship of public health is prone to become parasitic. If one is paid to address a particular health issue, and the issue is resolved through good management or a changing risk environment, there is a clear and urgent need to justify continuation of salary.

On a larger scale, whole public health bureaucracies have an incentive to find more issues that 'must' be addressed, make new rules that must then be enforced, and identify more risks to investigate. New international public health bodies keep emerging and growing, but they don't close down. People rarely choose redundancy and unemployment.

This is where the public health industry has a real advantage. In nature, parasites usually must concentrate on just one host to survive, adapting to maximize their gains. A hookworm is designed specifically to survive in its host's gut. The host, however, has a whole variety of parasites, illnesses, and other pressing concerns to deal with. A host must therefore ignore the hookworm as long as it does not pose an obvious immediate threat. The worm needs to milk the host of blood whilst seeming relatively innocuous.

A really smart hookworm would find a way to trick the host into thinking it beneficial – perhaps by promoting the benefits of medieval practices such as bloodletting, as we have seen with masks and curfews through the recent COVID response. The global health industry can use this approach by building a story that will benefit them, plausible enough to the public to pass rudimentary scrutiny. If it sounds sufficiently specialized, it will dissuade deeper examination. In the current rendering of this ploy, the public faces an ever-growing threat of pandemics that will devastate society if we in the public health industry are not given more money. They are given a story of urgency, and shielded from the historical and scientific realities that would undermine it.

International public health organizations solely concentrated on addressing pandemics already exist, such as CEPI, inaugurated by the Gates Foundation, Norway and Wellcome Trust at the World Economic Forum in 2017, and the new Financial Intermediary Fund for pandemics of the World Bank. Others such as Gavi, and increasingly WHO and Unicef, focus heavily on this area. Many of their sponsors, including large pharmaceutical companies and their investors, stand to gain very large profits off the back of this gravy train.

The average taxpayer, dealing with inflation, family life, jobs and myriad other priorities can hardly be expected to delve into the veracity of what 'experts' say in some far distant place. They must trust that a symbiotic, mutually beneficial relationship is still in place. They hope that the public health industry will 'do the right thing'; that it is still on their side.

White papers on pandemic preparedness don't have detailed cost-benefit analyses, just as these were not provided for COVID lockdowns, school closures or mass vaccination. Cursory calculations suggest poor overall benefit, so they have been avoided. We now see this playing out through declining economies, rising poverty and inequality. Diverting billions of dollars annually to hypothetical pandemics will add to this burden. Yet this is being done, and the public are acquiescing to this use of their increasingly hard-earned taxes.

A dead rhinoceros will not support many oxpeckers, and a hookworm will not survive bleeding its host to death. A public health industry that impoverishes its funding base and harms society through ill-advised policies will eventually be caught up in the outcome. But the short-term gains from parasitism are attractive and humans don't seem to have the instincts (or intelligence) that keeps the oxpecker in healthy symbiosis.

Thus, the public health industry will probably continue its current trajectory, increasing inequality and poverty, comfortably on the receiving end of the wealth redistribution it promotes. The money requested for pandemic preparedness will be paid, because the people deciding whether to use your taxes are essentially the same people asking for them. They run the international financial and health sector and they all meet at their private club called the World Economic Forum. Their sponsors now have more than enough spare cash swirling around to keep needy politicians and media on board.

Those working within the industry know what they are doing – at least those who pause long enough to think. But needs must, and there are enough people involved to dissipate the blame. This abuse will continue until the host, the parasitized, realizes that the symbiotic relationship they had been banking on is a fallacy, and they have been duped. There are ways to deal with parasites that are not good for the parasite. A really smart public health industry would adopt a more measured approach and ensure their policies benefit the public more than themselves. But that would also require a moral code and some courage.

https://essl.leeds.ac.uk/downloads/download/228/rational-policy-over-panic
https://documents.worldbank.org/en/publication/documents-reports/documentdetail/099530010212241754/p17840200ca7ff098091b7014001a08952e
https://iris.who.int/bitstream/handle/10665/329438/9789241516839-eng.pdf?ua=1
https://brownstone.org/articles/whos-driving-the-pandemic-express/
https://brownstone.org/articles/four-myths-about-pandemic-preparedness/
https://www.who.int/news/item/19-04-2022-delivering-on-the-g20-leaders-commitment-to-build-an-equitable-and-effective-financial-intermediary-fund-(fif)-for-pandemic-preparedness-and-response-(ppr)
https://www.worldbank.org/en/publication/poverty-and-shared-prosperity
https://www.nature.com/immersive/d41586-022-01647-6/index.html
https://wir2022.wid.world/

CHAPTER 22

Clean vs. Dirty: A Way to Understand Everything

Jeffrey Tucker

President at Brownstone Institute and
Senior Economics Columnist at the Epoch Times.

Jeffrey Tucker is Founder, Author, and President at Brownstone Institute. He is also Senior Economics Columnist for Epoch Times, author of 10 books, including Life After Lockdown, and many thousands of articles in the scholarly and popular press. He speaks widely on topics of economics, technology, social philosophy, and culture.

The other day, I listened to as much National Public Radio as I could stand and one point stood out to me. The experience was anodyne. The topics were nothing that mattered. It felt like a gentle ooze of news that always came to the proper conclusion at the end of the well-produced bit.

By proper, I hope you know what I mean. It confirmed the listeners' biases. And everyone knows who they are: wealthy, mostly white professionals in urban centers with high-end salaries to match their educational credentials. Probably 90 percent Biden voters last time and next time Kamala, not because he was a great president but rather because he inherited the anti-deplorable mantle of his predecessor nominee.

NPR was raising money on that particular day, which they do despite the taxpayer subsidies. If you give money, you can get an NPR umbrella or be given a bit of nature trail to adopt or perhaps acquire a coffee mug for your desk to proclaim your loyalties to your co-workers or just reinforce your opinions while eating your breakfast of Whole Foods granola and soy milk.

The experience happened even as I'm reading, with great joy, _Fear of a Microbial Planet_ by Steve Templeton. The book is about the ubiquity of germs, trillions of them everywhere. They can be a threat but they are mostly our friends.

Exposure, his thesis goes, is the path to health. Without it we will die. And yet, over the last three years, avoiding exposure has been the main goal of policy and culture throughout the world. "Stop the spread" or "Slow the spread" or "Socially distance" or "Stay home, stay safe" have been entrenched as slogans to govern our lives.

The phrases still have gravitas. It has been a maniacal fixation on a single pathogen to the exclusion of trillions of others that are truly everywhere in us and around us. It is like going back before the invention of the microscope when we didn't know that every surface of everything is covered in creepy crawling things. We further indulge the completely unscientific fantasy that by doing some hopping-around dance to avoid others, plus covering our face and getting a shot, would keep us forever clean, meaning free of the bad pathogen.

Dr. Templeton's view is that this is a potential disaster for human health. And he explains the point with great erudition and examples from all of history. He picks up on the extraordinarily keen insight of Dr. Sunetra Gupta, who has traced longer life expectancy in the 20th century to more exposure to a greater heterogeneity of pathogens as a result of transportation and migration. We don't just need to learn to live with COVID. We need to live with them all and orient social and political organization around the reality of their ubiquity.

Now, what precisely is the connection between NPR's sanitized "news" and the thesis of the Templeton book? It suddenly dawned on me. It is possible to understand nearly everything going on today – the COVID response, the political tribalism, the censorship, the failure of the major media to talk about anything that matters, the cultural and class divides, even migration trends – as a grand effort by those people who perceive themselves to be clean to stay away from people they regard as dirty.

And not just people but ideas and thoughts too. This goes way beyond some reemergence of Puritanism, though this is a species. The desire for purification extends to the whole of the physical and intellectual world. It's the reason for the cancellations, the purges, the demographic upheavals, the loss of liberties, and the threat to democratic norms. It covers everything.

Let me see if I can persuade you.

The attacks on Elon Musk's curbing of censorship on Twitter have been relentless. One might suppose that once he revealed that Twitter was operating as a censor for the Deep State, there would be outrage and a renewed celebration of free speech. The opposite has happened. As Musk opened the place up more and more, and non-conventional opinions started gaining traction, we saw panic ensue.

Sure enough, now we see all the usual suspects quitting the platform in a huff. More likely, individuals at these organizations are creating fake accounts so they can keep up with the news. Otherwise, they preserve their fan accounts on Zuckerberg and Gates's platforms.

Why might they be doing this? They do not want their organizations to inhabit (or be seen to inhabit) the same space with dirty opinions that they don't like. They believe their own platforms will do their best to avoid being infected by them. They would rather hide out in their country-club social spaces in which everyone is woke and everyone knows what to say and what not to say. At least the algorithms are skewed in their favor.

The line they use is that they want to be around those who are "house trained" but consider what that means. They don't want pet waste on their carpet, thus comparing ideas with which they disagree with a nasty pathogen. They are seeking to stay clean.

In this case and in every case, they are glad for the government to operate as the clean-up crew. It's dirty ideas and people who hold them that they oppose. They don't want to have friends who articulate them or live in communities where such people live.

They put out yard signs as signals to neighbors about where they stand. The issue in its particulars doesn't matter (BLM, Support Ukraine, Water Is Life [huh?]). All that matters is the signaling system: Team Clean instead of Team Dirty. We all know what those slogans are and what they really mean and for whom they are displayed.

The coronavirus panic played right into this. Stay home and get the dirty people to bring you groceries, leaving them on the doorstep to air out before you pick them up. If there is a pathogen on the loose, better that they get it than us. To be sure, the people on the front line are heroes so long as we can cheer them from our windows.

This is why when it came to the vaccine, the nurses had to get them too despite having natural immunity. Vaccines were seen as an extra bar of soap to make sure that the dirty people whom we might encounter are extra free of the bad germ itself. Everyone had to get them. Those who refused, what can they say? At least we know who they are.

The virus too was a metaphor for an infected country, a land soiled by a bad president. Of course there was an outbreak. That's why we had to lock down and wreck everything including our kids' education. Anything to rid the country of the pestilence of Trump. And can we really be surprised that it was South Dakota that never locked down? It's a dirty red state and they do dirty things like ride motorcycles, shoot animals with guns, and raise cows.

For the clean people, it was hardly a surprise that Georgia, Florida, and Texas opened first, since they were already intellectually infected by right-wing thought. And they were also places where vaccine uptake was low.

In the fall of 2021, the *New York Times* proved that red states that Trump won had lower vaccination rates: they are hopelessly blechy already. Look at the sheer number of evangelical churches, and AM radio stations, in those places where icky people gather to sing stupid songs about God.

The clean vs. dirty symbolism explains the whole of the vaccine push and even the mandates, since getting the shot was nothing but a gesture of tribal loyalties. This is why it didn't matter when it turned out that the vaccine protected neither against infection nor spread. Who cares, since the vaccine does what it is supposed to do: separating us from them?

For a while, the clean ruling classes in New York and Boston even sealed off their cities to dirty people by forbidding them from going to movies, libraries, restaurants, bars, and museums. What a blessed world it became for the sanitized among us that they could navigate their favorite institutions in absence of the untouchables! This was to them how life should be.

No need to elaborate on the wild fashion for sanitizer and plexiglass. The meaning of those are obvious. Everyone needs to douse themselves as a precaution, especially when others are watching. And as customers we don't want to be anywhere near the face of the merchant class. And for two years and more, every surface needed spraying with disinfectant after any human contact.

Then there is the sudden fetishistic longing for "contactless" menus, checkouts, and everything else in this corrupt and sinful world. Somehow it has become an ideal never to touch anything or anybody, as if we long to be followers of the Prophet Mani and evolve into Pure People of the Spirit. After all, only dirty people would pick up a menu or handle cash, because god only knows whom else has held it.

Remember the jars for clean vs. dirty pens at the hotel check in that still require signatures? No need to elaborate on that one. It's all part of the ethos of the untouchables, or the *Dalit* or *Harijan* in the old caste system. To inhabit a "contactless" world recreates the same thing under a different label.

Reflect on the masking practices for a moment. Why is it ok to take off your mask when seated but the server had to wear one when standing? Because the seated are already proving their cleanliness because they are paying customers and being served and hence well-to-do. It's the servers who have to work for a living who are in doubt. And then if you got up to go to the restroom, of course you had to mask up because you might accidentally have a brush with a cook, cleaner, or server.

When the inflation started, one might have supposed that the people who shop at Whole Foods would have shifted *en masse* to Aldi or WalMart. But this prediction misunderstands the whole point of shopping at Whole Foods for a certain class. The point is that we don't want to be around dirty people who buy dirty food. No need for the clean to buy in bulk to alleviate the inflation squeeze. Rather, the higher cost of groceries is worth it to stay apart from soiled, unvaccinated patrons, otherwise we could get infected.

Plus, to have the resources to spend 50 percent more on clean food bought by other clean people works to give off the all-important signal. All the better that the owner of Whole Foods was a huge supporter of lockdowns as a way to beat the competition.

Notice the way we talk about energy too: clean vs. dirty. Oil and gas, with their fumes and methods of processing, are contrary to the ethos of highly sanitized people. Electric cars make less noise so they are surely better, never mind that coal is also a fossil fuel and that batteries are a massive environmental hazard in disposal and even use more energy overall. Facts don't matter. Only symbolism and clean-class identity carry the day.

To be sure, it's not always obvious who is and who isn't clean enough for social interaction. That's why we need constant surveillance of ideas since views on matters like religion, politics, and even issues like trans rights are proxies to demarcate the difference between us and them. Surveillance makes the invisible visible and that enables the construction of whole systems to punish the unclean and reward the cleanly compliant.

All of this came to light with the pandemic of course since having a virus on the loose perfectly illustrates the core point that Anthony Fauci made in his August 2020 article in *Cell*. The emergence of migration thousands of years ago, and the building of cities over hundreds of years, mixed up the populations too much and created terrible epidemics of cholera and malaria. The solution was obvious to him: get rid of sports events, crowded urban conditions, pet ownership (blech), and mass population movements. Lockdowns were just the first step toward "rebuilding the infrastructures of human existence."

We've all been startled that there hasn't been more of a shift in mainstream media coverage despite the obvious failure of conventional "Covid science," the revelations of endless scandals of the Bidens and pharma, and even the plummeting profits of major media venues. Even when BuzzFeed News goes belly up, places like CNN, the *New York Times*, and *Vanity Fair* continue on their merry way as if nothing were happening.

The reason is simple. The clean people are convinced they are right. They have no doubt about it. And they simply will not soil themselves with bogus ideas like objective journalism or unbiased coverage of actual news. That would be the equivalent of wallowing in mud, wrecking all that they have worked for their whole lives and the whole agenda of their profession, which is to purge their institutions of infectious ideological disease.

This is also why the basics of cell biology that previous generations learned in the 9th grade seemed lost on these people. The idea that you would allow yourself to be exposed to germs in order to protect against more severe outcomes strikes at the very heart of their manichean worldview. The point is to stay away, not mix it up. Their germophobia applies not only to the microbial kingdom but to society and the world of ideas as well. The notion of sanitization is a worldview that admits not natural immunity via infection, since that would only mean that you have the bad thing inside of you.

The science be damned. It was long ago trumped by the cultural predisposition to live in a germ-free world: purged curricula, purged cultures, and purged politics. Of course the spread needed to be slowed and stopped. Of course the curve needed to be flattened. Of course there should be social distancing instead of random milling around. The elites need to minimize exposure to everything in a time when the masses are so obviously unwashed.

When the <u>Great Barrington Declaration</u> proposed focused protection based on age, while letting everyone else go about life as normal, that was nothing but a scandal. Anyone can and will get old, whereas they wanted class distinctions based on social and political rank in order to more closely approximate clean and unclean, which is their real ideal.

This is also, by the way, why protests against racism in the summer of 2020 got a pass: people gathering for the right cause are more likely to be among the ideologically clean. And today, this demarcation is all around us, both physically and intellectually. Salmon: farmed is dirty and wild is clean, so it is far more expensive. And with work: from home is clean, while going into the office is dirty.

What can we make of all of this? Dr. Templeton in his book tells the fascinating story of two cities in Finland, one on the poor Soviet side and one on the Western side. After the end of the Cold War, researchers were able to compare health between the two cities, one dirty and one clean.

> Although the two populations shared a similar ancestry and climate, there were some stark differences. The border between these two regions marks one of the steepest gradients in standard of living in the world, even steeper than the border between the United States and Mexico. Finland had become modernized as other countries in Europe after World War II, while isolated Karelia had remained impoverished under communism and stuck in the 1940s (and arguably wasn't in the 1940s during the 1940s).

The researchers in the Karelia Allergy Study noticed some striking differences in the data they collected and analyzed. In Finnish Karelia, asthma and allergies were over four times more prevalent compared to Russian Karelia. Positive skin prick tests, which measure rapid swelling and allergic inflammation in response to common allergens injected under the skin, were also much higher in Finnish people.

Differences in children were even more striking, with a 5.5-fold increase in asthma and eczema diagnoses in Finland, and a 14-fold increase in hay fever. Russian children with allergies, as well as their mothers, also had much lower soluble IgE levels, indicating a significant decrease in the antibody isotype that rapidly induces allergic inflammation.

Autoimmune diseases like type-1 diabetes were also 5-6 times higher in the Finnish population when compared to their Russian neighbors. Not surprisingly, the microbial environments of people living in Russian Karelia were markedly different from that of Finnish Karelia. Russian Karelians drank untreated and unfiltered water that exposed their guts to orders of magnitude more microbes than their Finnish counterparts. Household dust samples from both locations revealed that Russian house dust contained more Firmicutes and Actinobacteria species with a coincident 20-fold increase in the gram-positive cell wall component muramic acid and a 7-fold increase in animal-associated bacterial species. In contrast, Gram-negative species, mainly Proteobacteria, were predominant in Finnish household dust.

Clearly the Russians lived in a much more diverse and abundant microbial ecosystem than the Finns, and these environmental differences were associated with decreased allergies and asthma.

So the dirty people were healthier people in particular ways. Fascinating, right? It's only the beginning of what you will discover <u>in this book</u>. If I were to summarize, Templeton proves that there is no such thing as clean in the way that term is popularly understood, and every attempt to bring it about carries with it grave risks to human health. A naive immune system is a killer. This thesis could also be a metaphor concerning the attempts to clean up the public mind too: the more we censor, the more stupid we become. The more we cancel, the less fully human and safe are our lives.

The clean vs. dirty distinction was once an indicator of class, perhaps a desiderata of germaphobic pathology, even a harmless eccentricity. But in 2020, the obsession became extreme, an aesthetic priority that overrode all morality and truth. It then became a fundamental threat to liberty, self-government, and human rights.Today this demarcation has invaded the whole of our lives, and it threatens to create a horrifying caste system consisting of those who enjoy rights and privileges vs those who do not and serve (at a distance) the elites.

We need to see it clearly in order to stop it from happening. Freedom is rooted in an ethical presumption of equal rights, a cultural respect for the dignity of all human persons, a political deference to government by the people, and an economic experience of class mobility and meritocracy. Replacing those presumptions with a simplified, crude, aesthetic, and unscientific lurch into a neo-feudalism not only takes us back to pre-modern times; it overthrows basic postulates of what we call civilization itself.

(Brownstone Institute)

CHAPTER 23

How a False Hydroxychloroquine Narrative was Created, and much more.

Dr. Meryl Nass

Internal medicine physician

Meryl Nass is an internal medicine physician and was the first person in the world to prove that an epidemic (anthrax in Rhodesia) was due to biological warfare, which she did in 1992. She has given 6 Congressional testimonies regarding anthrax, biological warfare, Gulf War syndrome and vaccine safety, and has consulted for the Cuban Ministry of Health, the World Bank and the Director of National Intelligence.

Since the COVID pandemic began, she has written detailed articles regarding the suppression of hydroxychloroquine and ivermectin for treatment of Covid, the coverup of COVID's lab origin, corruption regarding the COVID vaccines and other vaccines, and how the WHO's proposed pandemic treaty and amendments will lead to more pandemics. She is an advisor to Children's Health Defense, and the founder of Door to Freedom. Her medical license was suspended in January 2022 for providing early COVID treatment and spreading alleged vaccine misinformation.

This is the most important article I have ever written, because it cracks open the plandemic nut. Perhaps more appropriate, it lances the pandemic boil so all can see and smell the putridness inside.

I began writing on this subject on my blog in May 2020 and kept adding items. It is remarkable that a large series of events taking place over the past months produced a unified message about hydroxychloroquine (HCQ), and produced similar policies about the drug in the US, Canada, Australia, NZ and western Europe. The message is that generic, inexpensive hydroxychloroquine (costing only $1.00 to produce a full course) is dangerous and should not be used to treat a potentially fatal disease, Covid-19, for which there are no (other) reliable treatments.

Hydroxychloroquine has been used safely for 65 years in many millions of patients. And so the message was crafted that the drug is safe for its other uses, but dangerous when used for Covid-19. It doesn't make sense, but it seems to have worked.

In the US, "Never Trump" morphed into "Never Hydroxychloroquine," and the result for the pandemic is "Never Over." But while anti-Trump spin is what characterized suppression strategies in the US, the frauds perpetrated about hydroxychloroquine and the pandemic include most western countries.

Why do I say "Never Over"?

I am expanding on this claim with a), b), c). Later in this essay additional evidence is provided.

a) Because if people were treated with HCQ at the onset of their illness, over 99% would quickly resolve the infection, avoiding progression to the late stage disease characterized by cytokine storm, thrombophilia and organ failure. Despite claims to the contrary, this treatment is very safe. (Yet outpatient treatment is banned in many US states.) The CDC forgot to rewrite its guidance on malaria and hydroxychloroquine during Covid. The CDC says hydroxychloroquine *"can be safely taken by pregnant women and nursing mothers..."* Only *"when it is used at higher doses for many years, a rare eye condition called retinopathy has occurred."*

b) If people were treated prophylactically with this drug (using only two tablets weekly) as is done in some areas and in some occupational groups in India, there would likely be at least 50% fewer cases after exposure. (Such treatment is currently banned in much of the US, including in my state of Maine.)

c) Protocols for in-hospital treatment (that were unknown during the initial peak of illness in the US and Europe) using HCQ and individually selected blood thinners, steroids, vitamins, zinc and other drugs such as used at NYU, have significantly reduced mortality of the very small number of people who might still progress to a serious illness. (The FDA, however, recommends against the use of HCQ outside of clinical trials, and the CDC and NIH recommend against it.)

If we had followed a), b) and c) the result would have been much briefer periods of infectiousness, lower viral loads, less severe illness and considerably less transmission. The R zero (average number of people each case infects) would drop below one and the pandemic would soon die out.

Were acts to suppress the use of HCQ carefully orchestrated? You decide.

Might these events have been planned to keep the pandemic going? To sell expensive drugs and vaccines to a captive population? Could these acts result in prolonged economic and social hardship, eventually transferring wealth from the middle class to the very rich? Are these events evidence of a conspiracy?

Here is a list of what happened, in no special order. I have penned this as if it is the **"To Do"** list of items to be accomplished by those who pull the strings. The items on the list have already been carried out. One wonders what else might be on their list, yet to be carried out, for this on-going pandemic.

1. You stop doctors from using the drug in ways it is most likely to be effective (in outpatients, at onset of illness). You prohibit use outside of situations you can control.

Situations that were controlled to show no benefit included three large, randomized, multi-center clinical trials (Recovery, Solidarity and REMAP-Covid), the kind of trials that are generally believed to yield the most reliable evidence. However, each of them used excessive hydroxychloroquine doses that were known to be toxic and may have been fatal in some cases; see my previous articles. And a 4th Chinese study that also used excessive doses (3.6 g HCQ in the first three days and 800mg/day thereafter, comparable to the above studies) also found no benefit from HCQ.

2. You prevent or limit use in outpatients by controlling the supply of the drug, using different methods in different countries and states. For

example, in New York state, by order of the governor, hydroxychloroquine could only be prescribed for hospitalized patients. In Nevada, the governor outright prohibited *both* prescribing and dispensing chloroquine drugs for a Covid-19 diagnosis. In New Jersey, the Department of Consumer Affairs required a positive test result before a chloroquine prescription could be dispensed or prescribed. Pharmacy boards coordinated to restrict its use.

France issued a series of different regulations to limit prescribers from using it. France's Health Minister also changed the drugs' status from over-the-counter (OTC) to a drug requiring a prescription.

3. You play up the danger of the drug, emphasizing side effects that are very rare when the drug is used correctly. You make sure everyone has heard about the man who died after consuming hydroxychloroquine in the form of fish tank cleaner. Yet its toxicity at approved doses is minimal. Chloroquine was *added to table salt* in some regions in the 1950s as a malaria preventive, according to Professor Nicholas White in his study for the Recovery trial.

4. You limit clinical trials to hospitalized patients, instead of testing the drug in outpatients, early in the illness, when it is predicted to be most effective.

Finally, you have Fauci's NIAID conduct a trial in outpatients, using hydroxychloroquine plus azithromycin, but you only enroll 20 patients, after planning for 2,000. You reduce the duration of followup from 24 weeks to 13 days post treatment. You cancel the study after only 5 weeks, claiming inadequate enrollments, even though you have 11 study sites to enroll patients.

5. You design a series of clinical trials to give much too high a dose, ensuring the drug will cause harm in some subjects, sufficient to mask any possible beneficial effect. You make sure that trials in 400 hospitals in 35 countries (Solidarity) plus most hospitals in the UK (Recovery) use these

dangerous doses, as well as additional sites in 13 countries (REMAP-Covid trial). There were additional Covid-19 trials that used similar excessive doses, such as PATCH, which I have not yet addressed.

6. You design clinical trials to collect almost no safety data, so any cause of death due to drug toxicity will be attributed to the disease instead of the drug.

7. You issue rules for use of the drug based on the results of the UK Recovery study, which overdosed patients. Of course the Recovery results showed more deaths in the hydroxychloroquine arm, since they gave patients 2.4 g in the first 24 hours, 800 mg/day thereafter. Furthermore, the UK has the 2nd highest death rate in the world for Covid-19 (Belgium is 1st), so simply conducting the trial in the UK may have contributed to the poor results.

8. You publish, in the world's most-read medical journal, the *Lancet*, an observational study from a massive worldwide database named *Surgisphere* (which includes 96,000 hospitalized Covid cases) that says use of chloroquine drugs caused significantly increased mortality. This was said to be the paper to end all controversy about HCQ and Covid-19. You make sure that all major media report on this result. This was to be the nail in the coffin for hydroxychloroquine. Then you quickly have three European countries announce they will not allow doctors to prescribe the drug. Soon additional countries ban its use for Covid.

9. You do your best to ride out any controversy over the veracity of this paper, never admitting culpability. Even after hundreds of people criticized this *Lancet* observational study due to easily identified fabrications--the database used in the study did not exist, and the claimed numbers of cases did not agree with known numbers of cases--the *Lancet* held firm for two weeks, which served to muddy the waters about the trial, until finally 3 of the 4 coauthors (but not the *Lancet* nor the author who purportedly owned the database) retracted the study. Neither the authors nor the

journal have admitted responsibility, let alone explained what it was that induced them to coauthor and publish such an obvious fraud.

You made sure very few media reported that the data were fabricated, the "study" was fraudulent, and the drugs were actually safe. Even though the story of the database company, Surgisphere, was full of scandalous details, most of the media ignored it. The story of the study's retraction went largely unnoticed by the public. You made sure most people remember the original (false) story: that chloroquine and hydroxychloroquine frequently kill patients.

10. You ensure federal agencies like FDA and CDC hew to your desired policies. Some examples: a) FDA advised use only in hospitalized patients (too late) and later advised use restricted to only clinical trials (which are limited, are difficult to enroll in, have been halted prematurely, or may use excessive doses).

b) you have FDA make unsubstantiated and false claims, such as: *"Hospitalized patients were likely to have greater prospect of benefit (compared to ambulatory patients with mild illness)"* and claim the chloroquine drugs have a slow onset of action. If that were really true, they would not be used for acute attacks of malaria or in critically ill patients with Covid. (Disclosure: I once dosed myself with chloroquine for an acute attack of *P. vivax* malaria, and it worked very fast.).

c) although providing treatment advice is a large part of its mission, CDC instead refers clinicians to the NIH guidelines, discussed below.

d) Despite the fact that Belgium's COVID treatment guidelines repeatedly mention that the doses of HCQ in the Recovery and Solidarity trials were four times the cumulative dose used in Belgium, you make sure the Belgian guidelines, paradoxically, only recommend use of HCQ within clinical trials.

11. You make sure to avoid funding/encouraging clinical trials that test drug combinations like hydroxychloroquine with zinc, with azithromycin, or with both, although there is ample clinical evidence that such

combinations provide a cumulative benefit to patients. For example, one study that did look at this combination had no funding.

12. You have federal and UN agencies make false, illogical claims based on models (or invention) rather than human data. For example, you have the FDA state that the dose required to treat Covid is so high it is toxic, after the Recovery and Solidarity trials have been exposed for toxic dosing. This scientific double-speak gives some legal cover to the clinical trials that overdosed their patients. According to Denise Hinton, RN, the FDA's Chief Scientist (yes, a registered nurse without scientific qualifications is the Chief Scientist at FDA), or perhaps a clumsy FDA wordsmith:

"Under the assumption that in vivo cellular accumulation is similar to that from the in vitro cell-based assays, the calculated free lung concentrations that would result from the EUA suggested dosing regimens are well below the in vitro EC50/EC90 values, making the antiviral effect against SARS-CoV-2 not likely achievable with the dosing regimens recommended in the EUA. The substantial increase in dosing that would be needed to increase the likelihood of an antiviral effect would not be acceptable due to toxicity concerns."

You have a WHO report claim toxic doses are needed. This is nonsense since:

- In 2005, CDC researchers showed strong effects against SARS-1 at safely achievable concentrations. Here is the relevant quote, *"The infectivity of coronaviruses other than SARS-CoV are also affected by chloroquine, as exemplified by the human CoV-229E [15]. The inhibitory effects observed on SARS-CoV infectivity and cell spread occurred in the presence of 1–10 μM chloroquine, which are **plasma concentrations achievable during the prophylaxis and treatment of malaria (varying from 1.6–12.5 μM) [26] and hence are well tolerated by patients**."* A reader asked me to note that this study was done in tissue culture.

- the drug at normal doses is being tested in over 30 different medical conditions (see clinicaltrials.gov), and
- reports from many different countries say that the drug is effective for Covid-19 at normal doses, while a high dose **chloroquine** treatment trial was halted in Brazil and a preprint of the study was posted, after finding that drug effects were causing ventricular arrhythmias and deaths. JAMA published the results in their April 24, 2020 edition.
- Toxicity in the Brazilian study was seen after only 3 days of treatment, during which 3.6 grams of chloroquine were administered. But the Solidarity (3.2 grams of hydroxychloroquine in 3 days), Recovery (3.6 grams of hydroxychloroquine in 3 days) and REMAP-Covid trials (3.6 grams of hydroxychloroquine in 3 days) **continued overdosing patients until June**, or probably longer in the case of REMAP-Covid, despite Brazil's evidence of deaths by overdose.

Tellingly, JAMA editor Gordon Rubenfeld wrote **in April**, after the Brazilian study came out in JAMA, *"if you are prescribing HCQ after these JAMA results, do yourself and your defense lawyer a favor. Document in your medical record that you informed the patient of the potential risks of HCQ including sudden death and its benefits (???)."*

13. You create an NIH Guidelines committee for Covid treatment recommendations, in which 16 members have or had financial entanglements with Gilead, maker of Remdesivir. The members were appointed by the Co-Chairs. Two of the three Co-Chairs are themselves financially entangled with Gilead. Are you surprised that their guidelines recommend specifically against the use of hydroxychloroquine and in favor of Remdesivir, despite a Chinese Phase III study showing no benefit, which was mistakenly posted on the WHO website, then taken down. The guidelines authors deem their

recommendations the new "standard of care." Additional Remdesivir studies have shown no clear mortality benefit.

You create an NIH treatment guidelines summary that cherry picks the literature to claim HCQ provides no benefit.

14. You frighten doctors so they don't prescribe hydroxychloroquine, if prescribing it is even allowed in their jurisdiction, because prescribing outside the new NIH "standard of care" leaves them open to both malpractice lawsuits and potential loss of license. For example, Michigan's Medical Licensing Board issued the following:

*"Prescribing hydroxychloroquine or chloroquine without further proof of efficacy for treating COVID-19 or with the intent to stockpile the drug may create a shortage for patients with lupus, rheumatoid arthritis, or other ailments for which chloroquine and hydroxychloroquine are proven treatments. Reports of this conduct will be evaluated and may be further investigated for administrative action... It is also important to be mindful that licensed health professionals are **required to report** inappropriate prescribing practices."*

In other words, Michigan pharmacists are **required** to snitch on doctors prescribing the drugs for Covid.

You further tell doctors (through the FDA) they need to monitor a variety of lab parameters and EKGs when using the drug, although this was never advised before, which makes it very difficult to use the drug in outpatients. You have the European Medicines Agency issue similar warnings. In Australia only physicians in certain specialties are allowed to prescribe the drug for Covid. And in Queensland, physicians or pharmacists who do not comply (for example, by prescribing the drug for prevention of Covid) face up to 6 months' imprisonment and a fine up to $13,000 Australian dollars.

15. You manage to control the conduct of most trials around the world by specially designing the WHO-managed Solidarity trials, currently conducted in 35 countries. WHO halted hydroxychloroquine clinical

trials around the world, twice. The first time, WHO claimed it was in response to the (fraudulent) *Lancet* study. The second time, WHO claimed the stop was in response to the Recovery trial results. Recovery used highly toxic doses of hydroxychloroquine in over 1500 patients, of whom 396 died. You stop the trial before the data safety monitoring board has looked at your data, a move that is unlikely to be consistent with trial protocol. WHO's trial in over 400 hospitals overdosed patients with 2.0 g hydroxychloroquine in the first 24 hours. The trial was halted three days after the toxic doses were exposed (by me). The trial involved doctors around the world typing minimal patient information into an online WHO platform, which assigned the patient a treatment.

The only "safety" information collected during the trial was whether patients required oxygen, required a ventilator, or died. This effectively masked the adverse effects of the drugs tested.

I should mention that WHO's initial plan for its Solidarity trial entirely omitted the chloroquine drugs, but they were added at the urging of participating nations. WHO's fallback position appears to have been to use toxic doses.

16. You have the WHO pressure governments to stop doctors prescribing hydroxychloroquine.

17. You have the WHO pressure professional societies to stop doctors prescribing hydroxychloroquine.

18. You make sure that the most-consulted US medical encyclopedia, UptoDate, advises physicians to restrict hydroxychloroquine to only clinical trials, citing the FDA.

19. You have the head of the Coronavirus Task Force, Dr. Tony Fauci, insist the drug cannot be used in the absence of strong evidence...while he insisted exactly the opposite in the case of the MERS coronavirus outbreak several years ago, when he recommended an untested drug combination for use...which had been developed for that purpose by his agency. And while

he was bemoaning the lack of evidence, he was refusing to pay for trials to study hydroxychloroquine, and cancelled two NIAID-sponsored trials of outpatient HCQ before completion. And he changed the goalposts on the Remdesivir trial, not once but twice, to make Remdesivir show a tiny bit of benefit, but no mortality benefit. Yet don't forget, Fauci was thrilled to sponsor a trial of a Covid vaccine (partly owned by his agency) in humans, before there were any data from animal studies. So much for Fauci›s requirement for high quality evidence, before risking use of drugs and vaccines in humans.

20. You convince the population that the crisis will be long-lasting. You have the second richest man in the world, and biggest funder of the WHO, Bill Gates, keep repeating to the media megaphone that we cannot go back to normal until everyone has been vaccinated or there is a perfect drug. (The Gates Foundation helped design the WHO Solidarity trial, which says only that it has multiple funders, helped fund the Recovery trial, and Gates is heavily invested in Covid pharmaceuticals and vaccines.)

21. You have CDC (with help from FDA) prevent the purchase of coronavirus test kits from Germany, China, WHO, etc, and fail to produce a valid test kit themselves. The result was that during January and February, US cases could not be tested, and for months thereafter insufficient and unreliable test kits made it impossible to track the epidemic and stop the spread.

22. You have trusted medical spokesmen lie to the public about the pandemic's severity, so precautions weren't taken when they might have been more effective and less long-lasting. Congress was repeatedly briefed about the pandemic in January and February, which scared several Congress members enough that they sold off large amounts of stock, risking insider trading charges. Senator Burr is one of them, currently under investigation for major stock sales.

Yet Dr. Fauci told USA Today that Americans should worry more about the flu than about coronavirus, the danger of which was "just miniscule." Then later, Drs. Fauci and Robert Redfield (CDC Director) wrote in the *New England Journal*:

"...the overall clinical consequences of Covid-19 may ultimately be more akin to those of a severe seasonal influenza (which has a case fatality rate of approximately 0.1%) or a pandemic influenza (similar to those in 1957 and 1968) rather than a disease similar to SARS or MERS, which have had case fatality rates of 9 to 10% and 36%, respectively."

23. You destroy the reputation of respected physicians who stand in your way. Professor Didier Raoult and his team in Marseille have used hydroxychloroquine on over 4,000 patients, reporting a mortality rate of about 0.8%. (The mortality rate of patients given hydroxychloroquine in the Recovery trial was 25.7%.) Raoult is very famous for discovering over 100 different microorganisms, and finding the long-sought cause of Whipple's Disease. With this reputation, Raoult apparently thought he could treat patients as he saw fit, which he has done, under great duress. Raoult was featured in a New York Times Magazine article, with his face on the magazine cover, on May 12, 2020. After describing his considerable accomplishments, the Times very unfavorably discussed his personality, implied he conducted unethical trials without approval, and using anonymous sourcing produced a detailed hit piece. Raoult is now considered an unreliable crank in the US. Raoult has now been legally charged with ethics violations in France for propounding and using HCQ in Covid patients.

You gather a group of Yale professors to dispute their Yale professor colleague Harvey Risch, an MD, PhD epidemiologist, on his publications and vocal support of the benefits of HCQ for Covid. Their first argument is that he is not an infectious disease doctor. Notably, the first signer of the statement opposing Dr. Risch is an economist.

Physician and state senator Scott Jensen of Minnesota was investigated by his state medical board due to anonymous complaints about 'spreading misinformation' and giving 'reckless advice' about COVID in interviews. Jensen was previously selected as "Family Physician of the Year" in his state. He was ultimately exonerated.

24. You have social media platforms ban content that does not agree with the desired narrative. As YouTube CEO and ex-wife of Google founder Sergey Brin, Susan Wojcicki (now deceased) said,

"YouTube will ban any content containing medical advice that contradicts World Health Organisation (WHO) coronavirus recommendations. Anything that would go against World Health Organisation recommendations would be a violation of our policy."

25. When your clinical trials are criticized for overdosing patients, you quickly have Oxford-affiliated, Wellcome Trust-supported scientists at Mahidol University publish papers (a literature review with modeling and a modeling study) purporting to show that the doses used were not toxic. You develop a new method to measure hydroxychloroquine in a handful of Recovery patients who were not poisoned. However, there are 2 problems you forgot with this approach:

- The Brazilian data, including 16 deaths, extensive clinical information and documented ventricular arrhythmias, are much more persuasive than a theoretical model of hydroxychloroquine pharmacokinetics.
- **Either** the drug is too toxic to use, even at normal doses, for a life-threatening disease, **or** even extremely high doses are safe. **You can't have it both ways.**

Oxford was the institution running the Recovery trial, and invented a Covid vaccine with AstraZeneca. The Wellcome Trust funded the Recovery trial.

26. You change your trial's primary outcome measures after the trials have started, in order to prevent detection of drug-induced deaths

(Recovery) or to make your drug appear to have efficacy (NIAID Remdesivir trial).

27. You stop manufacturers from supplying the drug. Shortly after the fraudulent *Lancet* paper came out, Sanofi announced it would no longer supply the drug for use with Covid, and would halt its two hydroxychloroquine clinical trials. One of the cancelled Sanofi trials was expected to test 210 outpatients early in the course of disease. You surely don't want a trial of hydroxychloroquine treatment early in the disease, since it might show an excellent effect.

Sanofi (a pharma company) began acting like a regulator. From the Australian DOH's Therapeutic Goods Administration website:

Sanofi, the supplier of one of the hydroxychloroquine products marketed in Australia (Plaquenil), has also written to health professionals reinforcing that hydroxychloroquine is not approved for use in Australia for treatment of COVID-19 outside the confines of a clinical trial. Sanofi also reinforced some of the known risks of prescribing hydroxychloroquine, in particular potentially serious cardiac issues. Globally, Sanofi has received an increased number of reports of serious cardiac issues, including deaths, in patients treated with hydroxychloroquine, This appears to be more common in patients also treated with other medicines that can affect the heart.

Then Sanofi started collecting information on all off-label use of hydroxychloroquine in New Zealand and Australia. Why is Sanofi, a drug manufacturing company, becoming a surveillance/enforcement mechanism intended to frighten medical providers from using the drug for Covid, which use is by definition «off label.» Sanofi alternatively suggests one may report (anonymously or not) others' off-label use to New Zealand's Pharmacovigilance Center or the Australian equivalent.

And see this: Novartis will supply HCQ only under certain conditions, and halted its HCQ trial due to lack of enrollments, although enrollment was not an issue for its other COVID trials.

28. You attempt to retract published papers that provide evidence to support use of hydroxychloroquine for COVID.

29. You have your 'bought' scientists conceal their financial conflicts of interest in their HCQ clinical trials and publications as well as in the guidelines they produce.

30. You can get your experimental, unlicensed drugs tested, much more expeditiously and cheaply than under ordinary circumstances, on Covid patients in large clinical trials, but only as long as no drug is designated effective for the condition. This opportunity only lasts while the "standard of care" for early Covid disease is nothing more than supportive measures, since no drug is deemed effective.

31. You have a research organization with big Pharma members (A.O.K.I.) pressure the Russian Ministry of Health to remove hydroxychloroquine from its treatment guidelines.

32. You stop use of hydroxychloroquine, allegedly in response to the fabricated Lancet study, in France, Italy and Belgium (countries with very high Covid mortality rates) then Portugal then Switzerland. But Switzerland restarted using HCQ 15 days later. This created a natural experiment in Switzerland. About 2 weeks after hydroxychloroquine use was halted, death rates approximately tripled, for about 15 days. Then, after its use was allowed again, two weeks later death rates from Covid fell back to their baseline.

33. You reverse an old trick of clinical trials, to mask the benefit of hydroxychloroquine. The trick was to replace the saline placebo with a substance that is being used by many clinicians and in many trials against Covid, thus by comparison likely to reduce the positive effect of your tested medication. This was done in trials both at NYU and at University of Washington, using vitamin C or vitamin C plus folate respectively as placebos.

34. You have the chief medical officers of Wales, England, Scotland and Northern Ireland, and the director of the UK's National Health Service,

write to UK doctors, a) urging them to enroll their Covid patients in one of 3 national clinical trials, two of which greatly overdosed patients with hydroxychloroquine, and b) stopping their use of "off license treatments" outside of a trial. Yet again, we encounter a veiled threat against clinicians actually attempting to treat the primary SARS-Cov-2 infection. The chief doctors wrote:

"While it is for every individual clinician to make prescribing decisions, we strongly discourage the use of off-licence treatments outside of a trial, where participation in a trial is possible... Any treatment given for coronavirus other than general supportive care, treatment for underlying conditions, and antibiotics for secondary bacterial complications, should currently be as part of a trial, where that is possible."

35. You have a state Pharmacy Board refuse to dispense hydroxychloroquine outside of clinical trials, citing the FDA recommendation for use only in trials. You issue this new regulation on the same day that FDA publishes its recommendation, indicating prior coordination. But when your regulation is exposed, you immediately rescind it.

36. You have the IMF offer rapid financing to Belarus, but only if it follows the recommended model of Covid response and imposes quarantines, isolation and curfews.

37. A group of doctors went to Washington. They called themselves "America's Frontline Doctors" and gave a press conference and livestream talks about the Covid-19 pandemic as well as about the need for physicians to be able to prescribe HCQ freely. While the media sparsely attended the press conference, the livestream got millions of views. And within hours, their livestream was banned by Google, YouTube, Facebook and Twitter. Twitter was said to additionally ban comments about its ban. Then Squarespace took down the Frontline Doctors' website.

Today, Bitchute is hosting their press conference. So is Brighteon. In those media that do discuss the event, the group is tarred for providing misinformation.

38. After the HCQ issue got so much attention on social media, you impose another ban on the prescribing of HCQ for Covid in Ohio, using its Pharmacy Board to dictate to physicians what they may not prescribe. (A repeat of #35 in a different state.) Ohio, with the governor's approval, had first limited hydroxychloroquine dispensing in March 2020. At least 3 other states limited its dispensing at the same time.

This ban got so much attention that Republican Governor Mike DeWine rescinded it the next morning. DeWine claimed to agree with FDA Commissioner Stephen Hahn, who said in a TV interview that the prescribing of HCQ is between a doctor and patient. This is in accord with FDA law; but then, why was FDA silent when pharmacy boards, governors and other state entities prevented the prescribing of this FDA-approved drug in their jurisdictions?

39. After having Google take down physician James Todaro's article on hydroxychloroquine for 4 months, you allow it to resurface right before Google's (and Facebook's and Amazon's and Apple's) CEOs testify before Congress on censorship and abuse of power. You have Twitter warn that Todaro's article is at an unsafe link.

40. After massive attention to the banning of the videos posted by the physician group 'America's Frontline Doctors' and its website, you make intense efforts to discredit the physicians involved.

MedPageToday claimed it *"could find no evidence that any of the speakers worked in hospitals with significant numbers of COVID-19 patients."* But the doctors claimed they used the drug early and prevented hospitalizations and deaths. With over 4.4 million Americans diagnosed with Covid, what doctor *hasn't* seen a Covid patient?

USAToday blared the headline: 'America's Frontline Doctors' may be real doctors, but experts say they don't know what they're talking about.'

You have USA Today review and publish detailed information on the licenses, practice locations and malpractice histories of the doctors who spoke out. USAT reporters claim these doctors are not experts and lack knowledge about the use of HCQ in Covid-19, despite the fact that most work in primary care, urgent care or emergency medicine and report using the drug for Covid. Yet no one asks how many years ago 'expert' Tony Fauci last treated a patient? 'Expert' Deborah Birx' medical license expired in 2014, so she hasn't treated a Covid patient either. BTW, she worked in Fauci's lab between 1983 and 1986.

41. Hydroxychloroquine use is truly the wedge issue for understanding and turning around the pandemic. If hydroxychloroquine works reasonably well as a prophylactic and treatment for Covid-19, it could potentially end the severity of the pandemic, greatly reduce transmission, and return us to life as we knew it. You must make use of the levers of government, plus mainstream media and social media, to stop that from happening.

So, just in case doctors thought the Frontline Doctors' video, or a new study from Spain showing the drug's usefulness meant they should use hydroxychloroquine to treat Covid, you must act fast. You use Representatives at a Congressional health subcommittee hearing to threaten doctors about one use of the drug, in veterans who were nursing home patients. Per the Washington Post:

"doctors at the 238-bed nursing home dosed [30] patients with what came to be called a "covid cocktail" for more than two weeks in April, often over the objections of nurses and without the full knowledge of residents' families. At least 11 residents received the drug even though they had not been tested for covid-19, The Post found."

I have treated patients in nursing homes, and one rarely discusses medication changes with family, unless the patient is seriously ill. When nursing home residents were dying like flies last April, when tests were hard to come by, and confirmed diagnoses few and far between, doctors used this medicine to try to prevent nursing home deaths during a pandemic. And now they are being scapegoated for doing so.

The WaPo article does not even tell us whether the patients survived, thrived or were harmed. The article hardly makes sense. Its only purpose is to blacken the drug and the physicians who use it.

Yet with respect to HCQ's use in nursing homes, Senators Warren, Wyden and Casey demanded that FDA and Medicare/Medicaid explain how they are tracking it, and also demanded an Inspector General investigation into its recent use in nursing homes. *"The Trump Administration owes us answers on the use of an ineffective drug like hydroxychloroquine in nursing homes — the epicenter of the pandemic,"* Elizabeth Warren said in a statement.

42. You use state Medical Licensing Boards to threaten doctors who claim there is a cure for Covid-19.

43. You have Dr. Fauci discredit published observational studies that show benefit during a Congressional hearing, demanding randomized controlled trials. Fauci never tells the Committee he has cancelled the one randomized controlled trial of HCQ that his agency, NIAID, had promised to conduct on HCQ. NIAID claimed that it could not enroll enough subjects, and the study was cancelled after only 20 were enrolled. However, Fauci told the Committee that 250,000 Americans have shown interest in participating in trials of a Covid vaccine. It is difficult to reconcile such extreme lack of interest in a treatment trial, and such massive interest in a vaccine trial.

Doctors who wrote studies showing HCQ benefit, even when used late (50% mortality reduction) have defended their work from Fauci's criticism of it to Congress.

44. You erode the doctor's primary responsibility to the patient, replacing it with the need to perform clinical research. This is the first time I have ever heard such a thing in the US: research physicians are pressuring frontline doctors not to veer from protocol-determined treatment, even when patients enrolled in treatment trials are at risk of death. 'Helping future patients' is the rationale provided.

Need I say this was the justification for the Nazi doctors' experiments? It was not accepted at Nuremberg and it shouldn't be accepted now. Medical ethics are no mystery. As published in the JAMA, and accepted worldwide, the World Medical Association's Declaration of Helsinki, a.k.a. "Ethical Principles for Medical Research Involving Human Subjects" states,

"While the primary purpose of medical research is to generate new knowledge, this goal can never take precedence over the rights and interests of individual research subjects."

One of the Nuremberg Principles says essentially the same thing.

45. You use the term "stellar" to describe the Recovery trial in the August 5, 2020 NY Times, but avoid any hint that the Recovery trial's hydroxychloroquine arm gave 1500 patients a toxic, potentially lethal dose, of whom over 25% died.

46. You censure and oust from the Detroit Democrats a state legislator because she credited HCQ for saving her life when she had Covid-19, and she publicly thanked President Trump for bringing the drug to her attention. It had been extremely difficult for her to obtain the drug, because her governor, Gretchen Whitmer, had banned use of the drug for Covid.

47. Despite assuring you control the outcome of the vast majority of randomized clinical trials of the chloroquine drugs, you have been thwarted by physician researchers in Detroit, Spain, Italy, France, Saudi Arabia who publish their observational results with hydroxychloroquine, showing the drug dramatically reduces mortality from Covid.

Doctors in Turkey, the US and Canada, show that HCQ's cardiac toxicity is negligible. So you have frontman Tony Fauci repeatedly dismiss this evidence from thousands of patients, since it did not come from randomized controlled trials. See c19study.com for a compilation of 99 (58 peer reviewed) studies of the chloroquine drugs in Covid-19, and convince yourself what the overall data truly show.

48. You have Wikipedia write the following about Covid and HCQ: *"all clinical trials conducted during 2020 found it is ineffective and may cause dangerous side effects."* The footnotes refer to only a handful of trials, while a compilation of all 99 studies (of different types, including meta-analyses and observational studies) on the drug in Covid-19 tells a completely different story.

49. You electronically disappear articles favorable to HCQ. A meta-analysis preprint of 41 studies of EARLY HCQ use, written by US physicians, is posted on the ResearchGate site, which hosts a collection of academic papers. **The article rapidly disappeared from the link.** Here is a brief description of the article:

Prodromos et al., Preprint, doi:10.13140/RG.2.2.29781.65765 (meta analysis)

Hydroxychloroquine is Effective and Safe for the Treatment of COVID-19, and May be Universally Effective When Used Early Before Hospitalization: A Systematic Review.

Meta analysis of 41 studies concluding: "HCQ has been shown to have consistent clinical efficacy for COVID-19 when it is used early in the outpatient setting, and in general would appear to work better the earlier it is used. Overall HCQ is effective against COVID-19. There is no credible evidence that HCQ results in worsening of COVID-19. HCQ has been shown to be safe for the treatment of COVID-19 when responsibly used."

50. Can we begin to connect the dots between those who fraudulently suppressed effective treatments for Covid-19, and those who wish to maintain the pandemic crisis to remake the world? Today, on 9/11, Oxford epidemiologist Dr. Peter Horby, a principal investigator for the Recovery trial in which 396 people who were overdosed with hydroxychloroquine died, retweeted a tweet from the World Economic Forum about the environmental benefits of using bicycles. Horby added, "This is where we need to be headed."

51. From Anthony Fauci, who has perhaps done more than any other person to besmirch the value of HCQ and prevent Covid patients being treated effectively, comes a statement that seems to hearken to the World Economic Forum sentiment in #50 above. Fauci blames the pandemic (which his actions prolong) on humans damaging nature. And he suggests we must learn to live differently, in harmony with nature.

And now, suddenly, I understand why it is so important to claim the pandemic came from human encroachment on bat territory, and not from a lab accident. Because human encroachment is being positioned to take the blame for Covid-19. (SARS-1, Ebola and SARS-2 are claimed to have arisen from humans living too close to bats, eating them and getting infected, starting epidemics--but this has not been proven for either SARS epidemic, nor proven for the Ebola epidemics.). This is not Fauci waxing eloquent about nature. This is Fauci, America's Doctor, starting the conversation about how the human population, not the bat virus, is the real underlying problem.

The quote below was published in the journal Cell, by Fauci and Morens:

"The COVID-19 pandemic is yet another reminder, added to the rapidly growing archive of historical reminders, that in a human-dominated world, in which our human activities represent aggressive, damaging, and unbalanced interactions with nature, we will increasingly provoke new disease emergences. We remain at risk for the foreseeable future. COVID-19 is among the most vivid wake-up calls in over a century. It should force us to begin to think in earnest and collectively about living in more thoughtful and creative harmony with nature, even as we plan for nature's inevitable, and always unexpected, surprises."

Are they hinting that a reduced human population will be less susceptible to pandemics? Or that rural populations need to move?

52. Even though the famous Mehra/Desai Lancet paper claiming HCQ and CQ caused hugely increased deaths was exposed as a total

fabrication by the Lancet editor and retracted, the Washington Post links to its favorable May story about the Mehra/Desai paper--using it as the sole evidence for yet another false claim of the danger of hydroxychloroquine.

This despite the fact that the WaPo reported about concerns regarding the paper's authenticity. The New York Times ran at least three articles about the fabricated Mehra/Desai paper and the WaPo reads what the NYT reports.

You neuter criticism electronically by making it hard to read. I commented on the 9/11 article in the WaPo, and its gratuitous slur against HCQ, in which WaPo cited as authority a fabricated paper. I used the online comment form. I am a subscriber. The WaPo printed my comment, but my comment seems to be the only one whose words extend beyond the right margin, and are chopped off. How odd.

53. When all else fails, would you really try to blow up much of the world supply of hydroxychloroquine?

According to the Taiwan English News:

An explosion at a pharmaceutical factory in Taoyuan City left two injured and caused a fire early this afternoon, December 20...

Liberty Times reported that the factory produces hydroxychloroquine APIs, and is the world's second largest HCQ raw material supplier.

Another source tells the same tale. The Pharmaceutical company is named Sci Pharmtech Inc. The explosion was huge and spread to five other companies.

54. Big mistake. You meant to expunge all official information about the safety of hydroxychloroquine. But you forgot to remove CDC's malaria treatment guidance, which still tells the truth about the drug. A two-page information sheet was available online on the CDC website. CDC's guidance states,

*"**Who can take hydroxychloroquine?** Hydroxychloroquine can be prescribed to adults and children of all ages. It can also be safely taken by pregnant women and nursing mothers.*

346 | Canary In a (Post) Covid World

What are the potential side effects of hydroxychloroquine? *Hydroxychloroquine is a relatively well tolerated medicine. The most common adverse reactions reported are stomach pain, nausea, vomiting, and headache. These side effects can often be lessened by taking hydroxychloroquine with food. Hydroxychloroquine may also cause itching in some people. All medicines may have some side effects. Minor side effects such as nausea, occasional vomiting, or diarrhea usually do not require stopping the antimalarial drug. If you cannot tolerate your antimalarial drug, see your health care provider; other antimalarial drugs are available.*

How long is it safe to use hydroxychloroquine? CDC has no limits on the use of hydroxychloroquine for the prevention of malaria. When hydroxychloroquine is used at higher doses for many years, a rare eye condition called retinopathy has occurred. People who take hydroxychloroquine for more than five years should get regular eye exams.

- *Overdose of antimalarial drugs, particularly hydroxychloroquine, can be fatal.*

55. Twitter censored the Brazilian Ministry of Health for tweeting to citizens that they should seek early treatment for Covid, as the sooner they get treated, the better the result. (The harmful US recommendation is to stay home and do nothing until you require hospitalization.)

This Tweet violated the Twitter Rules about spreading misleading and potentially harmful information related to COVID-19. However, Twitter has determined that it may be in the public's interest for the Tweet to remain accessible. Later it was completely removed. It used to be an illustration for this essay, but it's gone now.

56. You have the WHO issue guidance that HCQ should not be used for Covid, based on 6 multicenter trials that included over 6,000 patients. Six! Scores of trials using much larger numbers of patients demonstrated benefit, but these were omitted from the WHO review.

Of course, included in these six trials (and accounting for about half the patients in WHO's review) are the Recovery and Solidarity trials that overdosed subjects on hydroxychloroquine and caused 10-20% higher mortality than in the placebo subjects who received no treatment!

In effect, WHO is confirming that when you poison patients with excessive doses they do not do well. I concur that poisonous doses of HCQ or anything else should never be used in patients.

Will WHO comment on the only real question, which is the value of using therapeutic doses early in the course of illness? The results of over 200 studies speak for themselves.

Why aren't the families of subjects who died in these trials bringing charges? Was information on which drugs their family members received withheld from them to prevent that from happening?

57. The Bill and Melinda Gates Foundation is still up to their dirty tricks smearing hydroxychloroquine. Yet another paper has come out of U. Washington, paid for by BMGF, that claims HCQ isn>t helpful for early treatment. If you read the new paper carefully, you learn that HCQ actually did help, but the authors massaged the data to remove statistical significance... and shut the trial down prematurely.

58. It is important to keep banging the drum that says, not only the drugs don't work, but they are dangerous, to boot. And so we have a new meta-analysis designed to do just that.

After providing 58 anomalous incidents regarding squashing the use of HCQ, was this deliberate or accidental? You decide.

CHAPTER 24

A Retrospective
in Whys

by Margaret Anna Alice

Writer and blogger

Margaret Anna Alice writes about propaganda, mass control, psychology, politics, and health with a focus on COVID at her Substack, Margaret Anna Alice Through the Looking Glass. She is the author of the fairy tale The Vapor, the Hot Hat, & the Witches' Potion and has presented her research to the Corona Investigative Committee. Described as "COVID's Best Chronicler" by Dr. Meryl Nass and "my favourite writer anywhere" by Dr. Mike Yeadon, Margaret Anna aims to unmask totalitarianism and awaken the sleeping before tyranny triumphs.

The following chapter has been extracted from my notes for the Corona Investigative Committee presentation I gave on July 1, 2022. You can find the complete, hyperlinked notes as well as a video and transcript of my presentation at my Substack, Margaret Anna Alice Through the Looking Glass.

Since the beginning of this manufactured crisis, the Berlin Corona Investigative Committee has been conducting the exploratory work I would have expected every government and so-called public health organization to have undertaken from the outset.

The fact that this did not occur was one of the first signs that COVID represented a departure from all prior pandemic protocols, but the question I kept asking myself is, *Why?*

Here are some of the permutations of that question I started asking beginning in early 2020 and continuing through the present-day:

TOTALITARIANISM

- Why are governments, public health agencies, the media, Big Tech, and "experts" stoking fear instead of calmly assessing the data and attempting to dispel panic—like every responsible authority has done for genuine crises in the past?

- Why are all of these entities <u>speaking in unison</u> with a single voice as if everyone has been handed the same script?
- Why are they covering COVID <u>24/7 on every available outlet</u>, drumming up the death tallies and case counts and behaving as if it were the only newsworthy story on the planet?
- Why are people all suddenly parroting the same phrases like "social distancing," "<u>New Normal</u>," "Build Back Better," and the Orwellian double-think gem "together apart"?
- Why does it seem like everyone has <u>suddenly lost their capacities</u> for critical thinking, reasoning, logic, and scientific analysis?
- Why are they <u>encouraging discrimination</u> against those who refuse to comply with unscientific and nonsensical guidelines?
- Why did they turn the world into an <u>open-air prison</u>?
- Why are governments patterning their policies after <u>Biderman's Chart of Coercion</u>?
- Why does it feel like we're being subjected to a permanent <u>Milgram Obedience–Stanford Prison–Asch Conformity experiment</u>?
- Why are Big Tech and Big Media silencing people—especially <u>scientists</u>, <u>physicians</u>, and other knowledgeable individuals who are most qualified to speak about these matters?
- Why are <u>California</u> and the <u>federal government</u> threatening physicians with loss of their licences for spreading "<u>misinformation</u>," which happens to be based on scientifically demonstrable evidence and clinical experience?
- Why are such extreme measures being taken for a disease with an <u>infinitesimal fatality rate</u> that primarily only affects those who are already likely to die—namely the elderly and those with serious comorbidities?
- Why are governments <u>rewriting human rights policies</u> and <u>revising statutes</u> to allow the forced quarantining of healthy individuals?

- Why are <u>ordinary, working-class Canadians</u> who are bravely protesting authoritarian policies being vilified by the media and <u>their leaders</u>?
- Why are they pushing for <u>International Health Regulations (IHR) amendments</u> that would grant an unelected bureaucrat and accused genocidal war criminal control over the entire world's public health policy?
- Why is the <u>WHO drafting a pandemic accord</u> that would give it the ability to set a "OneHealth" policy for all member states and seize supranational powers in times of declared public health "emergencies"?
- Why are <u>Australians and New Zealanders</u> being bullied, abused, arrested, and quarantined like they're living in a police state?
- Why are so many <u>colluders</u> willingly serving as implements of tyranny?
- <u>Why aren't people worried</u> that the <u>ten stages of genocide</u> are <u>unfolding before our eyes</u>?
- Why do people think relinquishing their liberties in exchange for "safety" is temporary when it has never been so <u>in the past</u>?
- Why are so many people <u>belligerently bamboozled</u>?
- Why are values such as independent thought, integrity, ethics, freedom, transparency, and individuality being denigrated while groupthink, obedience, complicity, prejudice, collectivism, fear, rage, and hatred are being promoted?
- Why are governments and employers mandating vaccines and pushing for vaxxports when they have been proven both <u>unsafe</u> *and* <u>ineffective?</u>
- Why does it feel like we're living in a <u>dystopian fairy tale</u>?

HARMFUL & ILLOGICAL HEALTH POLICIES

- Why aren't health authorities making <u>dietary, lifestyle, and supplement recommendations</u> that would bolster people's immunity—like encouraging them to eat healthily; reduce their stress levels; get proper sleep; exercise; enjoy sunshine and fresh air; and practice other habits that help prevent illness?

- Why aren't they focusing on the conventional practices for preventing respiratory illnesses such as washing your hands and staying home when you have symptoms?

- Why are we being commanded to "Trust the Science" when scientific inquiry is a continually evolving process and requires transparency and diverse viewpoints to progress?

- Why are they <u>suddenly telling us asymptomatic spread exists</u> when there was <u>no evidence for such transmission</u> and no studies demonstrating this has occurred with past coronaviruses?

- Why are they pretending that there's no such thing as <u>natural immunity</u>?

- Why did they previously <u>redefine "pandemic"</u> to <u>exclude</u> "simultaneous epidemics worldwide with enormous numbers of deaths and illness"?

- Why did they <u>change the definition of "herd immunity"</u> to inject the idea that it is acquired through vaccination when it was previously understood by immunologists and virologists to be achieved naturally when a virus spreads throughout a community?

- Why did they change the definitions of "<u>vaccine</u>," "<u>fully vaccinated</u>," "<u>cause of death</u>," and "<u>case</u>," for that matter?

- Why did they <u>censor</u> Bakersfield doctors <u>Dan Erickson and Artin Massihi</u> when they provided sensible, experience-based, and reassuring textbook information about COVID transmission, treatment, and herd immunity at their <u>April 22, 2020, press conference</u>?

- Why are they using <u>PCR tests</u> to calculate case counts when their <u>Nobel-Prize–winning creator</u> said it <u>"allows you to take a very minuscule amount of anything and make it measurable and then talk about it in meetings and stuff like it is important"</u>?

- Why did Fauci—or as I like to call him, <u>Dr. Mengelfauci</u>—first tell the truth about masks not working, then lie about them working, and then say he lied when he'd originally told the long-established truth that masks are ineffective for respiratory viruses? And why did he <u>lie about so many other things</u>?

- Why are they telling us staying six feet apart will magically protect us?

- Why are they <u>counting deaths *with*</u> and not just *from* COVID?

- Why are they <u>putting infected patients in nursing homes</u>, where the population is the most vulnerable?

- Why are nursing home residents being isolated, tortured, neglected, eldercided with <u>midazolam</u>, and deprived of the <u>visiting rights</u> even prisoners enjoy?

- Why are they instituting policies the <u>WHO previously warned against</u>—from lockdowns to masking to disinfection to border closures—because they are known to cause mass-scale harm, poverty, and even death?

- Why are they closing schools (and later, <u>pushing injections on kids</u>) when children are at the least risk of contracting and spreading COVID?

- Why are they requiring children to mask, social-distance, and follow other ineffective rules that <u>impair their development; inflict psychological and emotional damage; and even cause physical harm</u>?

- Why are they continuing to use ventilation for COVID patients when it was <u>found early on to be causing deaths</u>?

- Why is so much <u>data not shared</u> or <u>being hidden</u> from the public?
- Why are they <u>financially incentivizing the administration of a drug</u> found to cause multiple-organ failure and with no clinical efficacy for COVID?
- Why are hospital staff getting away with <u>"bagging" COVID patients</u> with plastic equipment covers to "protect" the workers?

THWARTING OF EARLY TREATMENT PROTOCOLS

- Why didn't they immediately start searching for treatments and researching the effectiveness of repurposed drugs per standard operating procedure?
- Why aren't they providing recommendations for at-home care and instead telling people to wait until their lips turn blue and then go to the hospital?
- Why are <u>disinformation campaigns</u> being launched against <u>early-treatment protocols</u>?
- Why are the <u>doctors</u> who prescribe these life-saving treatments being smeared and <u>stripped of their licences</u>?
- Why is <u>scientific fraud</u> being committed to discredit a <u>Nobel-Prize–winning medications</u>?

GLOBAL MASS INJECTION EXPERIMENT

- Why are people okay with skipping long-term clinical trials for a novel gene therapy that has never been deployed on humans?
- Why are they embarking on a coercive global mass injection campaign when such a feat has also never been attempted—let alone with a genetic inoculation lacking long-term clinical safety data?
- Why aren't people bothered that pharmaceutical companies have zero liability for these products thanks to emergency use authorizations?

- Why aren't people being told they are experimental subjects and that the Pfizer clinical trials won't be completed until <u>March 31, 2023</u>?

- Why are they advising pregnant women to get injected with an experimental product when they <u>excluded pregnant and breastfeeding women from clinical trials</u>?

- Why did Pfizer and the FDA ignore the devastating injuries suffered by <u>twelve-year-old Maddie De Garay</u> as a result of their <u>clinical trial for adolescents</u>?

- Why did the FDA want to hide the Pfizer clinical trial data from the public for <u>seventy-five years</u>?

- Why isn't the media shouting from the rooftops about the 1,223 deaths, 158,000 adverse events, and 1,291 side effects <u>reported in the first ninety days</u> of Pfizer's clinical trial and only recently disclosed to the public due to the FOIA request resulting in their release at a rate of <u>55,000 pages per month</u>?

- Why, for that matter, aren't the media, government, or <u>regulatory agencies</u> concerned about the <u>1,314,592 adverse event reports</u> received by the CDC through June 24, 2022—including <u>29,031 deaths</u> and <u>50,400 child reports</u>?

- Why has the <u>CDC never monitored</u> its own adverse events reporting system for COVID injection safety signals—only discovered recently thanks to another <u>FOIA request</u>?

- Why isn't anyone concerned that they keep <u>moving the goalposts</u> for the injection—first promising that it <u>would set us free</u>, then saying it's not working because of the <u>evil unvaxxed</u>, then saying it loses efficacy after a few months and you need a <u>booster shot</u>, then saying you need <u>second booster</u>, then saying you need it <u>every four months</u>?

- Why are there so many <u>breakthrough infections</u>?

- Why are the <u>boosted contracting COVID more</u> than the uninjected?
- Why did <u>deaths attributed to COVID</u> *increase* instead of decreasing after the mass injection program was rolled out?
- Why does the immune system appear to suffer <u>progressive destruction</u> with each additional shot?
- Why are <u>cancers exploding</u> in the injected?
- Why are <u>birth rates dropping</u> around the world?
- Why are there so many <u>miscarriages</u>, <u>stillbirths</u>, <u>fertility problems</u>, and <u>disabilities in the babies</u> of injected mothers?
- Why are so many people developing <u>myocarditis</u> and having <u>heart attacks</u> after injection?
- Why do they make it <u>so difficult</u> for medical staff to report adverse events?
- Why are <u>children</u>, <u>millennials</u>, <u>athletes</u>, and other healthy people <u>suddenly dying</u> and <u>becoming disabled</u>?
- Why are pathologists finding that <u>93 percent of people who died</u> after injection were killed by it?
- Why are <u>embalmers</u> discovering mysterious <u>wormlike strings</u> in the corpses of the vaxxed?
- Why did such a cosmically unprecedented <u>mass fatality rate</u> start in 2021—so bad that they've had to make up <u>Sudden Adult Death Syndrome (SADS)</u> to cover for the reality that <u>massive numbers of people are unexpectedly dropping dead</u>?
- Why did life insurance companies pay out as much as <u>163 percent</u> more for 18–64-year-olds and <u>258 percent</u> more overall in 2021 over 2020?
- Why is one of the largest casket manufacturers in North America reporting that <u>sales of child-sized caskets have skyrocketed by 400 percent since December 2021</u>?

- Why is the <u>funeral industry</u> <u>booming</u>?
- Why did a <u>German insurance executive get fired</u> for reporting <u>alarming numbers of vaxx injuries</u>?
- Why aren't people being given informed consent about the risks of <u>antibody-dependent enhancement</u> (ADE), <u>blood clots</u>, <u>Bell's Palsy</u>, <u>Guillain-Barré syndrome</u>, <u>cardiac diseases</u>, and the innumerable other debilitating and fatal side effects?
- Why aren't the vaccine manufacturers making any efforts to improve their products to reduce mortality and adverse reactions?
- Why is it okay to <u>keep pharmaceutical products in circulation</u> despite historically unprecedented rates of deaths and injuries when, before 2020, such drugs would have been <u>recalled</u> as soon as a tiny handful of serious reactions had been reported?
- Why aren't the vaxxed more <u>curious</u> about what they've been injected with?

Finally, why are so few people asking these questions, and why are they censoring us for asking them?

After assessing and meticulously <u>assembling thousands of pieces of evidence</u> over the past two years, I have concluded the only logical answers to the above questions are:

1. **PROFIT:** accomplishing the <u>largest wealth transfer</u> from the middle class to the <u>super-wealthy/super-rich</u> in history;
2. **POWER:** setting the stage for <u>The Great Reset</u> and a <u>global technocratic one-world tyranny</u>; and
3. **DEMOCIDE:** <u>reducing the population</u> to "save the planet."

In his 1928 book *<u>Propaganda</u>*, masterful consent engineer <u>Edward Bernays</u> reveals:

"The conscious and intelligent manipulation of the organized habits and opinions of the masses is an important element in democratic society. Those who manipulate this unseen mechanism of society constitute an invisible government which is the true ruling power of our country.

"We are governed, our minds are molded, our tastes formed, our ideas suggested, largely by men we have never heard of. This is a logical result of the way in which our democratic society is organized. Vast numbers of human beings must cooperate in this manner if they are to live together as a smoothly functioning society....

"In almost every act of our daily lives, whether in the sphere of politics or business, in our social conduct or our ethical thinking, we are dominated by the relatively small number of persons—a trifling fraction of our hundred and twenty million—who understand the mental processes and social patterns of the masses. It is they who pull the wires which control the public mind, who harness old social forces and contrive new ways to bind and guide the world."

Most ordinary people cannot fathom the degree to which their beliefs and perceptions have been molded by the public-opinion engineers—especially if they watch television and consume other mainstream media. They are stuck in Plato's Propaganda Cave and stubbornly refuse to believe the tales of those who have escaped the cave and returned to rescue them. They call the ones trying to liberate them from their deception "conspiracy theorists," "anti-vaxxers," "right-wingers," and "fascists" because those are the scripts their programmers have installed to prevent them from questioning the illusion they are voluntarily imprisoned in.

They merely need to take five minutes to view the data that is hiding in plain sight at OpenVAERS, but they aren't even willing to do that. Their captors are so confident the hypnotized will never awaken, they don't bother to conceal their corruption.

You've heard of Turtles all the way down? Well, this is corruption all the way down.

Getting back to those three end goals I mentioned earlier: **profit**, **power**, and **democide**.

Bernays and his fellow social engineers knew they had to work from the end goal backward. Want to capture women as a new consumer audience for cigarettes? Stage a "Torches of Freedom" demonstration at the 1929 Easter parade with glamorous debutantes sporting cigarettes as a sign of women's liberation.

Want to orchestrate a massive transfer of wealth, get people to accept one-world authoritarianism, and knock off a good portion of the population while you're at it? Stage a pandemic and terrorize the public into relinquishing their liberties in the name of an illusory "safety" that will never arrive. Tell them the only way out is to accept a novel pharmaceutical product that governments (i.e., taxpayers) will be required to fork out billions of recurring dollars to fund. Decimate small businesses, evaporate jobs, wreck the economy, and force the vassals to depend on the State for survival. Make them think it's all for the "greater good."

Despite one sucker punch after another, the deceived will cling to their belief in their Stockholm saviors and attack those trying to free them from their enslavement until their dying breath. Those who don't die immediately will generate a fortune in revenue for the pharmaceutical-medical complex thanks to their lifelong vaxx injuries and ravaged immune systems.

Pfizer, for example, reported a 77 percent increase in sales of Vyndaqel®/Vyndamax®—its products for treating transthyretin amyloid cardiomyopathy—in second-quarter 2021. "Coincidentally," the injections appear to cause cardiac amyloidosis, or stiff heart syndrome, according to Dr. Jessica Rose.

Meanwhile, the noble liars will perpetuate the Problem–Reaction–Solution hamster wheel until the requisite number of people have been eliminated—or we stop the string-pullers from completing their democidal agenda.

They don't just want us to eat bugs—to them, we *are* bugs.

Great Reset co-conspirator Prince Philip famously said: "In the event that I am reincarnated, I would like to return as a deadly virus to contribute something to solving overpopulation."

In "Letter to a Holocaust Denier," I map the ten stages of genocide to the contemporary democide underway, citing menacing quotes from futurist and François Mitterand special advisor Jacques Attali under #9) Extermination.

Below are excerpts from a 1981 interview conducted by Michel Salomon in which Attali states (emphases mine): "I believe rather in **implicit totalitarianism** with an invisible and decentralized 'Big Brother.' **These machines for monitoring our health**, which we could have for our own good, will **enslave us for our own good**. In a way, we will be subjected to gentle and permanent conditioning."

"But as soon as you go beyond 60/65, **people live longer than they produce and they cost society dearly**."

"Indeed, from the point of view of society, **it is much better for the human machine to come to an abrupt halt** than for it to deteriorate gradually."

"**Euthanasia will be one of the essential instruments of our future societies** in all cases. In a socialist logic, to begin with, the problem is as follows: socialist logic is freedom and **fundamental freedom is suicide**; consequently, the right to direct or indirect suicide is an absolute value in this type of society. In a capitalist society, **killing machines**, prostheses that **will make it possible to eliminate life when it is too unbearable or economically too costly**, will come into being and will be common practice. I therefore believe that **euthanasia**, whether it is a value of freedom or a commodity, **will be one of the rules of future society**."

"Medicine is indicative of the evolution of a society that is moving towards a decentralized totalitarianism. We can already see a certain conscious or unconscious desire to conform as much as possible to social norms."

"It is clear that the discourse on prevention, health economics and good medical practice will lead to **the need for each individual to have a medical file** which will be put on a magnetic tape. For epidemiological reasons, **all these files will be centralized in a computer** to which doctors will have access."

"I believe that we are leaving a universe controlled by energy to enter the **universe of information**. If matter is energy, **life is information**. This is why the major producer of tomorrow's society will be living matter. Thanks in particular to **genetic engineering**, it will produce **new therapeutic weapons**, food and energy."

You will recognize echoes of these prophecies in the ominous prognostications of fellow futurist, Attali intellectual heir, and Klaus Schwab muse Yuval Noah Harari.

While these concerns about overpopulation were all the rage in the 1970s and 1980s, reality has not borne out their dire predictions. Contrary to the sky-is-falling Malthusian projections of the Club of Rome; philanthropath Bill Gates; inexplicably-unconvicted war criminal Henry Kissinger; and other tyrants and colluders, the "world's population is projected to nearly stop growing by the end of the century" according to Pew Research.

Whether these diehard depopulationists are forging ahead with their culling plans because they genuinely believe the human species is growing at a rate that threatens the planet or they simply want to hoard the Earth's resources for themselves is purely speculative—although betting on malicious, self-serving intentions has historically paid off.

Either way, they have used COVID as a cloak to achieve all three of these objectives—profit, power, and democide—in record time.

Chapter 25

My Journey:
The Freedom Convoy

Tamara Lich

Organizer of the Canadian Freedom Convoy

Tamara Lich is a Canadian political activist and key figure in the Freedom Convoy movement that took place in 2022. Born and raised in Saskatchewan, she is of Métis heritage and has spent much of her life advocating for the rights and freedoms of Canadians. Before becoming involved in the convoy, Tamara worked in various industries, including the oil and gas sector. Her leadership in the Freedom Convoy brought her national and international recognition as a champion for personal liberties and government accountability. Despite facing legal challenges, including arrest and incarceration, Tamara remains a steadfast voice for freedom, continuing to inspire people both in Canada and around the world.

I never imagined that one day I would be at the forefront of a movement that would capture national attention and become such a defining moment in Canadian history.

My name is Tamara Lich, and I was part of a grassroots movement that took on a life of its own—the Freedom Convoy. What started as a group of truckers opposing vaccine mandates, soon blossomed into a nationwide and even global symbol of resistance against government overreach. This movement grew far beyond our initial plans, capturing the hearts of Canadians and inspiring people around the world who felt the weight of their freedoms slipping away.

I did not come from a background of political activism. Like many, I was a regular citizen who found myself pushed to the edge by government mandates and restrictions that seemed to encroach more and more on our personal liberties. My story is not unique. It's the story of thousands, maybe millions, of people who felt the same way but never imagined they could make a difference. When I joined the Freedom Convoy, I found that standing up for freedom means that ordinary people like me, can create extraordinary change.

When the COVID-19 pandemic began, I, like many Canadians, followed the rules. I wore the mask, I stayed at home, and I kept my distance from loved ones. We all thought we were doing the right thing—doing our part to stop the spread of the virus. But as time went on, it became clear that these restrictions weren't temporary. Instead, they were becoming more severe and felt more like a form of control than a public health strategy. And it wasn't just me who felt this way. Thousands of others across Canada began to see the same cracks in the system.

The most infuriating part wasn't just the mandates themselves; it was the refusal of the government to listen to any opposition. If you dared to question the narrative being pushed by public health officials or the government, you were labeled as a conspiracy theorist or worse. Anyone who voiced concerns about personal freedoms or who wanted to ask if there were alternative approaches was dismissed outright. The media played a huge role in this, too. They fueled the fear and painted anyone who had doubts about the government's response as irresponsible or even dangerous.

By the time the vaccine mandates came into effect, it felt like the breaking point. The truckers, who had been heralded as heroes in the early days of the pandemic for keeping our supply chains moving, were now being told they couldn't do their jobs unless they complied with vaccine requirements. It was hypocritical and unfair. Many of us saw this as a clear case of government overreach, and we knew we had to act.

That's when the idea of the Freedom Convoy came to life. It started simply enough—a convoy of truckers driving across the country to Ottawa in protest at the vaccine mandates. But soon, it turned into something much larger. People from all walks of life began to join us—parents who were frustrated with the lockdowns that kept their children out of school, small business owners who had lost everything due to restrictions, healthcare workers who had been on the frontlines of the pandemic and felt betrayed by the very government they had trusted.

As the convoy gained momentum, so did the support. What started as a protest among truckers quickly turned into a movement for freedom. People from every corner of Canada wanted to stand up and say, "Enough is enough." The outpouring of support was overwhelming. People came out to cheer us on, to wave flags, and to offer us food and supplies as we made our way to Ottawa. By the time we arrived in the capital, the convoy stretched over 100 kilometers long. It was an incredible sight—a testament to the power of ordinary citizens united for a common cause.

When we reached Ottawa, it was clear that this was bigger than any of us had anticipated. Thousands of people joined us in the capital to peacefully protest the mandates. The energy was electric; there was a palpable sense that we were doing something important, something that could truly make a difference. But even as we stood there, united in our cause, the government's response was nothing short of dismissive.

Prime Minister Justin Trudeau refused to meet with us. He chose to call us a "fringe minority" and rejected our concerns outright. His government's refusal to listen only fueled the frustration that had brought us to Ottawa in the first place. We had come in peace, hoping for dialogue, but instead, we were met with silence and disdain. Other political leaders and some members of parliament did meet with us, recognizing that our message resonated with millions of Canadians. But Trudeau remained resolute in his decision to ignore us, to ignore the voices of everyday Canadians who had supported him in the past, but now felt betrayed.

We weren't asking for anything unreasonable. We wanted the mandates lifted so people could return to their jobs, businesses could reopen, and children could go back to school without restrictions. We even reached a deal with the City of Ottawa to address some of the concerns about the protest, but just as things seemed to be moving forward, Trudeau made a shocking decision—he invoked the Emergencies Act.

For the first time in Canadian history, the Prime Minister invoked the Emergencies Act, essentially declaring that peaceful protesters were a threat to national security. The Act gave the government sweeping powers to freeze bank accounts, seize property, and arrest people without cause. It was a move that many of us couldn't believe was happening in a democratic country like Canada. This was not how the government should respond to peaceful protest. We had come to Ottawa in peace, hoping for dialogue, and yet the government responded with force.

As the police moved in, the media quickly jumped on board, portraying us as dangerous extremists who were disrupting public order. The smear campaign intensified. The media painted us as everything from racists to white supremacists, ignoring the fact that our movement was diverse, including people from all backgrounds, including Indigenous communities, immigrants, and those who had supported Trudeau's government in the past.

I was one of many who were arrested. The charges? Mischief. It seemed absurd to be charged with mischief for standing up for something I believed in. I spent 49 days in jail, including 4 days in solitary confinement, for what the government deemed to be mischief. The conditions in jail were difficult, and being placed in solitary was one of the most trying experiences of my life. But despite all that, I never wavered in my belief that we were doing the right thing.

The Freedom Convoy was more than just a protest in Canada. It quickly became a global symbol of resistance. People in countries around the world looked to us for inspiration. Similar protests sprang up in New Zealand, Australia, Europe, and even the United States. What we had started in Canada had taken on a life of its own, inspiring others to stand up to their governments and fight for their freedoms. It was a powerful reminder that when people come together, they can create change on a massive scale.

Our movement also embarrassed the Canadian government. Trudeau's invocation of the Emergencies Act was widely criticized, both domestically and internationally. It exposed the lengths to which the government would go to maintain control, and it made it clear that our fight wasn't just about vaccines or mandates—it was about the fundamental rights of citizens in a free society.

And in the end, the movement was successful. Shortly after the convoy, mandates across Canada began to fall. The government, feeling the pressure from citizens who had had enough, started to lift restrictions. People were returning to their jobs, businesses were reopening, and life was starting to move forward again. Our movement had made a real, tangible difference. We had stood up, and the world had taken notice.

As I write this, I am still awaiting the verdict in my trial on charges of mischief. I know there are those who will never agree with what we did. There will always be critics who see the Freedom Convoy as nothing more than a disruption. But I also know there are millions of Canadians and people around the world who stood with us. They understood that this was more than just a protest—it was about holding the government accountable, about standing up for our rights, and about showing that when we come together, we have the power to create real change.

Looking back, I don't regret a thing. The Freedom Convoy was about so much more than vaccine mandates—it was about challenging the very foundations of government overreach. We made history, and we proved that even in the face of overwhelming odds, we can stand up and demand change.

Our journey isn't over. The fight for freedom continues, and I will keep standing for what I believe in, no matter the cost. What started as a convoy of truckers became a global movement, and that movement will continue to inspire others to stand up for their rights and freedoms. It's not about me—it's about all of us. It's about showing that when the people come together, we have the power to change the world.

CHAPTER 26

Mask Mania

Paul D. Thacker

Investigate journalist

Paul D. Thacker is an investigative journalist and founder of The DisInformation Chronicle, a newsletter that reports on corruption in science and medicine. He was awarded a 2021 British Journalism Award for a series in The BMJ that investigated the financial interests of medical experts advising U.S. and U.K. governments on COVID-19 pandemic policies. A separate BMJ investigation examined problems in the clinical trial for Pfizer's COVID-19 vaccine. That article was the finalist for an investigative journalism award and is the most highly viewed article in all of science in 2021.

Thacker has written on conflicts of interests and corruption in science and medicine for multiple outlets including The New York Times, Los Angeles Times, Washington Post, NEJM, The New Republic, Vice, Slate, JAMA, Environmental Science & Technology, and Mother Jones.

He is a former investigator for the United States Senate where he looked into corruption in science and helped pass reforms in medicine, and a former Fellow at the Edmond J. Safra Center for Ethics at Harvard. Thacker has lectured on journalism and corruption in science at multiple universities including Harvard, Georgetown, MIT, Brown University, NYU, the University of Toronto, and the University of West Virginia.

I can't tell you the exact day that I began to doubt what I was being told about masks, but it was sometime toward the end of the pandemic's first year in late 2020. I'm on an email list with over 100 different physicians, academics, and scientists, all sharing problems about drugs and the pharmaceutical industry. But when the pandemic started, much of the conversation shifted to COVID.

Several scientists expressed doubts on this list about masks effectively stopping viruses, pointing to studies that found masks didn't do much.

This was at a time when almost everyone, including myself, just fell in line and masked up when going out.

Over time, my doubts about what I was reading in the news began to grow, and I spent more time on social media trying to run down claims about the science supporting mask mandates. I couldn't help but notice a "follow the science" sentiment passed around among online Liberals in the media and academia. This sentiment among elites felt more like a public relations campaign than a scientific discussion, and Liberals' use of the term "anti-mask" reeked of politics.

I eventually chased down several stories in _Scientific American,_ _Wired, New York Magazine_ and _The Atlantic_ reporting that scientific studies found masks didn't seem to stop viruses.[1][2][3][4] But "follow the science" cheerleaders, I noticed, had drowned these articles out. I certainly hadn't noticed them when they were published, and only found them after I looked back to try and piece together what had happened during the pandemic.

Then, Cochrane published a review in early 2023 that looked at masks and found there wasn't much evidence supporting their use to stop viruses.[5] I had heard quite a bit about Cochrane and knew they were considered the "gold standard" of evidence in medicine, so I interviewed the review's lead author, Tom Jefferson.

My interest in the topic was to help readers understand some of the underlying science on masking and to cut through the controversy so people would be informed about the science of both masking and the relevance of mask mandates. I had noticed videos and news stories circulating on social media pointing out that several public health officials had done a 180 from the early months of the pandemic, first stating that masks don't work, before pivoting to advocate for masks. This included Canada's chief health officer, Theresa Tam, as well as the leading public health official in England, Jenny Harries.

Even Tony Fauci had done this, first arguing that masks didn't work, before pivoting into full on mask activist.

The interview with Jefferson about the Cochrane mask review was a bit of a slog. Jefferson loves going into all kinds of details about the hierarchy of evidence, how reviews are done, the contrasts between different types of reviews, and other tiny bits of medical information that only interest people with decades of expertise in clinical trials and medical research.

In short, very hard to follow.

As Jefferson kept rambling on with tiny details about how to perform medical reviews that nobody but an expert in medical reviews could really follow, and why certain types of studies have more credibility than others, I stopped him.

"Wait, did you just say that Cochrane has done this mask review several times?" I asked. "This isn't the first one?"

"Yes," he replied.

So we went down the list. The Cochrane mask review published in January 2023 wasn't the first time Cochrane scientists had examined the scientific literature to see if there was evidence masks work to stop viruses. Starting back in 2006, they had scoured the academic literature several times for similar reviews—all finding the same thing that masks don't seem to do much to stop viruses.[6]

So the evidence finding that masks didn't do much against respiratory viruses had been known for almost two decades. And nobody seemed to question this conclusion until after the pandemic started in 2020.

"Didn't you bother to notice," I asked Jefferson, "that none of these 'experts' argued that masks worked until after 2020 and governments made people wear masks and said they worked? That's the story."

For example, in their 2019 pandemic preparedness plan, the World Health Organization concluded: "There have been a number of high-quality randomised controlled trials (RCTs) demonstrating that personal protective measures such as hand hygiene and face masks have, at best, a small effect on influenza transmission."[7]

This is pretty much in line with the Cochrane review's conclusions.

But about a month after I published my February 2023 interview with Jefferson, walking readers through the best evidence on masks, the New York Times published an essay claiming "the science is clear masks work" attacking the Cochrane mask review, and quoting from the head of Cochrane, Karla-Soares Weiser, that changes would be made to the mask review.[8]

The article also denigrated several statements made by Jefferson about the pandemic, even though Jefferson was only one of about a dozen scientists who wrote the Cochrane review. Plus, Jefferson had been studying respiratory viruses for several decades. Why this need to attack him so personally?

The whole thing smelled fishy and I soon learned that Karla Soares-Weiser had rushed out the statement attacking Cochrane's own review and had spoken to the New York Times columnist, Zeynep Tufekci, without consulting the scientists who had actually done all the work and written the actual review.

While Soares-Weiser runs Cochrane, scientists with expertise in each specific subject matter write and edit the reviews. For Karla Soares Weiser to hurry out a statement attacking a Cochrane review without consulting the actual scientists, would be like the executive editor at the New York Times publishing a personal essay criticizing a New York Times investigation, without bothering to discuss the matter with the editors and journalists that conducted the actual investigation.

It was weird and very unprofessional. Again, it reeked of politics. Plus, Tufekci then began tweeting that she had gotten the Cochrane review "corrected."

I had never heard of New York Times columnist Zeynep Tufekci, so I decided to look into her past. I immediately noticed that Tufekci, like many others, had also done a 180 on masks.

"Don't worry if you cannot find masks," Tufekci wrote in a February 2020 article for *Scientific American*.[9] "For non–health care people, washing your hands often, using alcohol-based hand-sanitiser liberally and learning not to touch your face are the most important clinically-proven interventions there are." Promoting the article on X, Tufekci reiterated this point: "Clinical studies show hand-washing is the crucial step, not masks."

But the following month, Tufekci rocketed to fame when a *New York Times* media reporter praised her for reversing her former opinion in a 1 March tweetstorm and a 17 March essay for *The New York Times* that convinced the CDC to alter federal guidance and advise Americans to mask.[10]

What makes this all alarming is that Tufekci is an academic sociologist, with no training in medicine or public health. And yet, she managed to alter national health policy with a bunch of tweets and an essay. You don't need an advanced degree in epidemiology to be alarmed that the CDC sets pandemic policy because of Tufekci tweets and an essay, but Tufekci also tweeted that she promoted masks in two 2020 meetings with the World Health Organization.

Tufecki followed up a couple months later in 2020 by co-authoring a scientific preprint that promoted mask mandates. "We recommend that public officials and governments strongly encourage the use of widespread face masks in public, including the use of appropriate regulation," the review concluded.[11] The review's lead author is Jeremy Howard, a mask advocate and Australian software entrepreneur, who, like Tufekci, has no training in public health or medicine. The review was later published in a medical journal and remains the only article I could find that Tufekci has published in the scientific literature on masks.

Something weird was going on. None of this made any sense.

But then, during the summer of 2024, I got a bunch of emails from a person who had filed freedom of information requests with several academics affiliated with Cochrane. I also had several emails leaked to me by a whistleblower at Cochrane who was upset at apparent corruption inside the organization.

Those emails showed that Tufekci had spun the words of one person she interviewed for her essay and she apparently bullied Cochrane's Soares-Weiser into putting out that statement against Cochrane's own mask review.

One of the first things I noticed was that Tufecki had emailed Michael Brown, a physician at Michigan State University, on February 24, 2023. According to other emails, I learned that Michael Brown had been the sign off editor for the Cochrane mask review.

Why, I wondered, had Tufekci contacted Brown at this time?

Searching the news, I realized that Tufekci's New York Times colleague, Bret Stephens, had published an essay three days prior, ribbing mask advocates like Tufekci because of Cochrane's mask review: "The Mask Mandates Did Nothing. Will Any Lessons Be Learned?"[12]

Tufekci's rise in public prominence is tied so closely to mask advocacy that you can't separate her from the mask mandates movement. The thrust of Stephens' piece must have cut her like a knife:

> [W]hen it comes to the *population*-level benefits of masking, the verdict is in: Mask mandates were a bust. Those skeptics who were furiously mocked as cranks and occasionally censored as "misinformers" for opposing mandates were right. The mainstream experts and pundits who supported mandates were wrong.

Reading this column in the New York Times, where she also worked, must have felt threatening. I had dug into Tufekci's academic publishing record and found she had published little to no scientific studies. All of her credibility as an expert and "academic sociologist" seemed to ride on her essays in the New York Times.

But when she contacted Brown, Tufekci laid it on thick that she was an academic researcher, claiming expertise in statistics and causal inference, as well as scientific reviews. "I use and participate in reviews myself (I'm writing one in my own field soon) and thus am familiar with many of the challenges and issues," Tufekci emailed Brown.

This is something of an embellishment of Tufekci's bona fides. According to Google Scholar, she has published no academic articles this year, in 2024, and the only one she published in all of 2023 was an opinion piece.[13] As for the review article Tufekci told Brown she was writing?

It has never appeared.

Tufekci then contacted Karla Soares-Weiser, the woman running Cochrane. Apparently, Tufekci sent a slew of questions, because Soares-Weiser then emailed Lisa Bero, a professor of medicine at the University of Colorado and who serves as Cochrane ethics advisor.

"Lisa, I have been back and forth with NYT about the mask review. CAN I GET YOUR VIEWS ON THE FOLLOWING QUESTIONS?" Soares-Weiser emailed.[14] She then sent questions to Bero that she had gotten from Tufekci.

What makes this all comical is that Tufekci obviously knows nothing about reviews, yet Soares-Weiser freaked out because Tufekci writes a column at the New York Times.

It's science by essay writer.

After Bero answered the questions, Soares-Weiser thanked her. "Thank you, Lisa. I'm navigating a difficult situation and of course need to take these points into account. Help appreciated."

376 | Canary In a (Post) Covid World

I got a copy of the email Tufekci sent Jefferson for questions and it's dated March 9, the day before she published her 2000+ word essay. I've written for the New York Times. It's a rather laborious process dealing with editors and fact checkers. It would be impossible for Tufekci to contact Jefferson for comment and then slam out a 2000+ word essay, get that essay edited, deal with those edits, and then get it fact checked.

What those dates tell you is that Tufekci had the essay ready to publish *before* she contacted Jefferson for comment, meaning, she didn't even care what he had to say. Jefferson has been publishing scientific research on respiratory viruses for several decades, but Tufekci wasn't interested in listening to him because she already considered *herself* the expert.

The day Tufecki published her essay, Soares-Weiser then dashed out a statement claiming she was working to fix problems in the Cochrane mask review and sent an apology to the mask review scientists.

"You may have seen the New York Times article," wrote a Cochrane official in an email to the mask review scientists, adding that Tufekci had "blindsided" them. He then added, "On behalf of Cochrane, Karla [Soares-Weiser] has taken responsibility for the loose wording. This is made clear in our full statement, which we have decided to publish on Cochrane.org in light of its partial inclusion in the NYT coverage."[15]

If Cochrane has made clear that Karla Soares-Weiser was taking responsibility, then why did Tufekci need to drag Tom Jefferson in her essay?

"I will not speak for the others but am deeply distressed by this course of events which have occurred without our knowledge," replied Jon Conly, a professor and former head of the department of medicine at the University of Calgary.[16]

"There was no intention to 'throw you or anyone under the bus'," Brown responded, "since I would be throwing myself under the bus as the sign-off editor." Brown added that he had told Tufekci that he stood by the review and had asked her to contact the review authors for their statements.

Brown then sent an email to Soares-Weiser and several of the Cochrane editors reminding them that changes were being considered to the mask review language, even though it was the same wording as had been used in the 2020 update.

Why were changes being considered then? As Brown explained, it had nothing to do with science. "[I]t was only under intense media coverage and criticism that these revisions were suggested."[17]

Emails find that Soares-Weiser appeared to be in a bit of panic at the time, monitoring negative commentary about her decision to publish a statement without bothering to consult the scientists. "I had a challenging meeting with the [governing board] yesterday. I am holding on, stressed, but OK," she emailed Lisa Bero.

Bero then suggested to Soares-Weiser that Cochrane publish negative comments being submitted by outsiders criticizing the mask review. "That should be published as soon as possible (following screening for libel or profanity)," Bero emailed to Soares-Weiser.[18] "It is important for readers to know that criticism has not just come through the media, but through the formal channels that we have."

This email was a bit unbelievable. Experts had peer reviewed and gone over the mask review with an incredible amount of scrutiny, but Cochrane's ethics advisor now seemed to be inviting criticism from outside experts.

I also noticed an email that Brown sent out several months after he spoke with Tufekci for her New York Times essay. In that email, Brown made his views on the science of masking clear, explaining masks "likely" provide "some" protection but masks "do not make a major impact at the community level when promoted as a public health intervention."

This is pretty much the exact opposite of how Tufekci framed Brown's views.

In her article, Tufekci quoted Brown and followed up in the next paragraph implying that he supported the idea that "the evidence is really straightforward" that masks provide protection from COVID.

Here's the section of Tufekci's essay:

> Brown, who led the Cochrane review's approval process, told
> me that mask mandates may not be tenable now, but he has a
> starkly different feeling about their effects in the first year of
> a pandemic.
> "Mask mandates, social distancing, the other shutdowns we
> had in terms of even restaurants and things like that — if places
> like New York City didn't do that, the number of deaths would
> have been much higher," he told me. "I'm very confident of
> that statement."
> So the evidence is relatively straightforward: Consistently
> wearing a mask, preferably a high-quality, well-fitting one,
> provides protection against the coronavirus.

This is just sleazy.

When I contacted Brown, he said that Tufecki spun his words, because
the evidence is clear that masks don't seem to do much. He also told me
that he did not look her up before talking with her and did not know that
she had a history of mask advocacy and a poor publishing record in the
scientific literature.

"I'm a trusting person," Brown told me, explaining that he had never
looked up Tufecki's history before speaking with her. "She's definitely
more of a journalist than a scientist. I didn't agree with her, the way she
then spun it: masks work."[19]

"The bottom line is that [our] review was well-done," Brown added.
As for proposed changes to the review's language that the *New York
Times* reported on, Brown explained that the summary language had

been written by Cochrane staff reporting to Karla Soares-Weiser, not Tom Jefferson and the other review authors.

"She sort of got caught in the crossfire," Brown told me of Soares-Weiser, adding that colleagues pressured her because they didn't like the conclusions that there is no evidence masks work. "Which is really hard for her, for someone in her position as editor in chief."

Brown added that he had told Tufekci to contact the mask review authors because they were the experts who had looked at all the studies before publishing the review. But she hadn't done so and Tufekci did not respond to questions that I sent her.

Soares-Weiser's statement attacking Cochrane's mask review and Tufekci's "mask work" essay spurred several news articles as well as ridicule of the mask authors on social media. Pulitzer Prize-winning reporter and author of several books on pandemics, Laurie Garret, accused the mask authors of fraud. "[T]hese bozos have undermined public faith in [masks] & biz/govt willingness to promote use," she posted on X.[20]

This is the exact opposite of Garrett's former position on masks before the pandemic. In 2018, Garrett posted on X that masks don't work for influenza and other respiratory viruses. "We have also known for 100+ years that masks do no good."

Soares-Weiser's statement even reverberated throughout American politics. Testifying in her final appearance before Congress, CDC Director, Rochelle Walensky, cited Soares-Weiser's statement, falsely stating that Cochrane had "retracted" the mask review. Congressional staff were forced to correct her testimony: "The lack of trust in public health officials is becoming an enormous problem," a congressional staffer later wrote.[21]

Word of Soares-Weiser's actions also reached the highest levels of the British government. While she was in London for a 2023 Cochrane event, an MP invited her to Parliament's Portcullis House to explain her statement. A staffer in Parliament told me that Soares-Weiser dodged the invite and never appeared.

Throughout much of last year and into 2024, the mask review scientists demanded that Soares-Weiser explain her interactions with Zeynep Tufekci. Why had she collaborated with Tufecki when Tufekci had an obvious conflict of interest, having published a review that competed with Cochrane's conclusions while also lobbying government agencies for mask mandates?

Soares-Weiser never responded to these concerns. But in June 2024, Soares-Weiser relented, posting another statement that said Cochrane would make no changes to the mask review.[22] The entire episode raises questions about Zeynep Tufekci's ethics as well as whether the leadership at Cochrane is still fit for purpose.

Most importantly, this series of events proves beyond all doubt that politics played an outsized role in many pandemic decisions that were purportedly based on "science."

[1] https://www.scientificamerican.com/blog/observations/preparing-for-coronavirus-to-strike-the-u-s/

[2] https://web.archive.org/web/20200702004759/https:/www.wired.com/story/its-ridiculous-to-treat-schools-like-covid-hot-zones/

[3] https://nymag.com/intelligencer/2021/08/the-science-of-masking-kids-at-school-remains-uncertain.html

[4] https://www.theatlantic.com/science/archive/2021/12/mask-guidelines-cdc-walensky/621035/

[5] https://www.cochranelibrary.com/cdsr/doi/10.1002/14651858.CD006207.pub6/full

[6] https://disinformationchronicle.substack.com/p/researchers-find-no-evidence-again?utm_source=post-email-title&publication_id=264299&post_id=101303325&isFreemail=true&utm_medium=email

[7] https://iris.who.int/bitstream/handle/10665/329438/9789241516839-eng.pdf

[8] https://www.nytimes.com/2023/03/10/opinion/masks-work-cochrane-study.html?unlocked_article_code=Br3II3Oh7TS19AcwPx3r95LM9TKxjZ1vE15Ud_

nw00QafqHIvDxfuqqhV-PSw2JtqTmP_8P91YrrCDOJG0XU_5NImNh_cb0C5tjoFY5sN
5MKhoGjir075EY1ZuH7GBk6xn8VXU4sSHljQA_1qUZFyo2nlnbZVkpWUHjagArRQn
i3jRilZuKbcNAV63G6HPDDMIpFnCxugzqv-g3B6AW48sawlrjecIMC7WryP7En2GoZ2-
as6_-y8It7_dpaoTR861cWFtXCLq3GUiobHyRnwCQtXyt9Ok736lky_
MblwViUzYUr3rmgexKH-WKaTGFleAZVSniZ76bRzOalIWDIt88-SJw&smid=url-share

[9] https://www.scientificamerican.com/blog/observations/preparing-for-coronavirus-to-strike-the-u-s/

[10] https://www.nytimes.com/2020/08/23/business/media/how-zeynep-tufekci-keeps-getting-the-big-things-right.html

[11] https://www.preprints.org/manuscript/202004.0203/v2

[12] https://www.nytimes.com/2023/02/21/opinion/do-mask-mandates-work.html

[13] https://scholar.google.com/citations?user=XUODawIAAAAJ&hl=en

[14] https://www.documentcloud.org/documents/24776926-karla-asks-about-mask-trials

[15] https://www.documentcloud.org/documents/24776927-throwing-review-authors-under-the-bus

[16] https://www.documentcloud.org/documents/24776927-throwing-review-authors-under-the-bus

[17] https://www.documentcloud.org/documents/24776938-cochrane-editors-discuss-zeynep-tufekci

[18] https://www.documentcloud.org/documents/24776929-lisa-bero-says-publish-comments-quickly

[19] https://unherd.com/2024/08/how-the-nyt-undermined-mask-evidence/

[20] https://disinformationchronicle.substack.com/p/after-throwing-scientists-under-the

[21] https://disinformationchronicle.substack.com/p/congress-corrects-the-record-on-cdc

[22] https://www.cochrane.org/news/statement-physical-interventions-interrupt-or-reduce-spread-respiratory-viruses-review

CHAPTER 27

The FDA is not Your Doctor

Dr. Mary Talley Bowden

Otolaryngologist and sleep medicine specialist in Houston, Texas who treated over 6,000 COVID patients during the pandemic.

Dr. Mary Talley Bowden is an otolaryngologist and sleep medicine specialist in Houston, Texas who treated over 6,000 COVID patients during the pandemic. Her vast experience prompted her to become a fierce advocate for early treatment. After the FDA spread misinformation about ivermectin, she and Drs. Paul Marik and Robert Apter successfully sued them, forcing the agency to delete several misleading social media posts and web pages. Houston was ground zero for the COVID shot mandates, and Dr. Bowden was an early outspoken critic. The first hospital in the country to implement mandates, Houston Methodist, suspended her privileges and reported her to the Texas Medical Board in response to her tweeting "Vaccine mandates are wrong." The ensuing attacks prompted her to fight back, and she founded a nonprofit, Americans for Health Freedom, whose foundational project is to enlist politicians and other doctors to call for the COVID shots to be pulled off the market. She also serves as a Senior Fellow with FLCCC and is on the board of Vaccine Safety Research Foundation.

On March 5, 2021, the FDA invaded my exam room. No shots were fired, but casualties resulted nonetheless. I fought back, and after a series of attacks and a long occupation, the FDA finally retreated and fled back to Washington, DC. Reconstruction may take longer than the war, but FDA overreach into my office— and every doctor's office in America— was halted.

The Food and Drug Administration politicized the practice of medicine during the pandemic, unlawfully foisting itself between doctors and patients on COVID treatment decisions. Together with Drs. Robert Apter and Paul Marik, I took legal action against the agency and fought this injustice for ourselves, our patients, and our country.

As a licensed physician in Texas, I had one mission during the pandemic: help my patients. I offered access to testing when testing was hard to find. I provided treatment when other doctors told my patients to stay home. I kept over 6000 patients out of the hospital and maintained a successful treatment rate of 99.97 percent.

I relied on an array of medicines including ivermectin, an inexpensive drug the FDA approved for human use in 1996 but has since strenuously discouraged doctors from using to treat COVID. TheFDA's role is to approve the labeling for medications sold in America—period. It's a gatekeeper, not a doctor. It has no accountability for patient outcomes and no authority to advise patients on what drug treatments to pursue. Yet it repeatedly and unlawfully used its office to scare the public into thinking ivermectin is unsafe and unfit—even prohibited—for human consumption.

On its official website, the FDA published "Why You Should Not Use Ivermectin to Treat or Prevent COVID-19," and FAQs asking "Should I take ivermectin to prevent or treat COVID-19?" with a decisive answer "No." The fact that the FDA cannot tell physicians or patients what medications to use, or prohibit physicians from prescribing medications off-label was not included in these webpages.

On August 21, 2021, as COVID cases surged for the third time since the pandemic started, the FDA launched a missile strike against ivermectin, broadcasting the now-infamous tweet featuring an attractive health care worker nuzzling a horse.

The caption, "You are not a horse. You are not a cow. Seriously, y'all. Stop it," unequivocally directed the public not to use ivermectin to treat COVID. The media embraced the horse theme with gusto— the tweet went viral, and ivermectin became instantly branded as horse-dewormer. Reaching over twenty-four million people in less than a week, their tweet quickly became the most popular in FDA history.

Let's back-track nine months to understand where this started. The Pfizer- BioNTech COVID shot was unleashed on the market a mere nine months after COVID became a concern in America. Trump was still in office - this was December 11, 2020 - and the public was cautious. At this time, the shots were still EUA status, and despite three months of assertive encouragement, by March 2021, only 10% of Americans were considered "fully vaccinated." Monoclonal antibodies were still officially available, and as monoclonal antibodies became harder to access, ivermectin was gaining traction as an unofficial treatment option.

The Biden administration was outraged by how few people were willing to take the shot. Too much money, too much ego, too much power was at stake - the COVID vaccine was too big to fail. The government knew the public was less likely to take the shot if safe, effective treatment was available. Ivermectin was a clear obstacle and had to be eliminated.

On March 5, 2021, the FDA began its attack, adding a page on its website stating ivermectin should not be used for the treatment or prevention of COVID. While demonizing ivermectin, the government amplified its push for Americans to get the vaccine, announcing the deployment of a $1.5 billion PR campaign towards that effort ten days after the FDA added the ivermectin page to its website.

Two weeks later, on April 1, 2021, Houston Methodist Hospital - where I had privileges - announced all employees would be required to get the COVID shots, making history by becoming the first major employer and hospital in the country to impose a COVID vaccine mandate. On the very same day, HHS announced the launch of its $10 billion vaccine propaganda machine, COVID-19 Community Corps, which recruited a vast web of organizations and social media influencers to flood the internet with pro-vaccine propaganda. At this point, only 50% of Americans had taken one shot.

Meanwhile, COVID cases started to surge for the third time since the pandemic started. This was the summer of 2021, and at the time, I was collaborating with two ENTs on staff at Houston Methodist Hospital, Dr. Mas Takashima and Dr. Omar Ahmed. My clinic offered a contact-free saliva test for COVID and also treated patients with monoclonal antibodies, so I had a busy COVID practice sitting on mounds of data. With no spare time to process it, I asked the doctors at Houston Methodist to help, and we initially focused our research on ENT symptoms in patients with COVID.

As I was doing COVID testing, I was tracking patients by their vaccination status, and by August 2021, I realized the shots weren't working. Vaccinated patients testing positive outnumbered the unvaccinated and were just as sick if not sicker than the unvaccinated. I reached out to Mas and Omar and asked them if they were seeing what I was seeing. Only Omar responded... and barely. He simply stated he thought the shot was supposed to lower the severity of infection.

COVID cases surged hard that summer - the government responded by pushing their agenda harder. On August 21st, the FDA, with help from the media, launched a full-scale public relations campaign to gaslight the public into believing ivermectin is solely for horses. The FDA would later claim it was merely a "quip," but in reality, the horse tweet was the shot across the bow, setting off a cascade of human rights violations.

Two days following the horse tweet, on Aug 23, 2021, the Pfizer shot got full FDA approval, and a flurry of mandates followed. On August 24th, numerous large companies announced employee mandates, on Aug 26th, the Pentagon announced a military mandate, and on September 9th, Biden announced a mandate for all employers with 100 or more employees.

To complete their mission, the government needed to shut down all treatment options. A week after Biden announced the federal shot mandate, HHS seized distribution of monoclonal antibodies.Whereas I once was able to get an unlimited supply from the manufacturer, I was no longer able to get monoclonal antibodies to treat my patients. So I started using ivermectin.

Prior to using ivermectin, I went to the FDA's website to make sure it was safe. The original study submitted to the FDA when ivermectin was approved by the agency contains its LD50. "Lethal dose 50" is a benchmark number that describes a drug's toxicity and is the amount of drug, given in a single dose, that causes the death of 50% of a group of test animals. The LD50 of ivermectin proves ivermectin has a wide margin of safety - one would have to take 250x the amount prescribed to kill 50% of the test animals. I also performed a literature search for accidental and intentional overdoses from ivermectin and found no studies. Once I was assured ivermectin was safe, I began using it to treat patients, and when I could no longer obtain monoclonal antibodies, I relied heavily on it.

I treated almost two thousand patients with monoclonal antibodies and found them to work very well with no serious side effects. I was worried ivermectin would be less effective with more side effects, but in the late summer/early fall of 2021, when cases were surging the highest they'd ever been, I found ivermectin to work just as well as monoclonal antibodies. I still kept people out of the hospital and even had success when patients came to me late in the course of disease with severe hypoxemia. The only issue I had was getting it to my patients.

At the same time, I had numerous patients coming to me distraught over the mandates. While not imposed for all healthcare workers until November 4, 2021, mandates started at Houston Methodist in June. I also had patients telling me they were being mistreated by other physicians if they weren't vaccinated; one elderly woman with bladder cancer called me in distress after her urologist at Houston Methodist told her she would need to find a new doctor if she didn't get vaccinated.

In late September, Erin Jones reached out asking me to testify on her behalf in a lawsuit against Texas Huguley Hospital. Her husband, Jason

Jones, had been in a coma for over a month following infection with COVID, and the doctors and hospital Texas Huguley Hospital refused to let her husband try ivermectin. Along with Senator Bob Hall from Texas, I testified on his behalf, and the judge ordered the hospital to grant me temporary privileges so I could administer ivermectin to Mr. Jones. Despite the order, the hospital denied my privileges and delays ensued. The hospital appealed, and Mr. Jones was never allowed to receive ivermectin. His wife, however, covertly applied it topically, and he eventually made it out of the hospital alive. Unfortunately, he was never able to make a full recovery, and Jason Jones passed away on April 11, 2023.

In protest over the mandates and what was happening with Mr. Jones, I sent an email to my patients declaring I was prioritizing the unvaccinated and not going to accept new patients with routine ENT problems who were vaccinated. I explained I was hearing stories from unvaccinated patients that they were being refused care, using the example of the bladder cancer patient from Methodist. I never upheld the policy - I was seeing too many sick vaccinated people to ethically do that - but it caused quite a stir. I received a flood of responses, both good and bad, and was contacted by Mas to ask that I retract my comments about Houston Methodist refusing to see the unvaccinated. I sent a follow-up email to my patients with his comments - but days later I would discover that wasn't enough.

At the time, I was posting updates about what I was seeing in my clinic mostly on Facebook and Instagram, but as the tyranny ramped up, I decided to start tweeting.

On November 7, 2021, I tweeted out the same message twenty-five times - "Vaccine mandates are wrong," with a screenshot of a patient testimonial sent in response to my controversial email. A few days later I cautiously tweeted "Ivermectin works." I don't recall how many followers I had, but each post garnered only a dozen or so likes.

Five days later, on Nov 12, 2021, Houston Methodist hospital told a reporter at the Houston Chronicle that my privileges were suspended based on comments I'd made on social media. At the same time, the hospital posted on X that I was spreading dangerous misinformation harmful to the community. The media swarmed me, the story went global, and in response, I resigned from the hospital.

Publicly humiliating me was not enough. A month later, the hospital reported me to the National Practitioner Data Bank for resigning while under investigation, and on December 22, 2021, I received a letter from the Texas Medical Board (TMB) accusing me of quality of care violations, disciplinary action by peers and unprofessional conduct. Nearly three years later, I am still fighting these charges.

A week prior to me receiving the letter from the TMB, the FDA notified the Federation of State Medical Boards and National Association of Boards of Pharmacy with a warning against physicians using ivermectin. Like myself, doctors around the country received formal complaints from their state medical boards following the FDA's action.

These attacks prompted me, along with two other physicians experiencing the same difficulties, Dr.Robert Apter and Dr. Paul Marik, to take legal action against the FDA for their gross overreach. COVID was not the first global pandemic, nor will it be the last. We sued to prevent their unlawful actions from restricting doctors' ability to practice medicine in the future.

Apart from the threats to my license, the FDA's attack on ivermectin created daily hurdles I still must overcome to treat my patients. Pharmacists won't dispense it. Insurance companies won't pay for it. Patients want reassurance that it's safe—and I tell them it's the safest medication I've ever prescribed. Every time I prescribe ivermectin I am reminded how this government agency unlawfully interfered in the sanctity of the doctor-patient relationship.

Because I had a different point of view, no matter how well-informed, my medical license was put at risk, my livelihood in jeopardy, and my ability to help my patients significantly impaired. Countless doctors across the country were put in the same position.

The issue in our case was not whether ivermectin is an effective treatment for COVID. The issue was whether the FDA can interfere with the free flow of information and assume the role of a doctor. We must have healthy debate about best methods to combat the disease, especially with cases continuing to periodically spike.

Science and medicine are always changing. So should our willingness to consider alternative strategies. Consider how our base of knowledge has changed since the start of the pandemic. In March 2020, the Surgeon General was urging Americans to "STOP BUYING MASKS," describing them as "NOT effective in preventing general public from catching #Coronavirus," but less than a year later President Biden was signing Executive Orders mandating masks as part of "science-based public health measures." Similarly, Dr. Fauci once preached herd immunity, only to later abandon the idea.

Our battle started in the courts on June 2, 2022, and despite an initial setback, we kept fighting and eventually emerged victorious. After nearly two years and a resounding rebuke by the Fifth CircuitCourt of Appeals, on April 6, 2024, the FDA deleted its infamous "You are not a horse" tweet and retired other publications about the use of ivermectin to treat COVID following our landmark case, Apter v. Dep't of Health and Human Services. The damage the FDA inflicted will linger, but future patients are now protected from one meaningful government intrusion into their medical care.

I took an oath to practice medicine—"do no harm"—and the FDA prevented me from fulfilling that oath. That's why we stood up to protect every doctor's right to practice medicine without interference from politicized government agencies. Fighting the system should never be part of fighting the disease.

CHAPTER 28

The Financial Coup d'état Explained

Catherine Austin Fitts

Founder and President of the Solari Report

Catherine Austin Fitts served as Managing Director and Member of the Board of Directors of the Wall Street investment bank, Dillon, Read & Co., Inc. She also served as Assistant Secretary of Housing / Federal Housing Commissioner in the first Bush Administration. She is the Founder and President of the Solari Report which provides actionable intelligence on finance, geopolitics, health and more to help live a free and inspired life.

Catherine has a BA from the University of Pennsylvania, an MBA from the Wharton School, and studied Chinese at the Chinese University of Hong Kong.

In 2019 the G7 central bankers voted on a plan called The Going Direct Reset. And what we've seen for centuries now, is every 75 or 100 years or so when the currency system gets long in the tooth, you get a reset.

A reset is a recalibration of the governance and management systems, as well as the currency. Think of it as an economic event. They voted on The Going Direct Reset, and we went into a reset.

One way to do a radical re-engineering of how the financial system operates, both in governments and the private sector, is to announce it and try to insist that everybody does it. But that's not a terribly effective way to implement such a thing. But you could use, say, a healthcare crisis to further this agenda.

The COVID pandemic had a purpose that was not a health purpose. It was to facilitate the type of control system through a financial reset that we see every 75 to 100 years, this time with significant centralization of the economy and much more assertion by the bankers of control of national governments. What's very unique about the current reset is that digital technology now permits for phenomenal central control. We see the central bankers literally announce that they plan on changing us from a currency system to a financial transaction control grid that will allow them to make the rules centrally and control us centrally by controlling financial transactions.

They're planning on essentially ending financial transaction freedom and have clearly said so. The pandemic, whether it helps implement digital IDs or vaccine passports, is part of creating that financial transaction control grid.

I believe everybody in Canada knows what happened to the truckers, so they understand what can happen with a digital currency. A government simply decides the rules: that certain people can't transact, or others only within certain limits, or it seizes bank accounts and assets.

When the Canadian government was seizing the bank accounts of people who had donated to the truckers' convoy, it put an incredible chill on Canadians and their trust in the banks. It's done irreparable harm to the international banking sector.

We have digital currency already. If you use a credit card, you're using a digital currency. If you make a bank transfer, you're using a digital currency. If you're not using cash, you're probably using digital currency. What we see is an effort globally to implement something called central bank digital currencies [CBDCs], which according to the central bankers, will allow them to have much tighter control of individual accounts and set the rules as to how money in an account can be used.

They insist that any money in your bank account is not your money, it's theirs. They call it, "central bank liability," so they think of it as theirs. We've seen examples. Several years ago the *Vanderbilt Law Review* published an article saying: the great thing about central bank digital currencies, commonly known as CBDCs, is if we're concerned about inflation, you can just freeze everybody's bank accounts.

The most important issue that comes out in your financial transaction is, we in the Western world practice a policy of taxation with representation. So the bankers may manage the monetary policy but our legislative representatives manage our tax proceeds and federal and national credit.

Now, with CBDC you're talking about creating a financial transaction system where taxes can just be taken out of your account. You can't stop it, so you will have taxation without representation.

If you're a Canadian, it's akin to "We're all truckers now." You're putting together a system that can be policed and micromanaged, to control where and how you spend your money. So if they don't want you going more than five miles from your home, your money won't work more than five miles from your home. Or if they want to turn off the electricity on your car, if they want to turn off your bank account, they can do so and they can do it centrally.

They'll have complete control, and basically be able to move us into a social credit-style system much like the Chinese. What you need is a smart grid in place, with the energy and electrical system components to make that work. Part of this is achieved with satellites. Extraordinary efforts have been made in building this grid during the pandemic.

What happened in the United States during the pandemic was an explosion of wealth moving upward. In 1990 there were approximately 60 billionaires in the United States. By the start of the pandemic, there were 614. Within the first 12 months of the pandemic the number of billionaires grew by 56 and wealth of the billionaire class grew by over a trillion dollars, estimated in the U.S. to be $1.3 trillion.

Some of that came from the fact that, as part of going direct reset, the central bank injected approximately $5 trillion into the economy. It was notable the way it was done, because it was injected directly, instead of doing it through the reserve circuit, which is normally the way a central bank would inject money. What that did was create bubbles in certain areas of the economy at the same time that the pandemic shut down others.

I'm going to grossly oversimplify just to help you understand how this worked conceptually. When I inject an enormous amount of money printed by the central bank into one group of people and, at the same time, I shut down all the businesses and the income of another group of people, it becomes much easier for those in the first group to increase their market share and pick up assets cheaply. Approximately 75 million people lost their jobs in the first year of the pandemic, mostly from small and medium sized businesses. Now people without income must sell their assets to generate money to survive.

A very clear example of this in action was when small businesses were forced to close during lockdowns, but Costco continued to trade, all in the name of "science."

Apparently it was dangerous to be in the small businesses but it was safe to be in Costco.

We saw a double standard applied to the large publicly traded companies represented on Wall Street and small businesses.. It was devastating. After the first two years of the pandemic, 34 percent of U.S. small businesses had shut down, and in San Francisco it was as high as 49 percent. That's an extraordinary number of jobs, because small businesses are the job engine in the United States. This set up two classes of business: one with a huge advantage. We saw an enormous shift in market share accordingly.

Basically we saw an incredibly large concentration of wealth at the top by design, not just some consequence of a health pandemic that hit the economy. It's very difficult to come up with an explanation for the restrictions seen through the health lens, rather than for the re-engineering of the political and economic landscape.

* * *

From 1998 I was tracking mortgage fraud, due to the fact that large amounts of money started to go missing from the U.S. federal government. I had been told by one of the largest pension fund investors in the spring of 1997, "they've given up on the country, they're moving all the money out starting in the fall."

I thought he meant they're reallocating the equity investment in the pension funds to the emerging markets. I didn't understand. He meant, no, literally we're going to have a financial coup. Because at the beginning of the next fiscal year, which was October 1st, 1997, which is the beginning of the 1998 federal fiscal year, huge amounts of money started to go missing. And it got worse and worse and worse.

There was a real effort before 9-11 to get to the bottom of what was happening and stop it. 9-11 changed all of that and money continued to disappear, with the largest amount that we know of disappearing in fiscal 2015: $6.5 trillion. Dr. Mark Skidmore, who's a full professor at Michigan State University and does government budgets, heard me and thought I must be making a mistake. He went out and checked the financial statements and discovered that I was right. He called me and said, "What can I do to help?" I said, "If you and your students would do a survey, it would help tremendously."

So he went out and did a survey and discovered that $21 trillion was missing by 2015. The two agencies where money was going missing was HUD [Housing and Urban Development], which was my old housing agency, and the Department of Defense, which has run the pandemic. If you look at which departments really ran Operation Warp Speed and the pandemic in the United States, it was the Department of Defense.

I would call it a financial coup d'état. That's a change of governance system by the "just do it" method. It's a coup but it's by financial means. I liken it to: you get fed up with the old system, so you start a new system; you move all the money, the assets into the new system and you leave the liabilities in the old system.

If you look at what has been happening since the money started to go missing, if you look at all the policies in the United States, I call it the "Great Poisoning." We have seen a steady diminution of life expectancy. Now that has accelerated during the pandemic. I don't mean to sound callous, but if you look at the decisions of how we were going to fund retirement obligations, the money wasn't there. So if you cannot fund your obligations then how are you going to explain to the people that you're going to abrogate them or change them? Funding retirement obligations, including health care, is a mathematical formula and if you can't fund it financially then you need to change the parameters - make the retirement age higher - or change the population claiming benefits. It's a mathematical requirement for depopulation. .

In the United States, there's been a steady debasement of the food supply. Food has become steadily less nutritious. Part of this, I think, is a combination of things, whether it's genetically modified food or pesticides. We've seen a steady deterioration in the quality of the food. We've seen a significant rise in environmental pollution and toxicity. We've seen a deterioration in many parts of the country in the quality of the water and sewer systems. And with it, we've also seen inflation and monetary policy by the central bank squeeze many of the retirees and elderly in a way that, I think, reduces their quality of life and lowers life expectancy.

If you look at what I consider to be the Great Poisoning, I consider it to be lots of different things. But one of the ways to significantly reduce the population on a slow and steady basis is to increase toxicity levels and lower the immune system. Then each person dies of their own individual weakness, but really, it's a pandemic of toxicity.

So back to the missing money. "Okay, let's move the assets into a new system. We'll move the liabilities back, then when we're basically in a position to reset the old, we've protected the assets; the bankers will take control and run both houses." And so it literally is a financial coup d'état because you are ending national sovereignty and putting the world under a dictatorship of the bankers, so to speak. I think this was always the plan.

Now, what's interesting is the budget deal in 1995, did a crash and burn. It was literally the next month that the predatory lending took off like a rocket and the FDA approved oxycontin. If you look at the extent to which the pill mills and the predatory lending targeted the same neighborhoods;

we also saw the private prison effort target the same neighborhoods. I think this was the beginning of the Great Poisoning, and it was intentional.

I see the pandemic as an exercise in re-engineering the economy away from small business and concentrated into large corporations—mostly publicly traded companies. That creates a concentration of business market share and employment under central control, and a consolidation of capital. It's centralization of business market share, centralization of capital, but also enormous centralization of political powers.

Unfortunately, we have now built into the global financial system an extraordinary dependency on war and organized crime. You have way too many people making money from helping other people fail, as opposed to making money on helping other people succeed.

I looked at the vaccine mandates from a different point of view because, for many years, I worked as an investment advisor. Many of my clients came to me because they had been touched by what I would describe as healthcare fraud, a lot of it associated with vaccinations. They had had their finances terribly harmed by vaccine injury and the cost of vaccine injury. A vaccine injury in a family can literally wipe out generations of savings; that can be very, very destructive.

I had spent a lot of time researching and trying to understand why we wanted to inject poisons and why pharmaceutical companies were being allowed to do so much harm with less and less liability over time. At one point, the chief financial officer at Moderna described the mRNA technology used in both Moderna and Pfizer - the gene therapy shots - as an operating system. I truly believe that there is a good possibility that those who orchestrated the pandemic believe that they can use gene and mRNA technology to install an operating system in all of us and use viruses to get us to update them just like we do on our computers.

Here's a good question: If throughout the G7 nations, you've promised retirement savings to several generations, if you've promised them health care and they're watching billionaires lead more and more luxurious lives, how are you going to inform them that you're going to abrogate your obligations to them? One solution is to put in a system of financial and physical controls, including using mind control technology to influence how they feel. So when the World Economic Forum says it's 2030 and you have no assets and you're happy, how are they going to make you feel happy when they've stripped you of your assets? It's all about control, which can be accomplished with digital technology.

On my website at Solari.com, go read an article called "I Want to Stop CBDCs—What Can I Do?" Number 11 action is "bring transparency." I list five of my favourite videos that show you what the central bankers say about what they're going to do with CBDCs and the extent of the control they will have.

There is a May 2020 speech by Richard Werner, who's the top academic scholar in the world on central banking, describing one of the top central bankers in Europe, explaining to him that CBDC would be a chip implanted put it in your hand. They are talking openly about chipping humans to make them compliant.

There is also Agustín Carstens, who was the general manager of the Bank of International Settlements [BIS], which is leading the global push for CBDC worldwide. What he explained in October 2020 at an IMF payment panel, was that they will be able to make the rules about how you use your money, and they will be able to control and enforce them centrally. It's the same as the Chinese social credit system. If you make the wrong post on the internet, then all of a sudden you can't take the subway to work in the morning scenario.

As bleak as this sounds, I'm optimistic because clearly our economy and our financial system need a reset. One of my favorite performance artists is Tina Turner and she starts one of her songs saying, "We can do this nice or rough." I would describe the current reset as rough. I can see why the people who run the system find their idea to be safer for them.

But I also think there are ways of doing a reset which can be much more market-oriented in solutions and much more decentralizing.

The problem with a decentralized reset, although it has the potential to create far more wealth than the current reset, is that it is going to require our system be governed by meritocracy. And it is going to require transparency. So if you look at the extraordinary secrecy that the governance system on the planet has enjoyed for the last 50 years, that secrecy is going to have to give way to transparency, to lead to more meritocracy.

Having really studied the economy from the bottom up, community by community, I know it is possible to do a reset that is much more wealth-building and can result in a very human society. What it's going to require is rejecting the current reset. That means, if you look at all the centralization that's occurring, the building of the smart grid, the creation of CBDCs, the institution of all the different digital payment system controls, we must just say "No." We are the people building the systems for our own enslavement in a digital concentration camp, and we must stop and pull out of the control grid.

We can throw out our smartphones, we can refuse to adopt the digital ID. If you saw what happened with vaccine passports, there was an extraordinary effort to not comply and not to adopt. Every one of us can say, "You know something? I don't want to be in the control grid and I don't want to help build the control grid and I'm going to back out."

There are lots of things to do to stop CBDCs. One of the simple things we love to recommend is that everybody uses cash. Let's walk back the digital systems and start to rebuild some health into the analog systems.

What we're watching in our networks is an explosion of people using cash and rebalancing and saying, "Well, wait a minute, a healthy system is part digital and part analog, let's rebuild and protect the analog because we need both."

The other thing you can do is start talking about local solutions. A healthy reset rebuilds our decentralized economy. Where are the opportunities to build great local relationships with other people? This could be in the realms of food, energy, shelter, alternatives both for bartering real assets but also making financial transactions locally without your national currency. And finally, where are the opportunities with your local and regional governance to start protecting sovereignty? If you can't protect it at a national level, there is a great deal you can do at a regional or local level.

At Solari.com an article by Richard Werner called "Why Tennessee Should Start a State Sovereign Bank," speaks to the idea of local banking, protecting local citizens and businesses. It could apply anywhere. There are hundreds of actions you can do to protect yourself and your family. Remember, each person who backs out of the control grid and becomes more free makes it easier for the rest of us. Start with you and your family by protecting yourself from the incremental steps. One of my favourite quotes is from Bobby Kennedy who says, "Nobody ever stopped tyranny by complying."

The middle of the road is going away. And you have the most powerful people in the world who want to centralize complete control. Throughout society they have allies who see it in their best interest to help them. Then we have the rest of us who are busy; we are raising kids, we are running businesses, we don't have time for politics. But now we are starting to realize, "Wait a minute, I can't stay in the middle of the road. The road is parting and I've got to go with freedom or I've got to go with slavery." Which is it going to be? We are all going to have to get involved because this is going to be trench warfare at our local and regional governments and national governments and we need to find our allies and do everything we can to protect our freedom.

We are talking about global fascism. Some people call it a technocracy, implementing control at an invasive level. I call entrainment technology and subliminal programming, a form of mind control technology. The ability to do surveillance on people's thoughts and inside their homes with all the different surveillance systems. We're talking about something much more high-tech and invasive than old-fashioned fascism. Fascism used force to control people physically, now you're talking about using invasive technology to brainwash them in ways that were inconceivable 20 years ago. It's akin to slavery.

I think there's a tremendous advantage in facing how absolutely dark we have allowed it to get and then proceed to say, "Okay, where do we go?" If you look at how centralized this is, it's what the English poet Shelley said, "They are few and we are many."

I would say two things; first, if you study the economy, one of the reasons for my profound optimism is words cannot express to you how expensive tyranny is. Our economy is so poor compared to what it could be if we were free to just optimize economically. The wealth potential of freedom combined with new technology, if we get the risk management right, is extraordinary. Second, centralizing this way is very destructive of wealth. I'm an investment banker, I love to create wealth, and the thought of building a society where you could let that wealth really grow is very exciting to me. I have a mathematically conceptual understanding of what is possible in terms of wealth creation. That's one of my reasons for optimism.

Tyranny is just fantastically expensive, as is secrecy. I mean, it's very profitable for the billionaires but it's very wealth-destroying.

One other thing is, I think the closer and closer the people running the centralized systems get to their end game, the more and more they're going to risk killing each other. They're not creating a culture, at least not a homogenous one. They're creating a very psychopathic environment and it's not the kind of culture that holds together through thick and thin over long periods of time. It's the antithesis of community.

The road ahead may be difficult, but there is power in numbers. If we resist building the control grid and encourage others to do the same, we can steer this reset toward a more decentralized, wealth-generating, and transparent system.

CHAPTER 29

'Trusting the Science' in an Era of Marketing-Based Medicine

Dr. Peter Parry

Associate Professor of Psychiatry

Dr. Peter Parry is an associate professor of psychiatry whose career encompasses that of a medical officer in the Royal Australian Navy, and GP and palliative care, prior to training in psychiatry from 1990. He was until recently a senior psychiatrist with Children's Health Queensland, a position terminated for not being able to conscientiously consent to a gene-based vaccine based on the information he was aware of (the principle of informed consent) and he currently works as a locum psychiatrist with private and interstate health services that recognise the protein-based vaccine Spikogen he received in a clinical trial and/or have dropped the mandates.

He has research and teaching interests in developmental psychology, lifestyle factors in mental health, the history and politics of psychiatric nosology, and conflict-of-interest issues between psychiatry-medicine and the pharmaceutical industry.

In recent decades, pharmaceutical vested interests extended their influence over medicine[1] at all levels: journals, research, academic institutions, guidelines committees, and clinical practice. Even though ethical well-intentioned professionals predominate, such systemic influence is insidious, starting with control of research data upon which Evidence-Based Medicine relies.

From January 2000 to March 2024, the pharmaceutical industry paid US$116 Billion in criminal fines[2] for felonies[3] such as off-label marketing, data suppression and 'kickbacks and bribery'.[4] This does not include vast sums in class action settlements[5] (including for the recent US opioid crisis[6]) to patients injured but insufficiently forewarned of adverse events. Data suppression has prevented clinicians from providing appropriate informed consent to patients. These billions of dollars are referred to as the cost of business, as pharmaceutical revenue over the same period exceeds US$20 trillion.[7] This is the era of Marketing-Based Medicine.[8]

In this global corporate context[9] modern medicine finds itself now cornered and ushered into narratives conducive to prescribing lucrative on-patent drugs and novel 'warp speed'-developed mRNAvaccines that bolster the industry's bottom line. 'Evidence-Based Medicine' has generally been reduced to what large randomised controlled trials (RCTs) find statistically significant. Only Big Pharma can afford to conduct them, outsourcing to contract clinical and contract research organisations[10] (CROs) which outsource data management to medical writing firms who ghost author[11] first drafts. Academic and clinical role authors for papers on the RCT often receive ghost-written drafts to edit for final manuscript submission to journals. For Big Pharma's big new RCTs these will be prestigious journals like *The New England Journal of Medicine (NEJM)* or *The Lancet.*

Even a little boy watching a naked emperor parade by can see the corruption such a scenario enables.[12] Although CROs and medical writing firms employ well-meaning people, 'who pays the piper calls the tune' still applies. Lack of transparent data[13] is the root rot infesting the whole tree of modern medicine and pharmacy. Articles[14] in the *British Medical Journal*[15] *(BMJ)* indicate this is not a fringe perspective. As I discovered in my doctoral research and have lectured on for years, substantial academic medical literature[16] contends that we cannot trust the academic medical literature.

One of the most cited papers in Medicine is titled 'Why most published research findings are false'.[17] The author John Ioannidis, professor of four faculties at Stanford University, Medicine, Epidemiology, Statistics, and Biomedical Data Science, argued this conclusion was due not only to flaws in statistical analyses and trial design, but inherent bias – from both favoured perspectives of researchers and commercial conflicts of interest.

Fellow of the Canadian Academy of Health Sciences emeritus professor Joel Lexchin and colleagues published in the *BMJ* a meta-analysis finding a four-fold odds ratio of a clinical trial finding favourable results for a drug if that trial was sponsored[18] by the pharmaceutical manufacturer, compared to an independent study of the same drug. Thus, peer-reviewed published research demonstrated that peer-reviewed industry-sponsored research literature cannot be trusted.

Chief-editors of major medical journals have addressed the commercial bias problem. Marcia Angell resigned as chief-editor of the *NEJM* to write what she had gleaned. Her book, *The Truth About the Drug Companies: How They Deceive Us and What to Do About It*[19] described the financial and persuasive marketing power of the pharmaceutical industry she witnessed at the helm of the *NEJM*. She noted the capture of academic medicine and the profession via corporate-sponsored research and medical education, and this capture extended to the agency charged with regulating the industry – the Food and Drugs Administration (FDA). Angell followed in *JAMA* with 'Industry sponsored research: a broken system',[20] and a 2009 media piece 'Drug Companies and Doctors: A Story of Corruption'.[21]

The *NEJM* is where Pfizer,[22] Moderna,[23] AstraZeneca,[24] Janssen[25] and Novavax[26] all published their COVID-19 vaccine clinical trial papers. The current editor-in-chief, Eric Rubin, was on the FDA's Vaccine & Related Biological Products Advisory Committee (VRBPAC), and as VRBPAC voted on 29 October 2021 approving Pfizer's COVID-19 vaccine for children,[27] he noted the risk of myocarditis stating, 'We're never gonna learn how safe the vaccine is until we start giving it.'

Richard Horton, chief-editor of *The Lancet* in an editorial 'How tainted has medicine become?'[28] answered his rhetorical question, 'heavily, and damagingly so.' He expanded on this in 'What is medicine's 5 sigma?',[29] referring to the physics standard for accepting a result as not due to chance being 5 standard deviations or 1 in 3.5 million. Medicine relies on a p (probability) value of 0.05 or 1 in 20 risk of chance and as Horton described, many factors can enable erroneous research over that low bar:

The case against science is straightforward: much of the scientific literature, perhaps half, may simply be untrue. Afflicted by studies with small sample sizes, tiny effects, invalid exploratory analyses, and flagrant conflicts of interest, together with an obsession for pursuing fashionable trends of dubious importance, science has taken a turn towards darkness.

Despite the chief-editor's sceptical eye, *The Lancet* suffered an egregious example of his description. 'Lancet-gate' refers to a large study from over 600 hospitals worldwide that purported to find hydroxychloroquine, a 60-year-old off-patent medication, had no benefit in COVID-19. But most patients did not exist. The study, largely fiction, was retracted.[30] The fraudulent data had been contrived by a CRO and writing company, Surgisphere.[31] The WHO halted all trials of hydroxychloroquine, only to do a 180-degree turnaround. However, a media narrative had damned hydroxychloroquine, which then posed no further risk to Marketing-Based Medicine.

It is a truism of Marketing-Based Medicine that off-patent drugs can threaten pharmaceutical industry profits from on-patent products. Former *BMJ* chief-editor Richard Smith titled a paper, 'Medical journals are an extension of the marketing arm of pharmaceutical companies'[32] where he noted RCT methodologies designed to disparage old off-patent competitor drugs.

Following hydroxychloroquine, another such competitor was ivermectin,[33] an antiparasitic with broad antimicrobial properties[34] whose discoverers won the 2015 Nobel Prize[35] in Medicine for ivermectin's safety and efficacy record. Although a review[36] indicated likely efficacy for COVID-19, ivermectin was disparaged by drug regulators and media as dangerous and ineffective. This website details all the studies on ivermectin for COVID-19[37], overwhelmingly positive but for a few large well-funded RCTs, which the website reviews[38] as having critical methodological flaws. The FDA appears to have conceded defeat in a legal settlement,[39] and ordered to withdraw all critical commentary[40] the agency made against ivermectin.

The TGA restricted ivermectin in September 2021;[41] one concern was its use could increase 'vaccine hesitancy' to the gene-based COVID-19 vaccines. Australian doctors lost practising licences over this. Getting a manuscript[42] reviewing favourable evidence for ivermectin's use in COVID-19 accepted in journals became nigh impossible.

A Pittsburgh and Carnegie-Mellon university-funded survey[43] in early 2021 found 'vaccine hesitancy' towards the lipid-nanoparticle encased modified mRNA (LNP-modRNA) and adenovectorDNA gene-therapy technologies used in Pfizer, Moderna, AstraZeneca and Janssen's COVID-19 vaccines was (in terms of education qualifications) highest among medical PhD holders for those with post-high school qualifications. In terms of occupation, paramedics with 45.6%[44] hesitancy were the highest among all healthcare workers.

In my case, having completed a PhD – 'Paediatric Bipolar Disorder': Why did it occur, the iatrogenic consequences, and the implications for medical ethics and psychiatric nosology[45] – on a pharmaceutical industry-funded academic child psychiatry-driven overdiagnosis epidemic of bipolar disorder in hundreds of thousands of prepubertal children including toddlers, where many children died of adult psychiatric medication regimes, I was a hesitant medical doctorate holder. As work colleagues were hospitalised shortly post-vaccine with myo-pericarditis my hesitancy increased.

During my doctoral research, I coined the term 'Marketing-Based Medicine' in a 2010 paper, 'From Evidence-Based Medicine to Marketing-Based Medicine: Evidence from internal industry documents'.[46] In the wake of multiple Big Pharma corruption 'of ' medicine scandals,[47] legal discovery exposed internal company documents disclosing data suppression and manipulation. My co-author and I read over 400 documents concerning antipsychotic and antidepressant medications from six major pharmaceutical companies. I recall a journey of cognitive dissonance through shock and outrage as to the level of systematic fraud. I have lectured on these documents for 15 years; a 2014 version is onYouTube;[48] more documents are compiled at this webpage,[49] and the UCSF library has a large Drug Industry Documents Archive[50] (DIDA).

I had not always been so sceptical. As a GP straight from a mid-1980s three-year stint as a medical officer in the Royal Australian Navy, I was keen to see pharmaceutical sales representatives who could tell me about medications for geriatric and paediatric patients I'd not experienced during Navy service. As well as accruing free pens, notepads, and coffee mugs, I was likely being profiled by pharmaceutical companies[51] for marketing strategies.

I believed, erroneously like the majority of clinicians,[52] I would see through any marketing spin and glean important information to save me reading time.

To some extent I possibly did, but I was naïve and likely fooled on several points but with no way to know which. That realisation grew early in my career as a child and adolescent psychiatrist in a tertiary referral mood-disorders clinic for young people. I was confronted by clear cases of selective serotonin reuptake inhibitor (SSRI) antidepressant-induced agitation and suicidality in adolescent and young adult patients.

Initially the marketing narrative was that this exacerbation of suicidality was either a very rare side effect, or simply the underlying illness. While at times it probably was the depression, temporal proximity of agitation-akathisia[53] and increased suicidality to SSRI dose initiation, change and stoppage was often obvious, and not dissimilar to reports these days of serious adverse events to COVID-19 vaccines. A prominent NIH study of fluoxetine for adolescent depression[54] seemed to suggest safety, but our letter to the *BMJ*[55] outlined methodological flaws obscuring suicidality. By 2004 under pressure of compelling case reports from clinicians and bereaved parents, the FDA issued a black box warning[56] label that this adverse event was indeed real. SSRIs have not met their marketing hype[57] though can be effective for high anxiety and severe depression. Informed consent and judicious prescribing on a risk-benefit basis particularly in young people remains, and evidence supports the black box labelling.[58]

GlaxoSmithKline (GSK) was convicted of data fraud that included its SSRI drug paroxetine in two GSK (formerly SmithKlineBeecham SKB) RCTs for adolescents with depression: studies 329 and377. Internal SKB/GSK documents[59] revealed the company suppressed study 377 where paroxetine' failed [to] demonstrate any separation of Seroxat/Paxil [paroxetine] from placebo', and cherry-picked secondary endpoint data in study 329 which 'failed to demonstrate a statistically significant difference from placebo on the primary efficacy measures'. These secondary data were published in 2001[60] in *The Journal of the American Academy of Child & Adolescent Psychiatry (JAACAP)*, touting paroxetine as 'generally well tolerated and effective'.

However, following a US$3 billion fine, as a sign of goodwill, GSK allowed restricted access to raw data from study 329[61] to an independent group of researchers; several of these I knew and could follow their work. In 2015 these independent researchers published their analysis of the study 329 RCT data in the *BMJ*.[62] Key findings were that paroxetine showed 'increased harms' (specifically a four-fold increase in suicidality) and 'no efficacy'.

RCT studies summarise data in clinical study reports (CSRs) that are submitted to regulators such as the FDA and from which data are extracted to write manuscripts to submit to peer-reviewed journals. Raw participant level data are held in the form of case report forms (CRFs). The hidden paroxetine suicidality data were in the CRFs – normally not shared with regulators like FDA and TGA, named authors, peer-reviewers and editors of journals.

The *JAACAP* has declined repeated calls to retract or correct[63] the RCT paper. Thus, based on the same RCT data, two papers in prestigious peer-reviewed medical journals present contradictory results.

Something similar has happened with the Pfizer and Moderna mRNA vaccine RCTs published in *NEJM*. The papers claimed 95% and 94% 'efficacy in preventing COVID-19' and adverse events were 'similar in the vaccine and placebo groups'[64] and 'no [serious systemic] safety concerns were identified'.[65] Primarily because of these two papers, and similar RCTs in *NEJM* concerning the AstraZeneca, Janssen and Novavax RCTs, echoing what regulators say they saw of the data, governments instituted vaccine mandates, with significant economic and psychosocial consequences.[66]

However, both RCTs' summary data had been posted to www. clinicaltrials.gov website, a recommended practice to allow some degree of independent vetting, even though mainly CSR not CRF level data. An independent group of researchers including senior *BMJ* editor Peter Doshi analysed these Pfizer and Moderna RCT data and published on the safety data in the journal *Vaccine*, not as prestigious as *NEJM* but nonetheless the leading vaccinology journal. Their analysis found:

> Pfizer and Moderna mRNA COVID-19 vaccines were associated with an excess risk of serious adverse events of special interest of 10.1 and 15.1 per 10,000 vaccinated over placebo baselines of 17.6 and 42.2 (95 % CI −0.4 to 20.6 and −3.6 to 33.8), respectively. Combined, the mRNA vaccines were associated with an excess risk of serious adverse events of special interest of 12.5 per 10,000 vaccinated.

Doshi was involved in the *BMJ*'s editorship of GSK study 329 rewrite and was aware of the need for raw patient level data to truly know the safety risks. They concluded:

> Full transparency of the COVID-19 vaccine clinical trial data is needed to properly evaluate these questions. Unfortunately, as we approach 2 years after release of COVID-19 vaccines, participant level data remain inaccessible.

Aware that this data credibility issue applies to the COVID-19 vaccines, Doshi along with immediate past and current *BMJ* editors-in-chief Fiona Godlee and Kamran Abbasi published an editorial titled 'COVID-19 vaccines and treatments: we must have raw data, now'.

Access to the FDA's copies of the Pfizer and Moderna RCT data has been achieved by US court-ordered enforcement of a FOI request by Public Health and Medical Professionals for Transparency, and volunteers have started analysing and publishing these data. The FDA had made its EUA decision within weeks based on these data, but argued (unsuccessfully) in court for 75 years to release it to PHMPT. Such resistance to transparency adds weight to the questioning title of a *BMJ* article: 'From FDA to MHRA: are drug regulators for hire?'

A key Pfizer-FDA document showed voluntary reports of suspected adverse events collected by Pfizer between mRNA vaccine launch in December 2020 and end of February 2021 included 1,223 reports of fatal adverse events among 42,086 cases. Reports of serious adverse events to national pharmacovigilance databases like the US VAERS, Australian DAEN, UK Yellow Card and others, or to the WHO VigiAccess, all show gene-based COVID-19 vaccines suspected adverse events are orders of magnitude above normal antigen-based vaccines, including antigen-based COVID-19 vaccines. In the past, product market recall would have occurred. This has indeed now happened for adenovector-DNA vaccines AstraZeneca and Janssen, but not as yet for the mRNA vaccines. Could this relate to sunk cost investments in mRNA technology, or the Bill Gates statement about the ease and cheapness of mRNA manufacturing?

Ease and cost-efficiency are desirable, but ethically should not be prioritised above safety and efficacy.

The Vioxx scandal was a prominent medicinal product withdrawal for adverse events reasons, among around 500 such market recalls. The FDA approved Vioxx, an anti-inflammatory analgesic in 1999, based on Merck's data and *NEJM* RCT paper. Despite a paper in *JAMA* (like that in *Vaccine*) showing greater safety risk than the *NEJM* paper, the FDA only recalled Vioxx in 2004 after further data suppression of heart attacks exposed by an FDA scientist who published in *The Lancet* despite FDA pressure on *The Lancet* to reject the paper.

Estimates of global strokes and heart attacks were 160,000 per 10 million, and an estimated 80 million were prescribed Vioxx. Cardiovascular deaths were around 60,000 in the USA although only 6,638 were reported to the FAERS pharmacovigilance database (Figure 1). This like all other pharmacovigilance research indicates these databases have under-reporting biases, yet inexplicably regulators argue there has been over-reporting of COVID-19 mRNA and adenovector DNA vaccines, the TGA only affirming 14 (1.5%) of 1006 death reports.

Reported Deaths for Major Drug/Vaccine Recalls
(Data Obtained from VAERS and FAERS)

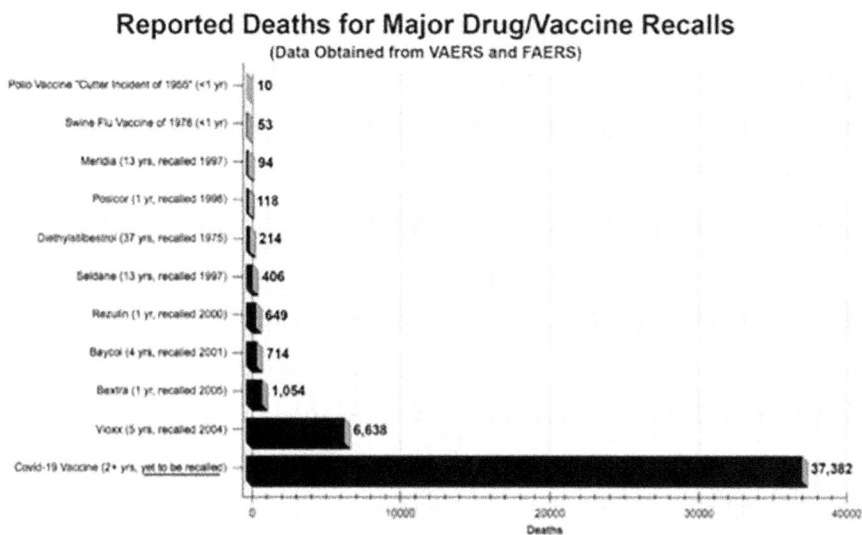

	Deaths
Polio Vaccine "Cutter Incident of 1955" (<1 yr)	10
Swine Flu Vaccine of 1976 (<1 yr)	53
Meridia (13 yrs, recalled 1997)	94
Posicor (1 yr, recalled 1998)	118
Diethylstilbestrol (37 yrs, recalled 1975)	214
Seldane (13 yrs, recalled 1997)	406
Rezulin (1 yr, recalled 2000)	649
Baycol (4 yrs, recalled 2001)	714
Bextra (1 yr, recalled 2005)	1,054
Vioxx (5 yrs, recalled 2004)	6,638
Covid-19 Vaccine (2+ yrs, yet to be recalled)	37,382

Figure 1. Major drug and vaccine recalls(FAERS & VAERS data).
As of 23 Feb 2024, www.vaersanalysis.info

Merck settled a class action and internal documents revealed plans to harass and silence dissenting doctors and scientists and create a fake journal touting Vioxx. In this pandemic, Merck has criticised its Nobel Prize winning but now financially worthless off-patent ivermectin, which could compete with its lucrative on-patent antiviral molnupiravir.

Similar to the *NEJM* RCT that failed to report three heart attacks on Vioxx, four subjects with serious adverse events were not reported in the *NEJM* COVID-19 vaccine RCT papers. These were: Augusto Roux (peri-myocarditis, hepatic injury; Pfizer); Brianne Dressen (chronic demyelinating polyneuropathy; AstraZeneca); Catherine Olivia Tesinar (shoulder inflammation, tendon rupture near injection site, axillary lymphadenopathy, neurological symptoms and rapid T-cell lymphoma; Moderna); and Maddie de Garay (neurological injuries including paralysis; Pfizer adolescent trial). The first three were excluded from the

RCTs and their adverse events were not recorded in the *NEJM* papers despite correspondence with the editor-in-chief; the fourth was recorded as 'functional abdominal pain'.

Roux and Dressen are co-authors of a peer-reviewed paper on their RCT experiences. Doshi in the *BMJ* reports FDA documents show that an inexplicable excess of Pfizer subjects over placebo subjects (311 v 60) were excluded. Roux claims he knew another unreported exclusion with cardiac adverse effect; Tesinar says she knew another Moderna RCT participant with stroke. Could these exclusions include others? Doshi also noted out of approximately 22,000 in each of Pfizer and placebo arms, only 8 Pfizer and 162 placebo were PCR-positive participants (hence '95%' effective) but over 3,000 other participants had COVID-like symptoms, and PCR false negatives could have skewed the efficacy rate downwards.

Brook Jackson, trial site manager for a CRO running one of Pfizer's RCT trial sites, along with two anonymous whistleblowers informed the *BMJ* of serious irregularities including unblinding of whether participants received Pfizer or placebo. She was sacked by her CRO soon after reporting the irregularities to the FDA. Whether such unblinding relates to the imbalance in exclusions is an unanswered question.

The *NEJM* is the most prestigious medical journal, but dependent on pharmaceutical industry funding. An opinion paper in a medical ethics journal argued that the *NEJM's* 'commercial conflict of interest' influenced its handling of the Vioxx RCT paper for which Merck paid $697,000 US for preprints. The author concluded:

> Indeed, as the Vioxx scandal illustrates, the stakes are too high to either downplay or turn a blind eye to the problem of commercial COI. What is disconcerting is that the conditions that gave rise to the Vioxx scandal remain intact.

The AllTrials campaign, led by the *BMJ* and other eminent British medical institutions, sought to bring transparency and honesty back to medical research. This was so we could truly trust it when a clinical trial published in a medical journal proclaimed a medicine 'safe and effective'. Following scandals like study 329 and Vioxx, AllTrials had momentum, garnering signature support from over 700 medical organisations and colleges, including our own RANZCP after a group of us lobbied it in 2014-2015. Unfortunately, AllTrials appears to have run out of steam, and has not updated since the start of COVID.

As there is dissipation of the mass fear and group-think from the COVID pandemic, magnified via media and social media strategies coordinated by the Trusted News Initiative and psychological strategies from 'nudge units', more people are realising that Marketing-Based rather than Evidence-Based Medicine skewed our public health responses. This realisation can reinvigorate the goals of something like AllTrials towards true patient-level (with privacy protections) RCT data transparency. Only then does Evidence-Based Medicine have a chance, resulting in true informed consent on risk and safety decisions for all clinicians and patients, as well as properly informed public health directives.

Key References

Angell, M. *Industry-sponsored research: a broken system. Journal of the American Medical Association* 2008, 300 (9), 1069-1071. DOI: 10.1001/jama.300.9.1069.

Demasi, M. *From FDA to MHRA: are drug regulators for hire? BMJ* 2022, 377, o1538. DOI: 10.1136/bmj.o1538.

Doshi, P.; Dickersin, K.; Healy, D.; Vedula, S. S.; Jefferson, T. *Restoring invisible and abandoned trials: acall for people to publish the findings. BMJ* 2013, 346, f2865. DOI: 10.1136/bmj.f2865.

Doshi, P.; Godlee, F.; Abbasi, K. *COVID-19 vaccines and treatments: we must have raw data, now. BMJ* 2022, 376, o102. DOI: 10.1136/bmj.o102.

Fraiman, J.; Erviti, J.; Jones, M.; Greenland, S.; Whelan, P.; Kaplan, R. M.; Doshi, P. *Serious adverseevents of special interest following mRNA COVID-19 vaccination in randomized trials in adults. Vaccine* 2022, 40 (40), 5798-5805. DOI: 10.1016/j.vaccine.2022.08.036.

Healy, D.; Germán-Roux, A.; Dressen, B. *The coverage of medical injuries in company trial consentforms. International Journal of Risk and Safety in Medicine,* 2023; Vol. Pre-press, pp 1-8.

McDonald, C. I.; Parry, P. I.; Rhodes, P. *Economic and psychosocial impact of COVID-19 vaccine non-compliance amongst Australian healthcare workers. Journal of Psychiatry and Psychiatric Disorders* 2024, 8, 40-50.

Parry, P. I.; Lefringhausen, A.; Turni, C.; Neil, C. J.; Cosford, R.; Hudson, N. J.; Gillespie, J. *'Spikeopathy': COVID-19 spike protein is pathogenic, from both virus and vaccine mRNA. Biomedicines* 2023, 11 (8). DOI: 10.3390/biomedicines1108228.

Rhodes, P.; Parry, P. Gene-based *COVID-19 vaccines: Australian perspectives in a corporate and global context. Pathol Res Pract* 2024, 253, 155030. DOI: 10.1016/j.prp.2023.155030.

Scholkmann, F.; May, C. A. *COVID-19, post-acute COVID-19 syndrome (PACS, "long COVID") andpost-COVID-19 vaccination syndrome (PCVS, "post-COVIDvac-syndrome"): Similarities and differences. Pathol Res Pract* 2023, 246, 154497. DOI: 10.1016/j.prp.2023.154497.

Smith, R. *Medical journals are an extension of the marketing arm of pharmaceutical companies. PLoS Med* 2005, 2 (5). DOI: 10.1371/journal.pmed.0020138.

Spielmans, G. I.; Parry, P. I. From *Evidence-based Medicine to Marketing-based Medicine: Evidence from Internal Industry Documents. Journal of Bioethical Inquiry* 2010, 7 (1), 13-29. DOI: 10.1007/s11673-010-9208-8.

Thacker, P. D. COVID-19: *Researcher blows the whistle on data integrity issues in Pfizer's vaccine trial. BMJ* 2021, 375, n2635. DOI: 10.1136/bmj.n2635.

1 https://davidhealy.org/pharmageddon-is-the-story-of-a-tragedy/

2 https://violationtracker.goodjobsfirst.org/summary?major_industry_sum=pharmaceuticals

3 https://projects.propublica.org/graphics/bigpharma#:~:text=In%20the%20last%20few%20years,the%20 Food%2and%20Drug%20Administration.

4 https://violationtracker.goodjobsfirst.org/violation-tracker/-pfizer-inc-10

5 https://www.smh.com.au/world/merck-reaches-485-billion-dollar-vioxx-settlement-deal-20071110-197n.html

6 https://www.npr.org/2022/02/25/1082901958/opioid-settlement-johnson-26-billion

7 https://www.statista.com/statistics/263102/pharmaceutical-market-worldwide-revenue-since-2001/

8 https://www.croakey.org/evidence-based-medicine-or-marketing-based-medicine/

9 https://violationtracker.goodjobsfirst.org/summary?major_industry_sum=pharmaceuticals

10 https://guides.clarahealth.com/top-clinical-research-organizations/

11 https://www.ncbi.nlm.nih.gov/pmc/articles/PMC3190555/

12 https://www.center4research.org/ghostbusting-exposing-drug-company-hired-ghostwriters-medical-journals/

13 https://www.alltrials.net/find-out-more/why-this-matters/

14 https://www.bmj.com/content/346/bmj.f2865

15 https://www.bmj.com/content/345/bmj.e7303

16 https://journals.plos.org/plosmedicine/article?id=10.1371/journal.pmed.0050217

17 https://journals.plos.org/plosmedicine/article?id=10.1371/journal.pmed.0020124

18 https://www.bmj.com/content/326/7400/1167

19 https://www.ncbi.nlm.nih.gov/pmc/articles/PMC521592/

20 https://jamanetwork.com/journals/jama/article-abstract/182478

21 https://www.nybooks.com/articles/2009/01/15/drug-companies-doctorsa-story-of-corruption/

22 https://www.nejm.org/doi/full/10.1056/nejmoa2034577

23 https://www.nejm.org/doi/full/10.1056/nejmoa2035389

24 https://www.nejm.org/doi/full/10.1056/NEJMoa2105290

25 https://www.nejm.org/doi/full/10.1056/NEJMoa2101544

26 https://www.nejm.org/doi/full/10.1056/NEJMoa2107659

27 https://www.theepochtimes.com/health/fda-adviser-explains-why-he-abstained-from-vote-on-pfizers-covid- 19-vaccine-for-young-children-4074913

28 https://www.thelancet.com/journals/lancet/article/PIIS0140-6736(02)08198-9/fulltext

29 https://www.thelancet.com/journals/lancet/article/PIIS0140-6736(15)60696-1/fulltext

30 https://www.thelancet.com/journals/lancet/article/PIIS0140-6736(20)31324-6/fulltext

31 https://www.theguardian.com/world/surgisphere

32 https://journals.plos.org/plosmedicine/article/info:doi/10.1371/journal.pmed.0020138

33 https://www.nature.com/articles/ja201711

34 https://www.sciencedirect.com/science/article/pii/S0168365920305800?via%3Dihub

35 https://link.springer.com/article/10.1186/s40249-015-0091-8

36 https://www.sciencedirect.com/science/article/pii/S2052297521000883?via%3Dihub

37 https://c19ivm.org/

38 https://c19ivm.org/meta.html

39 https://www.courthousenews.com/fifth-circuit-sides-with-ivermectin-prescribing-doctors-in-their-quarrel- with-the-fda/

40 https://covid19criticalcare.com/wp-content/uploads/2024/03/Stipulation-of-Dismissal.pdf

41 https://www.tga.gov.au/news/media-releases/new-restrictions-prescribing-ivermectin-covid-19

42 https://www.drphilipmorris.com/repurposed-drugs-to-treat-covid-19-ivermectin/

43 https://www.medrxiv.org/content/10.1101/2021.07.20.21260795v2.article-info

44 https://www.sciencedirect.com/science/article/pii/S221133552100259X?via%3Dihub

45 https://theses.flinders.edu.au/view/e8c15152-a279-4e61-88ce-e96080a908da/1

46 https://www.researchgate.net/publication/225663511_From_Evidence-Based_Medicine_to_Market- ing-Based_Medicine_Evidence_from_Internal_Industry_Documents

47 https://www.enjuris.com/blog/resources/largest-pharmaceutical-settlements-lawsuits/

48 https://www.youtube.com/watch?v=AXS_oiEzeTw&t=2s

49 https://www.healthyskepticism.org/global/news/int/hsin2009-12

50 https://www.industrydocuments.ucsf.edu/drug/

51 https://www.acpjournals.org/doi/10.7326/0003-4819-146-10-200705150-00008

52 https://link.springer.com/article/10.1007/s11606-009-0989-6

53 https://rxisk.org/akathisia/

54 https://jamanetwork.com/journals/jama/fullarticle/199274

55 https://www.ncbi.nlm.nih.gov/pmc/articles/PMC534889/

56 https://antidepressantsfacts.com/2004-10-15-FDA-Black-Box-SSRIs-suicide.htm

57 https://www.mja.com.au/journal/2016/204/9/unfulfilled-promise-antidepressant-medications

58 https://www.frontiersin.org/journals/psychiatry/articles/10.3389/fpsyt.2020.00018/full

59 https://www.industrydocuments.ucsf.edu/docs/#id=xrfw0217

60 https://www.jaacap.org/article/S0890-8567(09)60309-9/abstract

61 https://study329.org/

62 https://www.bmj.com/content/351/bmj.h4320

63 https://study329.org/request-to-retract-study-329/

64 https://www.nejm.org/doi/full/10.1056/NEJMoa2034577

65 https://www.nejm.org/doi/full/10.1056/NEJMoa2035389

66 https://www.fortunejournals.com/articles/economic-and-psychosocial-impact-of-covid19-vaccine-noncom- pliance-amongst-australian-healthcare-workers.html

CHAPTER 30

Pandemic Free Future

Professor Ian Brighthope

Physician and Agricultural Scientist

Professor Ian Brighthope graduated in Agricultural Science in 1965 and then in 1974 graduated with a Bachelor of Medicine and Bachelor of Surgery. As founding president of Australasian College of Nutritional and Environmental Medicine (ACNEM) and president for over 26 years.

The Brighthope clinics Biocentres Australasia were developed in the 1970's. They specialised in Nutritional Medicine, Environmental Medicine and intravenous therapies for acute and chronic medical and psychiatric conditions. Professor Brighthope has acted as an advocate for doctors practicing Integrative Medicine for over 42 years. He has had training and extensive experience in Crisis Management, Risk Management and Public/Government Relations. He has also had extensive experience in the pharmaceutical manufacturing and exporting industry as the managing director of a TGA licensed natural products manufacturing facility. He is no longer directly involved in the industry.

Professor Brighthope has consistently spoken about how seriously unprepared and uninformed we, as a global species, are regarding epidemics and pandemics. In late February 2020, with the advent of SARS-COV-2, the COVID-19 pandemic had been affecting countries around the globe. Professor Brighthope realised that there would be a need for people to improve their state of health and increase their resistance to this new and novel coronavirus. From previous experiences with SARS-COV-1, Bird Flu and Swine Flu, and based on the scientific literature, he initiated a prophylactic and treatment protocol titled "The CD Zinc Campaign". It consisted of the use of vitamin C, vitamin D and Zinc as oral supplements and the use of high dose vitamin D for deficiency states and high dose intravenous vitamin C for acutely and severely ill patients, either as outpatients or inpatients.

Nutritional medicine could save hundreds of millions of lives and create new wealth for the globe. The world will be free of future pandemics only when we come to the understanding that the known scientific fundamentals have not been applied to the pandemic of SARS-CoV2 (COVID-19) and we react positively. Whilst the social distancing, hygiene, testing, tracking and tracing have not been effective, this approach is a reflection of the failure to plan and manage infectious disease. Waiting and hoping for effective, safe vaccines and antiviral drugs is farcical. The question must be asked 'are we going to continue to wait for vaccines and drugs when the next, and possibly highly lethal viral pandemic strikes?'

Currently, the innate strength of the human immune system is completely ignored. It is the most powerful defence we all have against Coronaviruses and every other pathogenic microbe.The function of the immune system depends mostly on the individual's nutritional status and genetic makeup. It's the basic building blocks of amino acids, fatty acids, vitamins, mineral and trace elements that determine how powerful the immune system will respond to an infectious agent such as a virus, bacteria or fungus. Any deficiency or imbalance of a single nutrient will weaken the response and permit invasion, infection, multiple organ damage, severe disease and death.

Doctors practicing nutritional medicine understand how important diet, nutritional supplementation and the elimination of excesses such as sugar, alcohol and saturated fats are to preventing most diseases. For decades now, nutritional medicine (NM) experts have been quietly defeating infectious diseases especially when orthodox medicine has failed. They have been successfully preventing and treating influenza, severe Herpes simplex I and II, coronavirus infections, intractable bacterial infections and pneumonia for over five decades using nutrients that are essential for improving the immune response and suppressing the viral load, including killing the viruses responsible.

The advent of COVID-19 saw panic, pandemonium, economic destruction and death. The world's health authorities failed to manage it. They should have had strategies of defence for individuals rather than the application of simple epidemiological tools. The scientific evidence and experience that NM has accumulated over the decades has been and still is, completely ignored. Practitioners of NM have universally attempted to make the authorities aware of how powerful it is, but the preference of hoping and waiting for safe and effective vaccines and antivirals has dominated their thinking. Meanwhile, unnecessary deaths, sickness and destruction of social values has prevailed.

January 2020 saw the commencement of the 'CD-Zinc Campaign' in Australia, a campaign based on previous decades of experience. It consisted of public health recommendations for the entire population to take vitamins C and D and the trace element zinc, the most critical, effective, safe and readily available nutrients for optimal immunity and virus elimination.

The common cold and seasonal influenza are caused by respiratory viruses. Regular oral supplementation with vitamin C has been found to reduce the duration and severity of these illnesses in adults and children. Vitamin C deficiency results in impaired immunity and higher susceptibility to all infections. Also, infections have a significant impact on vitamin C levels due to enhanced inflammation and metabolic requirements. Supplementation with vitamin C both prevents and treats respiratory and systemic infections.

COVID-19 caused more serious conditions such as pneumonia, acute lung injury (ALI), acute respiratory distress syndrome (ARDS), septic shock and multiple organ failure. Some patients develop serious co-infections of bacteria and fungi. ARDS is characterised by severe low-blood oxygen, uncontrolled inflammation, oxidative damage and damage to the air sac barriers leading to death. Infections and sepsis cause the 'cytokine storm'. This leads to fluid accumulation in the airways. Increased oxidative stress is a key factor in pulmonary injury including ALI and ARDS.

Vitamin C has many functions for COVID-19 prevention and treatment. It can reduce the incidence and severity of bacterial and viral infections, it increases white blood cell activity which hinders the replication of viruses. It aids in the production of interferons, enhances killer and helper cell proliferation and increases antibody formation. It is a very powerful antioxidant that can protect cells and tissues. Its antiviral effects have been demonstrated in influenza, herpes viruses, pox viruses, coronaviruses and many other microorganisms. Vitamin C can ameliorate hyperoxia-induced ALI and attenuate hyperoxia-induced white blood cell dysfunction. Vitamin C prevents the cytokine surge damaging the lungs. It eliminates alveolar fluid by preventing the activation and accumulation of neutrophils, special white blood cells.

High dose intravenous Vitamin C (HDIVC) is instrumental in both early treatment and recovery from influenza and ARDS and other serious complications of acute viral infections. Patients on life support (ECMO) with a poor prognosis have been rapidly and successfully recovered using HDIVC, with no evidence of lung fibrosis . IV Vitamin C use in septic shock reduces mortality. It also reduces the length of stay in ICU and significantly shortens the duration of mechanical ventilation. HDIVC does not cause kidney stones or kidney damage, an excuse used by opponents to justify the routine refusal to use the treatment. A rare side effect is preventable; a breakdown of some of the red blood cells.

In March 2020, the Shanghai government announced its official recommendation that COVID-19 should be treated with high doses of IV Vitamin C. The experience of thousands of doctors around the world who have used HDIVC is that this molecule is one of the most powerful in virtually all human conditions, including physical and mental illnesses and trauma. It should be used as the treatment of first choice in every epidemic.

Vitamin D is the sunlight vitamin. When ultraviolet light falls on the skin, it manufactures a precursor of vitamin D that goes to the liver then kidneys to make active vitamin D; more accurately described as a hormone called calcitriol. Deficiency of vitamin D results in rickets in children, bone disease in adults such as osteoporosis and a greatly weakened immune system. Cod liver oil is a rich source of vitamin D. It was used extensively for children in the past during the winter to protect against colds and the 'flu. This 'sunlight' vitamin is essential for strong immunity in virtually every instance in which the immune system is called into action, including infections, some cancers if not all, neurological diseases and diabetes.

Lack of exposure to sunlight in winter increases the prevalence of vitamin D deficiency. The seasonal decrease in vitamin D deficiency amplifies the risk from respiratory viruses, including the COVID-19 coronavirus.

A large number of clinical trials of vitamin D supplementation for the prevention of acute respiratory tract infections have been conducted over the last 2 decades. Hundreds of randomised controlled trials and many meta-analyses have shown an overall protective effect of vitamin D supplementation against acute respiratory tract infections including influenza and coronaviruses. In fact, the benefits are greater in those receiving daily vitamin D than the benefits from influenza vaccination. The protective effects against acute respiratory tract infections are strongest in those with high levels of vitamin D. However, even those with low levels have greater protection when supplemented.

People with vitamin D deficiency are much more likely to suffer serious outcomes and death from exposure to respiratory viruses than people with optimal vitamin D levels. In particular, elderly people, especially those in aged-care, are at risk from the consequences of vitamin D deficiency, unless given adequate vitamin D supplementation to maintain optimal levels. Others who cannot manufacture enough include people of colour, people restricted to indoors, the obese, diabetics and others with chronic diseases.

The Nordic countries have public health policies for vitamin D supplementation and food fortification. They also have among the lowest mortality rates attributed to the SARS –COV2 coronavirus.

Thus, vitamin D adequacy in the general population resulted in much lower mortality. Countries that do not have any public health policy of vitamin D supplementation in winter and spring create at-risk groups for viral respiratory infections. Accordingly, further surges in cases and deaths from influenza-like viruses including COVID-19 occur. Public health programmes of vitamin D supplementation protect elderly people and healthcare workers from serious illness and death and allow for much less severe lockdowns and much less economic hardship. In fact overall, supplementation leads to greater productivity and economic gains.

Vitamin D supplementation is extremely safe, effective, cheap and readily available. No toxicity has been reported with doses of 10,000 IU or less per day. The myriad of mechanisms of action of vitamin D are understood. In fact, it has now been reclassified as a hormone (Calcitriol). Logically, if that is the case, then routine testing of people at risk of insufficiency and deficiency states should be conducted. If the level of hormone D (calcitriol) is low, it should be medically corrected with supplementation, just as is done with insulin for diabetes and thyroid hormone in hypothyroidism. Imagine if vitamin D was a drug with such a profound range of effects, it would be prescribed extensively by the medical profession. Doctors would be falling over one another to prescribe it.

The immediate introduction of public health measures to improve vitamin D status globally is essential, particularly in settings where insufficient levels and profound vitamin D deficiency is common. Unfortunately, because it has properties enabling it to successfully compete with vaccines and antivirals, the world's medical health authorities prefer to ignore it.

Finally, to zinc, a critical trace element in the fight against COVID-19 and future pandemics. It plays a fundamental role in protecting us against invaders. It is like the moat, turrets, gates and locks to the fort. Without it we are completely unprotected. Zinc creates killer mucous lining our airways from the nose to the airway's final passages and air sacs. It holds our lining cells together. Without zinc, our white cells cannot produce adequate antibodies and our genes cannot express and repair themselves from any viral onslaught. It has been shown to be effective in COVID-19, as have vitamins C and D.

There is absolutely every reason for the global health authorities to execute a CD-Zinc supplementation world-wide program. There is no excuse to deny the people of the world this cheap, readily available scientifically proven approach and to be pandemic and pandemonium free. We cannot wait for the medical profession's leaders to switch from drugs and vaccines to nutraceuticals when the extensive global experience around the current nutraceutical science is proof. We cannot wait and watch the bodies drop.

'Discovery consists of seeing what everybody has seen and think what nobody else has thought' (Albert Szent-Gyorgyi, the discoverer of vitamin C)

Having mentioned my preference for the best of health care, I cannot avoid the subject of vaccination to achieve induced immunity. Therefore I will attempt to restate the key facts about vaccination in a neutral tone. Vaccines are a diverse class of medicines, with some being slightly effective but unsafe, while others have proven defective or unsafe. It is seriously inaccurate to claim all vaccines are categorically "safe and effective."

Historically, most vaccines have demonstrated toxicity and caused harm through various mechanisms like contamination, unintended immune responses, contracting the targeted disease from the vaccine itself, or unknown causes, probably hyper-oxidation reactions.

Vaccine manufacturers have immunity from product liability lawsuits, based on government authorities recognising vaccines as "unavoidably unsafe" products. Since 1986, the number of vaccines on the childhood/adolescent schedules has increased from 7 to 21 in 2023. Only a minority of vaccines on the current schedule, like measles and chickenpox, are capable of providing herd immunity, albeit controversial. No vaccines can justify population-wide mandates.

The pharmaceutical industry wields enormous influence through lobbying, advertising to the medical profession, funding medical groups, and incentivising and rewarding doctors. The COVID-19 mRNA vaccines underwent less testing than usual, were authorised initially on shaky grounds, for emergency use only, utilised a new technology platform, and have generated high rates of reported deaths and adverse events compared to traditional vaccines. Yet they were quickly added to the childhood schedule.

Extremely high numbers of reported deaths and adverse events from COVID-19 vaccines have not been systematically accounted for by health authorities, who continue to strongly promote these products.

Calling the mRNA shots "vaccines" has broadened the definition of a vaccine, potentially shielding manufacturers from liability to an unprecedented degree.

Vaccine mandates can compel medical interventions, classified by law as "unavoidably unsafe," from manufacturers with liability protections, which have been proven to be anything but "safe and effective." Hence I argue for reevaluating the central dogma that all vaccines are fundamentally "safe and effective," and propose reforms to repeal liability protections, prohibit all mandates, and investigate all vaccines thoroughly. We remain ignorant while the drug and vaccine companies are profiteering. As such, we become sicker, weaker and poorer.

In the meantime, we have the CD and Zinc protocol.

Ensuring that new governments prioritise public health over corporate interests requires a multifaceted approach that includes policy reforms, transparency, accountability, and active engagement with civil society. Transparency and accountability are crucial for ensuring that public health policies are not influenced at all by corporate interests. Governments should adopt mechanisms to enhance transparency in decision-making processes and hold officials accountable for their actions. Implementing mandatory disclosure of financial and other conflicts of interest for policymakers and public health officials can help identify and remove these individuals from public office and positions of influence.

Ensuring that data related to public health policies, funding, and decision- making processes are publicly accessible will foster transparency and allow for independent scrutiny. Civil society organizations (CSOs) and non-government organisations (NGOs) play a critical role in advocating for public health and holding governments accountable. To enhance their impact, governments should institutionalize the involvement of CSOs in health policy-making processes, ensuring that their input is considered at all stages, from agenda-setting to implementation and evaluation.

Providing resources and training to CSOs and NGOs can enhance their ability to effectively advocate for public health and monitor government actions. Governments should establish and enforce regulatory frameworks that prohibit corporate influence on public health policies. The removal of the profit incentive for all individuals and corporations is the only way we can eliminate the influence of cartels and cowboys.

Implementing regulations to cease the lobbying activities and political donations from corporations will stop their ability to sway public health policies in their favour. Ensuring that public health policies are based on independent research and evidence is essential.Governments shall allocate funding for independent public health research and eliminate reliance on industry-funded studies, which are definitely biased until proven otherwise. Also, policies should be grounded in robust scientific, medical and natural health evidence with mechanisms in place to regularly review and update them based on the latest research findings. Anecdotal evidence must play a first ranking position in all individualized health care decisions.

International collaboration can help set global standards and best practices for public health governance. Governments should adopt and implement international frameworks outside any private-public organization such as the WHO. The Australian government of the future will not support the WHO and argue that there are cheaper and better systems for world health and peace. Engaging in local-global health partnerships can provide access to resources, expertise, and support for implementing effective true public health and medical care policies. These are already well established as a consequence of the catastrophic failure of the WHO COVID crisis.

Raising public awareness about the importance of prioritizing public natural health and medicine over corporate interests can build support for necessary reforms/replacements.Governments and CSOs should conduct public awareness campaigns to educate citizens about the impact of corporate influence on public health and the need for transparent and accountable governance. Mobilizing public support through advocacy efforts can pressure governments to adopt policies that prioritize public health.

By implementing these strategies, a new system of Australian governments can prioritize public health over corporate interests, ensuring that policies are designed and implemented in the best interest of the population. Transparency, accountability, civil society engagement, robust regulatory frameworks, independent research, international collaboration, and public advocacy are all essential components of this effort.

The future is ours to determine; not governments and corporations. Health and peace require work and passion.

CHAPTER 31

They Want One World; Dictated by Bureaucrats and Elites

Dr. Kat Lindley

Family Physician

Dr. Kat Lindley is a board-certified family physician with a direct primary care practice in Brock, Texas. She became a family physician because she loved caring for and seeing the family grow. Later in her career, she became interested in helping find solutions to improving the overall healthcare system at the State and federal levels. Doctor Lindley is the President and co-founder of the Global Health Project and Director of the FLCCC International Fellows program. She is also the Past President of the Texas Osteopathic Medical Association and Texas American Academy of Osteopathic Family Physicians. She has been involved in healthcare policy since 2015 and is a passionate advocate for her profession, patients, and children. Her recent work focuses on restoring trust in medicine and highlighting the dangers of globalism and global governance by the World Health Organization and the United Nations.

I was born in Split (in my eyes, one of the most beautiful places in the world), on the Dalmatian coast, in a small country called Croatia. I grew up under the communist rule of Josip Broz Tito, and as life would have it, our region of the world found itself at war again in the early 90s. Just as the Balkan war started, I left for Italy aged 18 and lived there for several years, working as a nanny. Eventually, I found my way to the States, where I went to college and became a physician. My life has been the ultimate testament of what the American dream represents.

I still remember clearly the day I became an American citizen in 2004. This country of ours founded on the shoulders of giants has stood proudly as the ultimate beacon of hope for people like myself who have lived through tyrannies.

The COVID era has exposed the global agendas and has cracked open the false belief that we are a free nation under God. As many of us have been censored and some lost their jobs due to mandates and coercive policies, I often think of the words of Ben Franklin when he was asked after the convention what they had decided. His words are etched in my mind. "The Republic if you can keep it." And the question is, "can we?" This is one of the reasons I have been very vocal about the World Health Organization, United Nations, WEF, and world events. The lockstep march towards globalism had me concerned early on.

This idea of "global governance" has been insidiously introduced into our society. An example often ignored is the European Union. The EU was formed in 1993 and it seemed that everyone was excited about creating this Europe-centric union of nations working together for the betterment of its people. Over time, as the EU became governed by bureaucrats instead of the nations' representatives, it became clear that the EU's priorities had changed. As bureaucrats continued to gain more power, they started erasing nations' national pride and identity and replaced it with the Euro, EU values and goals, no borders, etc. By accepting their values, member states have allowed bureaucrats to dictate to member nations what their country should be like according to the EU, instead of what it should be according to their history and values.

One must wonder why there is a big push toward global governance, not only in the EU, but around the world. As I write these words, the United Nations and its 193 member states have agreed and signed the Pact for the Future. As per AP News, "The 42-page "Pact of the Future" challenges leaders of the 193 U.N. member nations to turn promises into real actions that make a difference to the lives of the world's more than 8 billion people. The pact was adopted at the opening of the two-day "Summit of the Future" called by U.N. Secretary-General Antonio Guterres, who thanked leaders and diplomats for taking the first steps and unlocking "the door" to a better future. "We are here to bring multilateralism back from the brink," he said. "Now, it is our common destiny to walk through it. That demands not just agreement, but action."

According to the UN, global governance would allow a coordinated, controlled approach to solving shared problems: pandemics, wars, and financial crises. The question that needs to be answered is, who would lead the charge? The United Nations, the World Economic Forum, or the Council for Foreign Relations? How would they accomplish this?

With the Pact for the Future, is the UN trying to create "the one world government"? Do sovereign nations need a Pact for the Future?

The Pact for the Future is a central initiative of the United Nations' Summit of the Future, which took place on September 22-23, 2024. This pact aims to redefine global governance and cooperation in response to contemporary and future challenges, including but not limited to climate change, pandemics, technological advancements, and geopolitical tensions. It reaffirms commitments to existing frameworks like the Sustainable Development Goals (SDGs) and the United Nations Charter.

Key Components are:

1. Global Governance Reforms: There›s an emphasis on transforming global governance, including reforms in international financial architecture, new mechanisms for managing global crises, and a more integrated approach to global decision-making processes.

2. Sustainability and Climate Action: The pact is expected to turbocharge the implementation of the 2030 Agenda, focusing on sustainability in its environmental, economic, and social dimensions.

3. Technological and Digital Governance: Addressing the implications of digital technologies, artificial intelligence, and possibly the governance of outer space, aiming for a balanced approach that maximizes benefits while managing risks.

The most concerning policy brief is the Emergency Platform that would give the Secretary-General authority to "convene and operate an

Emergency Platform in the event of complex global crises," whether that be another pandemic, an environmental crisis, disruptions in global flows of goods, people, or finance, or some other "black swan" event. Under this platform, Guterres would be given "standing authority to convene and operationalize automatically an Emergency Platform" with minimal consultation from governments. What impact will the Pact have on continued censorship and surveillance? There's genuine concern that the Pact might encourage or legitimize forms of content regulation under the banner of combating misinformation or protecting public health, as seen with discussions around "chat control" laws in the EU. This could lead to broader censorship, where governments or large tech companies might suppress information or viewpoints deemed controversial or contrary to state interests, stifling free speech.

Each country will have to figure out its own path towards fighting this latest UN initiative. For the United States, we can do this in Congress by supporting and passing bills to abolish the UN. Also, by using the 10th amendment, the individual states can pass legislation to protect their citizens from UN influence in each state. Ultimately the answer for all 193 UN member states is to defund and exit once and for all.

They want **"global governance."** They want **control**. They want **One World** dictated by the elites and bureaucrats, with the loss of national identity, pride, and eventually individualism. They do not like the power of one person, the power of nations and people, because they realize our strength is knowing who we are and who we want to be. That will be their downfall. The arrogance to think they know what we want.

We do not need global governance and a one-world government: **Remember. Exult (be proud). Reclaim.**

Remember our history, **be proud** of who you are, cut ties with the EU, the United Nations, the WHO, the WEF, etc, as they are simply supranational, unrepresentative, corrupt entities trying to control your destiny. **Reclaim** your future.

Choose your family and friends, love your country, and care for your children's future.

We are the 8 billion, and we say NO!

NO to censorship.

NO to tyranny.

NO to globalism.

CHAPTER 32

National Citizens Inquiry – A Light on the Hill

Shawn Buckley

Constitutional lawyer and founder
of the National Citizens Inquiry in Canada.

Shawn Buckley is a constitutional lawyer who has spent the last 30 years of practice defending the constitutional rights of Canadians. He has spent his career trying to stop the constant erosion of our rights. Mr. Buckley is a founding member of the National Citizens Inquiry. He is the lead counsel for the NCI and is dedicated to establishing ongoing hearings to bring truth to Canadians.

In his 30 years of practising law Mr. Buckley has defended more natural health companies in Court than any other Canadian lawyer. He has an enviable track record in Court against Health Canada charges. Outside of Court Mr. Buckley has assisted natural health companies and practitioners to navigate and deal with Health Canada.

We have now had a couple of years without lockdowns, without mask mandates, without having to show our identity papers (vaccine passports) and without the media viciously dividing the 'vaxxed' against the 'unvaxxed'. If Canada was a person, she would be in the denial phase of the grieving process. Canadians are trying to pretend the madness of the past four years did not happen. Unfortunately this will not work. The COVID experience runs deeper than we are wanting to accept.

At two lectures I gave in Alberta in the Spring of 2023, I asked the audiences to put up their hand if, in the middle of the dark days, they honestly believed that the army would be going door-to-door dragging 'unvaxxed' people out of their homes and forcefully injecting them against their will. Almost every arm went up. How does a Nation recover from this level of tyranny? How did the citizens respond when this level of coercion was happening?

Sadly, most of the citizens participated enthusiastically with the lockdowns, the police state ritual of needing identity papers, the masking, and the division. Anyone who spoke out against the mandates and measures was vilified and/or punished. Most of the nation was paralyzed with fear. And then the truckers stood up. Their courage in driving across the country and protesting in Ottawa changed history. They inspired a Nation by showing that we can stand up. They made many of us who were still acting in fear, ashamed. They inspired us to be better.

The truckers bought the nation a reprieve. We were not locked down the next Fall. In that reprieve a group of citizens banded together to create the **National Citizens Inquiry** (the "NCI"). The NCI is a citizen run, a citizen organized, and a citizen funded initiative. It has no major donors. It was and is almost exclusively volunteer. It was and is a miracle!

For three months from March - May 2023, the National Citizens Inquiry travelled across Canada, visiting 8 major cities and conducting three full days of hearings in each city, a total of 24 days. The hearings were conducted in the style of judicial hearings where four independent Commissioners heard the sworn testimonies from 305 witnesses. Witnesses ranged from world renowned experts in dozens of disciplines to everyday Canadians. The testimonies ranged across every aspect of Canadian society.

The listing of expert witnesses included: Drs Peter McCullough, Pierre Kory, Byram Bridle, Patrick Phillips, Laura Braden, Robert Malone, Mark Trozzi, Jessica Rose, Jay Bhattacharya, Francis Christian, Eric Payne, Chris Shaw, Charles Hoffe, Steve Pellech, Denis Rancourt, Daniel Nagase, Chris Shoemaker, Jordan Peterson, Lt. Col David Redman, Bruce Pardy, Catherine Austin Fitts and many more.

All witnesses were questioned by legal counsel and the Commissioners. The body of evidence collected was substantial - the largest collection of testimony given under oath in the world pertaining to the impact of the government's and other institutions' response to COVID. It is a formidable library of information that reveals the true effects of the government's measures on businesses, families, communities, individuals, economy, and health including social, economic, mental and spiritual well-being.

The principles guiding the NCI included:

1. **Independent**– The Inquiry must be truly independent. Inquiry Commissioners shall be selected on the basis of experience, competence, and credibility and not for any pre- conceived positions they might hold on the issues to be dealt with by the Inquiry.

2. **Citizen Supported**– The authority of the Inquiry must rest on a mandate received from significant numbers of Canadian citizens across the country who have made repeated calls for an independent and objective review of governments' pandemic measures. This mandate is to be further reinforced by such citizens adding their names to the Petition of Support for a National Citizens Inquiry provided on the Inquiry's website.

3. **Open and Transparent**– The Inquiry's investigation and related activities must be open and transparent, free of biases or preconceived conclusions.

4. **Truthful**– All persons participating in the Inquiry may only submit oral or written testimony under oath, dutifully sworn before a Commissioner of Oaths.

5. **Evidence Based**– The deliberations and conclusions of the Inquiry must be evidence based, with any and all testimony received (including that containing extreme claims and conspiratorial charges) being subject to cross examination. The submitted evidence for all arguments, claims, and/or positions shall be made publicly available through the Inquiry's website.

6. **Respectful**– The Inquiry shall insist that all participants exhibit mutual respect for the contrary opinions and positions of others, to facilitate reconciliation, rather than further polarize Canadians.

The objectives of the hearings were the following:

1. To inquire into and undertake dialogue with Canadians. To listen to Canadians concerning the impacts of government health and policy measures impacting their personal lives, including their physical and mental health, families and communities (particularly children and seniors), jobs and livelihoods, businesses, and their fundamental freedoms and civil liberties as guaranteed by the Constitution.

2. To invite Canadians to pose to the Inquiry any unanswered or unclear questions concerning COVID-19 and governments' responses thereto, and for the Inquiry to make all reasonable efforts to secure answers to those questions.

3. To receive and evaluate testimony from medical, legal, scientific, and other relevant experts concerning the governments' pandemic measures and strategy, what information was known or knowable by governments, and what alternative approaches could have been taken.

4. To receive and evaluate testimony from legacy and independent media to understand what information was known or knowable and why information was conveyed to the public as it was.

5. To invite input from healthcare officers and other governmental officials as to the rationale behind the health care protection measures adopted – including mandates, lockdowns, and similar orders and actions – and the strategies employed to secure public compliance.

6. To invite and secure testimony as to the appropriateness, efficacy, legality and constitutionality of governments' responses to COVID-19.

7. To investigate public sector expenditures, grants, and any other subsidies or financial support programs and their distribution related to the governmental responses to COVID-19.

8. To consider the issue of civic and criminal liability for any damages or harms caused by governments' response to COVID-19.

9. To make publicly available to Canadians all findings, submissions, and testimonies certified by and formally presented through the Inquiry.

10. To identify any mistakes, negative impacts, or mismanagement that the Inquiry may determine have occurred and, if it does so, to recommend appropriate measures for more appropriate and effective government responses in the future.

The Truth is Out There

The Government and mainstream media messaging during COVID was exhausting in both its uniformity and prevalence. Phrases like *"follow the science"* and *"safe and effective"* were drilled into us. Contrary narratives were heavily censored.

The testimony at the NCI was shocking in countering the "official truth" of Governments and the mainstream media. Anyone who watches all 24 days of hearings will conclude they have been lied to by the Government and the media.

Ted Kuntz, Chair of the National Citizens Inquiry, summed it up this way in his closing remarks to the hearings held in Regina, Saskatchewan on May 30, 31 and June 1, 2024. Kuntz stated – *"There are two groups of people in the world. Those who want to know the truth, and those who don't. And those who want us to know the truth, and those who don't."* Kuntz also stated that what we are engaged in is primarily an invisible war, and what the NCI does is *"make the invisible visible"*.

People are visibly shaken by the testimony delivered at the NCI. The disconnect between the government's mantra of *"safe and effective"* and the reality of vaccine injury and death, medical malfeasance, and outright deception is deeply disturbing. The testimony underscores that we cannot trust our governments, health agencies and media to tell us the truth. This deception ruptures, possibly beyond repair, the trust in our institutions. Without trust, our society will fail.

Not a single institution stood against the monolithic Government and media narrative. Governments infringed on our rights more than they had during wartime. And yet, at the end of 2023, I was not aware of a single Court decision that would put a brake on any level of government from taking our rights away again.

Of particular note is that only one standing elected representative, of the many thousands across the country, responded to the request to testify before this citizen-led inquiry. Governments at every level refused to acknowledge the invitation to testify and justify their measures and mandates. Not one government body has formally acknowledged the NCI and its body of evidence in their legislative halls.

The silence of our governments and media is deafening. What should have been front page news and public debate in our legislatures has been systematically and intentionally ignored. A treasure trove of information and evidence is waiting for those with the courage and integrity to see and learn.

The inquiry revealed how those who stood up and defended fundamental rights and freedoms and adhered to ethical foundations as informed consent and bodily sovereignty were viciously attacked by their own regulatory agencies and oversight bodies. Doctors, nurses, scientists and others who saw through the lies and deceptions and revealed the real world consequences of the mandates and measures were hunted down and punished for their commitment to a moral code and evidence based response.

Similarly, those citizens who refused to take the vaccine were removed from their positions of employment and further punished by being denied unemployment benefits. Many lost their homes, marriages and social network. And many who did participate lost their health and their lives.

The Potential of the NCI

The evidence presented at the NCI has the potential to inform governments, media, regulatory agencies, health institutions and the public who want to understand the impact of the government's response to COVID. The library also serves in developing legal recourse against governments and other institutions who imposed and enforced mandates by identifying the impact and witnesses, both expert and lay, who can testify in lawful proceedings.

At the conclusion of the 2023 hearings, the Commissioners were tasked with preparing a comprehensive report which summarized what the inquiry did, what the witness testimonies revealed, and to make recommendations to prevent a repeat of the mistakes made during the COVID experience.

On November 28, 2023, in a virtual press conference the NCI Commissioners presented their final report titled: *"Inquiry into the Appropriateness and Efficacy of the COVID-19 Response in Canada"*. The result was an astonishing 5,342 page report, comprising 643 pages of in-depth analysis, discussion, and approximately 400 transformative recommendations, along with over 4699 pages of sworn witness testimony transcripts. The goal of the NCI was and is – **Listen, Learn, Recommend**.

Mini-reports have been developed which identify specific areas of focus and recommendations. Topics of the mini-reports include:

- Canada's Justice System
- Freedom of Expression
- Coercion does not equal consent
- Neglect and isolation of seniors
- Vaccine testing and authorization
- Undermining Democratic Institutions

More mini-reports are being developed.

The NCI witness testimony has been captured in hundreds of hours of video recordings and transcripts and is available for viewing on the NCI website. The testimony is searchable by location, date, and witness. An invitation is extended to those who have yet to experience the power of the NCI testimonies to select three testimonies at random and view them. The claim is – *You will never be the same*. And you will be challenged to stop at three testimonies.

The experience of a citizen-led, citizen funded inquiry into the actions of government and others has revealed the power of citizen engagement and accountability. Canadians now recognize that our governments and mainstream media are no longer reliable sources of truth, and that instruments of accountability independent of government funding and influence need to be established. As a consequence, the NCI is committed to serving in an on-going capacity. Additional hearings were held in 2024, and future hearings are being planned. The topic of inquiry is expanding beyond the government's response to COVID to other areas demanding accountability.

A Life Changing Experience

We had no idea when we began that we had set out to do something we could not do. We were a small group with no experience. We naively decided to hold 24 days of hearings in 8 cities in a short period of time and with no resources. Now I see the insanity of it. I also see God's hand in it. Time and time again the entire enterprise was on the verge of collapsing and then was saved at the last minute. As an example, at the Quebec City hearings we had no lawyers a week before the hearings. And then they appeared.

In 2023, many witnesses were afraid to testify. They were afraid of economic consequences. They were afraid of social consequences. They were afraid of losing privileges. Several backed out at the last minute. But many overcame their fear and shared their story. Their courage inspired us and the other witnesses. The fear was overcome.

When we were organizing the NCI I was expecting the hearings and witness testimony and was hopeful we could get Canadians to watch. I was not at all expecting what happened. We did hold hearings and had amazing testimony. But something else happened. We began to hear each other. We became a community again. The divisions faded. Starting with the Toronto hearings, anyone who watched a couple of full days (the full day videos, not the separate witness ones) will understand. We learned we are not alone. We learned we can overcome our fear. We learned we need to love each other. And we learned to be a proud community again.

Transcending Politics and Ideology

Within the pages of the NCI report lies a poignant and heartbreaking tapestry of stories from everyday Canadians. These testimonies offer a stark and unfiltered view of the profound and devastating impact that government actions had on Canadians from all walks of life. Their stories are not just statistics; they are the lived experiences of individuals who faced unimaginable challenges. They lost their jobs, their families, their communities, their health, their reputations, and tragically, many lost their lives.

These stories transcend politics and ideology; they resonate with the shared human experience of resilience in the face of adversity. The NCI report serves as a contemporary historical document, bearing witness to the trials and tribulations of our time. Its pages will undoubtedly be studied and remembered by generations to come. It is a testament to the power of citizen-led initiatives and the resilience of ordinary people striving to uphold democracy, transparency, and accountability. Their mission is a shining example of what can be achieved when concerned citizens come together with a shared purpose, and the enduring strength of the human spirit.

The implications of this inquiry go far beyond Canadian borders. In a world grappling with the challenges posed by ever occurring emergencies and increasing government overreach, the NCI's findings are of global significance. It delves into the complexities of pandemic management, human rights, and the responsibilities of government in times of crisis. This is a remarkable opportunity to engage in a fresh and comprehensive look at the challenges humanity faced during the crises and the pursuit of truth and accountability.

The NCI Final Report and video testimonies are available in their entirety on the NCI website: https://nationalcitizensinquiry.ca

I invite you to watch three testimonies and witness how your life is changed. Shawn Buckley, Lead Counsel National Citizens Inquiry

CHAPTER 33

A Personal Experience in Covid Institutional Corruption

Ivor Cummins

Chronic disease researcher and podcaster

Ivor Cummins BE(Chem) CEng MIEI completed a Biochemical Engineering degree in 1990. He has since spent 30 years in corporate technical leadership positions. His career specialty has been leading large worldwide teams in complex problem-solving activity. Since 2012 Ivor has been intensively researching the root causes of modern chronic disease. A particular focus has been on cardiovascular disease, diabetes and obesity. He shares his research insights at public speaking engagements around the world, revealing the key nutritional and lifestyle interventions which will deliver excellent health and personal productivity. He has recently presented at the British Association of Cardiovascular Prevention and Rehabilitation (BACPR) and also at the Irish National Institute of Preventative Cardiology (NIPC) annual conferences. Ivor's 2018 book "Eat Rich, Live Long" (co-authored with preventative medicine expert Jeffry Gerber MD, FAAFP), details the conclusions of their shared research, available at Amazon. Ivor hosts the popular Fat Emperor Podcast.

Most critical thinkers with a platform who tried to counter the sinister madness of the Covid Program were widely harassed and defamed. I managed to avoid some of the more serious repercussions of this globalist-led attack. I was the victim of a large hit piece in The New York Times (Sept 2020)[1]. And another in The Belfast Telegraph in which I was accused of having some responsibility for the death of a politician (Sept 2021)[2]. There were plenty of other sleazy articles seeking to impugn me.

In another bizarre incident the Dublin County Sherrif's staff turned up at my door to enforce a 'Final Seizure of Property' order – just the morning after I had received the first letter informing me of this fraudulent charge. I defeated that rap over several days with the aid of the chartered accountancy firm which manages all my accounts; not too hard as the whole incident was a fiction and manifest government corruption. But, enough of that. In this essay I'd like to relate one particular episode of globalist villainy, one I documented quite carefully at the time. It afforded me an opportunity to really summarize the reality of Covid – to parse out the key data and hence reveal the astonishing absurdity of the whole thing. So here we go folks.

In 2022 I received an email from a certain Ms Aoife Gallagher, who worked for the global 'think tank' The Institute for Strategic Dialogue (ISD)[3]. This globalist propaganda group was set up in 2006, supposedly to counter "extremism, hate, disinformation and polarization". In 2020 however, they (unsurprisingly) launched themselves wholeheartedly into defending the absurdities of the Covid 19 response measures. I was well familiar with this sinister outfit, as they had placed me in their "Covid Disinformation" annual reports a couple of times already. Always their wording was slimy, and careful to avoid direct libel as such – and always it was total nonsense.

In this latest scam, Gallagher informed me via email that she was featuring me in her upcoming book. She would not reveal details of the book, but did provide several passages of absurdity and misinformation – to which she was offering me the right to respond. I replied promptly and addressed all of her weasel words, debunking them with little effort. A couple of months later I got an email showing that "Web of Lies" would soon be published. Of course they had not corrected the material that included me. Okay then; I decided to send a letter to each member of the publisher's board by registered post. It began as follows:

"The writer Ms A Gallagher of ISD (see below and attached) has notified me of an intent to publish defamatory statements in a publication through your firm. The purpose of this registered letter is to provide you with advance notice that should this premeditated defamation be published, this notice will be used in the High Court to recover costs against you including for punitive damages under Defamation Act 2009. Be clear that giving me

sight of intended comments in no way mitigates the damages which will be sought, and this communication to you as the intended publishers firmly closes that off.

Outlined below in brief is a synopsis as to why such publication would amount to premeditated defamation. I trust your defamation lawyers and insurers will guide your firm to safety on this matter and that such references will not be published by you, but you need to be very clear that my intention is to issue legal proceedings against all parties involved, for reasons that are self-evident and laid out in detail here"

I then went on to expose how they were the very essence of corrupt charlatans, and I will paraphrase the letter here.

Firstly, I told them that the preface for their penny dreadful book highlighted explicitly the nature of the characters who would be included therein:

"Web of Lies presents a history of conspiracy theories and their roots in anti-Semitism, xenophobia and white supremacy"

"...examination of the rising threat of far-right extremist thought in Ireland and internationally"

I pointed out that even being included in such a book is de facto defamation, especially a book from a writer whose concurrent activity was focused on extremists like Qanon and other such twaddle.

I then went on to briefly summarize the actual facts in several of the statements they were intending to print. References were offered for all, and all material was available online and was also safely archived by me. The following passages are taken verbatim from my registered letter:

First statement: "[Cummins] general take on the pandemic was that Covid-19 wasn't as serious as it was being made out to be"

When read in context the book implies that these statements are false, particularly in light of the charges of badly sourced science etc. that follow – this is therefore defamatory. I have been proven correct on this point, from the actual published data. Dr. John Lee was in the UK media extensively during 2020, and repeatedly emphasized (correctly as it turned out) that the impact of Covid19 was "in the envelope of a bad/severe flu". It is also notable that Bill Gates (who publicly drove a narrative of quasi-hysteria over the past two years) has now acknowledged publicly in his May 2022 interview on 92NY network, and I quote: *"we didn't understand that it [Covid19] has a fairly low mortality rate, and it's a disease mainly of the elderly - kind of like flu is...".*

The data has in fact shown this clearly all along; from the landmark Diamond Princess cruise ship analysis back in February 2020, through to the WHO-acknowledged papers of Stanford Professor John Ioannidis and many others. The latter analyses show an infection fatality rate of 0.15% (and much lower than this for the under 70's). A recent WHO analysis shows that the hard-hit UK had approximately 0.1% excess mortality in 2020, a number similar to the world average. Ireland with a younger demographic had *no notable excess mortality in 2020* - and this is clearly apparent from the official CSO figures, with no ambiguity whatsoever.

Second statement: "...that lockdowns were doing more harm than good"

Again, the book implies that these statements are false, which is defamatory when read in the context of this book particularly. I have been proven correct on this point also - from the actual published data. There are now literally scores of published papers clearly illustrating that lockdown policies have had little, or indeed no measurable beneficial effect. The reasons for this non-intuitive reality are complex, but the actual reality cannot be denied. I include a draft document on the lockdown evidence base (Attachment A)[4], which references some of the major published papers establishing this fact; however, there are many,

many more which have demonstrated the same outcome. Importantly, I can present published papers and analyses that put the societal cost of lockdown policies at 10 to 30 times the (putative) benefit gained.

I mentioned above that the aged-demographic UK had approximately 0.1% excess mortality in 2020. However, in the same WHO report the similarly aged-demographic Sweden experienced approximately half of this impact. The fact is that Sweden achieved this with no lockdowns, no masks and with children under sixteen years of age maintained in school throughout the whole pandemic. Crucially, Sweden also did not come anywhere near its ICU capacity - even at the peak of the first (and primary) wave. The conclusion is dramatic and clear. Myriad other inter- and intra-country analyses verify this reality, time after time (again, see Attachment A). Because the negative impact of the lockdown policies was so catastrophic – unquestionably so - the conclusion that "lockdowns did more harm than good" is cast-iron solid. Again, I draw your attention to the attached draft document on the lockdown evidence base. In short, I simply share this correct view with approximately 63,000 medical and public health scientists who have signed The Great Barrington Declaration (www.gbdeclaration.org)[5].

Third statement: "...and that the vaccines were 'the scam of the century'."

I have furnished Ms Gallagher with my 2021 tweet which this libelous claim was based upon. In contrast to the claim shown here, I was clearly calling out the lack of transmission mitigation apparent with this new drug technology. Thus, the "scam" was to force vaccine passport systems, and it was misinformation to push the idea that the drugs would meaningfully impact transmission and "keep us all safe". In short, the drugs were acting primarily as a therapeutic for the individual themselves. Many analyses have now demonstrated that the vaccine has not prevented transmission to any meaningful extent, certainly nothing near the threshold that would justify mandates and passports; the apparent associational linkage rapidly falls away with time.

This has now been publicly acknowledged by Fauci, Gates, and many other previously powerful proponents of vaccine mandates and passport systems. Are they "right-wing conspiracy theorists" also? Just the other day on 25th July, the highly influential White House Coronavirus Task Force Coordinator Dr. Deborah Birx admitted openly on mainstream US television: "*I knew these vaccines were not going to protect against infection, and I think we overplayed the vaccines*". Is she now a "right-wing conspiracy theorist" also? On July 29th last, Florida's Surgeon General Dr. Joe Ladapo stated in a news conference: "*How can you force people to take a vaccine in order to stop transmission, when that vaccine is not effective in stopping transmission?*" Is he now a "right-wing conspiracy theorist" also? I can provide myriad more references and data showing that I was entirely justified in my comments on this topic.

Fourth statement: "He regularly said that his claims were based on science, data, logic and facts, often repeating this throughout his videos to assure people. But Cummins's posts have been widely debunked and noted to be based on flawed reasoning, poor data interpretation, cherry picking and badly sourced research."

No-one has actually debunked the substance of my positions; they have only made claims that do not stand up to scrutiny and would not stand up on cross-examination under oath. The reality, illustrated by my earlier clarifications, is that I have been overwhelmingly correct in my key analyses throughout the pandemic. Pimenta, the 33-year-old cardiologist referenced by Ms Gallagher has been incorrect, having no expertise in the relevant branches of data and science. These false accusations in the book are damaging to my established technical prowess, which has been a lifelong trademark of mine. Crucially, note that I have always verified my analyses against an extensive network of technical specialty experts. I have also published interviews with many of the latter relating to Covid19 data inference, and we all largely concur on the primary aspects of what I have been sharing over the past two years; a small sample below:

· Stanford Professor Michael Levitt, 2015 Nobel Prize winner (the true mortality impacts of Covid19)

· Professor Beda Stadler, former director of the Immunology Institute, Bern (the immunology of Covid19)

· Pathology Professor John Lee (retd) (all relevant aspects of Covid19)

· Stanford Professor of Public Health Jay Bhattacharya (all relevant aspects of Covid19)

· Professor Gordan Lauc, official advisor to the Croatian Government on Covid19 policy (all relevant aspects of Covid19)

My research sources include the people listed, who have confirmed the soundness of my analyses and concur with them. My position and methods are clearly within the range of reasoned and evidence-based debate within professional science. There are likewise countless more experts in my network, with many of whom I have published interviews – but the key point is that my material on Covid19 data has been overwhelmingly on point, and this has been borne out by the emerging reality over the past two years. You have now been notified of the defamatory nature of Pimenta's claims, and repeating his defamatory statements would constitute defamation.

Fifth statement: "Cummins claimed that the virus had run its course by June 2020 and that herd immunity had been reached. This is quite clearly untrue, as the two years following the release of his video would prove ... ICU doctor Dominic Pimenta pointed to the copious flaws in his claims, including cherry picking data to prove that masks and lockdowns were ineffective while ignoring evidence that showed the opposite. Cummins regularly used scientific language and phrases in the wrong way and made up his own definitions for certain words. He compared incompatible data sets to attempt to predict the trajectory of the virus, and he also frequently contradicted himself. Generally, his claims were scientifically baseless."

This relates to my commentary on the UK situation, and is highly misleading. In the summer of 2020, I called out that there would of course be a *winter resurgence of the virus.* I predicted generally that there would be a much lower excess mortality when compared to the 2020 season. The latter I hypothesized would occur due to substantial community immunity having been gained in the 2020 season, following consultations with Professor of Immunology Beda Stadler (Switzerland) and many other experts. I published interviews in the summer of 2020 which capture this and are on the record. It turned out that I was essentially correct, and the UK Actuarial Society proved me so in a May 2021 publication. The latter showed clearly that 2021 cumulative mortality for the period January-May was in line with many prior years such as 2015 and 2018, as predicted. I have all of the data and publications archived of course, should you need further references. The "cherry picking" accusation is nonsense – please see my earlier comments on lockdown, and the Attachment A on the lockdown evidence base. The rest of the comments, as in the last section, are defamatory in nature. *I also attach a brief summary of my technical track record (Attachment B), and it is important also that you are fully appraised of the same.*

Finally, attached is a document outlining some funding and other details around Ms Gallagher's organization, ISD (Attachment C)[6]. This document was prepared for me by an Irish network associate, who investigated the ISD organization due to their many attacks on freedom of speech and scientific discourse. Their particular modus operandi appears to be cleverly worded impugnation, keeping just inside the line of defamation. The ISD is attacking freedom of speech within the established parameters of good faith scientific discourse. Again, that I am even being included in a book of this nature (and by this particular author) is de facto defamation.

I will add that it is shocking to me that a company such as Gill Books[7], with a long history of ethical business in Ireland - would publish a smear campaign against an Irish professional such as myself.

In light of the above, please confirm by return that you will not publish the intended defamation.

Sincerely,

Ivor Cummins

BE(Chem) CEng MIEI

So there you have it folks. They went ahead and included some of the nonsense in their globalist propaganda 'book', but my evisceration of their knavery resulted in it being toned down considerably from the original. I made a video on the debacle, but it was immediately flagged, no doubt by ISD goons, and removed from Youtube. It's still available to view on X and other platforms[8]. While the entire episode was frustrating, it was more amusing than anything else. But make no mistake, these people are unscrupulous in their methods.

If you are interested, *Web of Lies* is still available on Amazon and other platforms, languishing at 10,000th position in the "Religious Studies (Books)" section. It has attracted a smattering of authentically penned bad reviews. And of course some five star reviews, provided no doubt by ISD staff. [9]

[1] https://www.nytimes.com/2020/09/29/health/coronavirus-herd-immunity.html

[2] https://thefatemperor.com/interesting-email-from-belfast-telegraph-reporter-see-here/

[3] https://www.isdglobal.org/

[4] https://thefatemperor.com/wp-content/uploads/2022/09/Evidence-For-and-Against-the-Effectiveness-of-Lockdown-Policies-DRAFT-RevC.pdf

[5] https://gbdeclaration.org/

[6] https://thefatemperor.com/wp-content/uploads/2024/09/ISD-Aoife-Gallagher-Summary.pdf

[7] https://www.gillbooks.ie/

[8] https://x.com/FatEmperor/status/1830752593645011100

[9] https://www.amazon.co.uk/Web-Lies-Fiction-conspiracy-theories/dp/0717195120

CHAPTER 34

The Weaponization of Mass Communication

Joshua Walkos

Journalist and researcher

"Josh Walkos is an independent journalist and researcher known for his incisive work uncovering forgotten histories and exposing institutional corruption. As the founder of We The Free, a popular Substack newsletter, Walkos has established himself as a formidable voice in investigative journalism. His writing skillfully synthesizes complex historical narratives for modern audiences, challenging conventional wisdom and shedding light on overlooked truths.

His work is characterized by its depth, originality, and commitment to challenging the status quo. The ability to distill intricate historical patterns into compelling, accessible narratives has earned him a dedicated following and established his credibility as a thought leader in alternative media circles. His work can be found on his Substack "We The Free" at wethefree.substack.com and he can be followed on Twitter/X at @JoshWalkos."

The psyche of the American public is under siege, assaulted by forces both within our borders and beyond. These forces, indifferent to humanity, aim only to bring us to our knees. Since the turn of the century, a series of incremental, deliberate, and continuous assaults have eroded our ability to take stock of our situation. This slow and steady encroachment on our liberties and perceptions brings to mind Milton Sanford Mayer's reflections in his book "*They Thought They Were Free: The Germans 1933-1945.*" He captures the subtlety of societal manipulation and the difficulty of recognizing it while it happens.

"To live in this process is absolutely not to be able to notice it—please try to believe me—unless one has a much greater degree of political awareness, acuity, than most of us had ever had occasion to develop. Each step was so small, so inconsequential, so well explained or, on occasion, 'regretted,' that, unless one were detached from the whole process from the beginning, unless one understood what the whole thing was in principle,

464 | Canary In a (Post) Covid World

what all these 'little measures' that no 'patriotic German' could resent must someday lead to, one no more saw it developing from day to day than a farmer in his field sees the corn growing. One day it is over his head."

Today, I fear we are in a similar state of oblivion, with the corn now over our heads. As we approach the November 2024 US election, the world watches, and we must ask ourselves: how did we get here? This essay explores the path that led us to this point, marked by extreme polarization, media manipulation, and a culture of deception.

So how did we get here? The question is a bewildering one, the world has been through a lot and I believe there is a sort of collective PTSD coursing through the population's veins.

The extreme polarization that characterized the COVID years still persists. Many, particularly in the media, are now in full-on gaslight revisionist mode, insisting that no one was forced to do anything.

They say things like, "It's all in our heads", "everyone had a choice" and this is repeated by people in their everyday lives who perpetuate the gaslighting.This dynamic, where weaponized mass communication flows from the media and government to the public, explains how we arrived at this point.

Generally speaking propaganda is nothing new, it has been a valuable tool for governments since governments have existed. It is defined as "the effort to spread information, ideas, or rumours for the purpose of helping or injuring an institution, a cause, or a person". It doesn't have to be false information but the defining factor is its attempt at persuasion. The public mind was primed for COVID and the groundwork for such an event had been laid for decades via mass media messaging.

When Obama won the White House, inheriting an economy on the brink of collapse and emerging from a war that was started under false pretences as well as the ongoing "war on terror", the country was fed up with the neo-cons and elected him by a wide margin in 2008.

Obama's campaign was brilliant, cultivating an anti-war message of 'hope and change.' This message was used to rehabilitate America's image, which had been tarnished by the War On Terror that proliferated conflicts worldwide.

This of course was just that, an image carefully cultivated by the campaign and then perpetuated by a media class who had become enamoured with the new president.

The only problem was that Obama not only continued the wars of his predecessor, but he also expanded the war theatre to include Syria, Libya, and Yemen. The fawning press barely reported on the many failures of the administration and instead treated him as a celebrity president who could do no wrong.

During Obama's first term, I began to notice the seeds of what would eventually become the blind belief in "authority" seen during COVID. I had been extremely critical of both Bushes and then I saw the continuation of their foreign policy under Obama, yet heard nothing but silence from those around me. Those same people who just months prior were outraged by the same policies acted as if I was crazy for criticising them and that is when I knew something was happening from a social psychology perspective. It was as if en masse people were deliberately ignoring the obvious to avoid cognitive dissonance, clinging fearfully to the "hope and change" mantra.

This phenomenon persisted in the media, elite circles, and the managerial class throughout both of Obama's terms. During this time, American culture had changed dramatically and I would argue that in part, it was changed deliberately via the help of a small amendment tucked into a piece of legislation.

On December 31, 2012, President Obama signed the National Defense Authorization Act (NDAA), an annual bill that determines the budget and expenditures for the Department of Defense (DOD). For

2024, the NDAA authorized $883.7 billion for the DOD. While some funding for defence is necessary, the NDAA is frequently used as a vehicle for policy and political manoeuvring.

In 2012 Republican Mac Thornberry and Democrat Adam Smith introduced an amendment to the Smith-Mundt Modernization Act and attached it to the NDAA. The original Smith-Mundt Act, passed in 1948, allowed the State Department to develop methods for spreading propaganda internationally. This Act prohibited the targeting of Americans, however that changed with the 2012 amendment and just like that it was transformed into a program targeting American citizens. The justification for this was the "war on terror" of course, citing threats from foreign terrorist organizations, such as al-Qaeda, which aimed to "undermine American values".

Thornberry, one of the amendment's sponsors, argued that the update was needed to "communicate effectively in a credible and transparent manner." Despite these assurances from lawmakers, recent events have shown a different reality. The Russiagate controversy, which accused President Trump of being a Russian agent, serves as a notable example.

In 2017, the Alliance for Securing Democracy (ASD) was established, primarily composed of former senior US Intelligence and State Department officials. This organization significantly influenced the media, feeding stories to the press that were often published with minimal scrutiny. The ASD developed the "Hamilton 68 Dashboard," which claimed to track social media accounts associated with Russian influence campaigns. Journalist Matt Taibbi later exposed the dashboard's flawed methodology and lack of transparency.

Remember when suddenly, the topic of racism was thrust into the limelight during Obama's tenure? A series of viral police shooting videos were seized upon politically to create division. Notably, the Trayvon Martin case seemed to be the spark used when he was killed on February 26, 2012. Also around this time academia was showing the first major signs of the critical race theory (CRT) takeover of administrations all over the country. Words and phrases like "diversity, equity and inclusion", "intersectionality", "queer theory", "black lives matters" were becoming mainstream and a wider socio-political conflict was stepping into the culture war as the focus.

By 2017 the #MeToo movement achieved vitality online by exposing serious wrongdoing in Hollywood and corporate America. It then morphed into a cultural phenomenon that strained interpersonal dynamics between the sexes, framing women as victims of "the white patriarchy".

Accusations of sexual impropriety were used as weapons and catch phrases like "believe all women" became widely adopted regardless of their validity. Then seemingly out of nowhere the topic of transgenderism started to be mainstreamed and the mantra of "believe all women" turned into "men are women" and if anyone challenged this notion, they were labeled "transphobic bigots".

This climate, a cultural cauldron, bubbled to the surface at the end of Obama's tenure. It set the stage for the 2016 election and the emergence of Donald Trump.

Each one of these issues, CRT, #metoo, intersectionality, BLM, the War On Terror and Transgenderism were, I would argue, all the result of weaponized mass communication.

They are all cultural pressure points that exploited people's perceptions through propaganda perpetuated by the mainstream media and then adding social media to the mix was like adding gasoline to the fire of discontent.

The big problem with all of this is that all of these issues forced into the cultural milieu were largely based on deception. Things like Iraq had "weapons of mass destruction", "men can be women", "all cops are bastards (acab), and "America is fundamentally a racist country" were used to manipulate the public and sow division.

All were objectively and proven to be false notions but nonetheless were inculcated so successfully within the public mind via mass propaganda that they became the truth to a large portion of the population. Importantly many leaders and individuals of influence believed these lies or at least they acted like they did. Everyone of them gearing up for the first woman president to be elected in a landslide, all but cementing their progressive cultural dominance into the future.

Then Donald Trump won perhaps the most surprising presidential victory in history, edging out Hillary Clinton by the slimmest of margins. The progressives were in disbelief and refused to accept the results, it had to be a mistake. This is when I believe the weaponization of mass communication went into overdrive. The entire establishment amassed forces to undermine Trump's presidency and made it their mission to trot out an endless parade of non-stop media propaganda and outright lies.

All the while the "liberal" establishment and their primed voters ate it up because to them it didn't matter if the accusations were true or not because they wanted to believe it.

They had to believe it because otherwise they would need to face the fact that their leadership and agenda was rejected by Americans, millions of whom voted for Barack Obama twice beforehand.

This was the real indictment, a rejection of the Neo-liberal and Neo-conservative policies that have fleeced the poor and middle class of this country for decades. At the same time across the pond in Great Britain, a similar sentiment was taking place and Brexit shocked the entirety of Europe's elite who could not admit the European Union had turned into a failed experiment.

This perfect storm of populist revolt was simply too much for the men and women who have no allegiances to countries and only care about maintaining their power while furthering their agenda worldwide. The agenda is quite simple, the gradual dissolution of sovereignty and rights both on the national scale and the individual scale. With Trump and

Brexit happening, these traitors to the human race decided they needed to take action fast and they were not about to let the plebs whom they have such abject hatred for, derail all the progress they had achieved over the last half century. Democracy be damned, the people do not know what's good for them.

It's quite amazing that even today in 2024, if you were to randomly stop to talk with a self professed liberal or democrat about Russiagate, I would wager 90 percent would still say Trump is a "Putin Puppet" or "Russian Agent". This, despite the inarguable proof that agents of their very own party and the FBI, along with the undying support of the media, orchestrated the entire story.

They will argue until they are blue in the face that Mueller confirmed all of their suspicions, but won't be able to give you details. And if they do give you details, they will be details that have long since been laid to rest as factually incorrect. Try telling a true believer that it was the Clinton campaign that paid for the Steele Dossier and worked with the FBI to disseminate the lies contained within throughout the press in order to delegitimize the Trump presidency.

They will laugh in your face and call you with certainty an "alt-right conspiracy theorist". If this isn't proof that the principles our constitution lays out have been all but completely abandoned by a large portion of the American public then you too might have abandoned them. This is the power of mass communication and offers valuable insight into the mindset of at least half of the public going into 2020, another election year.

When coronavirus emerged, those who ignored what their own eyes had seen and believed, the lies and deception of the past 20 years were primed for the fear-based propaganda that was ratcheted up to unprecedented levels worldwide. They were ready to give up their rights and view their fellow citizens as 'superspreaders' undeserving of fundamental human rights. Think about this; according to the New York Times, approximately 72.3 percent of the global population received at least one dose of the

COVID-19 vaccines with about 67 percent considered fully vaccinated, meaning they took two doses. This represents over 13.27 billion doses administered globally, or 5.5 billion people.

In the United States, based on the numbers provided by the CDC, 81 percent of the public took at least one dose with 68 percent considered fully vaccinated. I can't think of a better example to illustrate the power of mass communication and propaganda. We can debate the providence of those figures but even if they are mostly correct it is astounding to think that so many people, based solely on what the media and government were telling them, willingly rolled up their sleeves and had a liability free, novel technology injected into their bodies for "the greater good".

Yet today, in 2024 a large percentage of the public still believe that they did the right thing and that all of the measures taken, such as the lockdowns and masks, were the proper steps to take. This is despite the fact that we know that masks do not stop viral spread and the lockdowns had historical negative repercussions that we are still learning about today. Nearly half of parents (47 percent) reported that the pandemic had a negative impact on their child's mental health. The gap in feelings of hopelessness and sadness between adolescent females and males widened from 2019 -2021. Drug overdose deaths increased sharply across the total population coinciding with the pandemic, more than doubling among adolescents, and alcohol induced death rates also increased substantially.

While people suffered, the total wealth of 644 billionaires increased from $2.95 trillion to $3.88 trillion between March 18, 2020 and October 13, 2020, a rise of 31.6 percent. The total number of billionaires grew during this time as well from 644 to 745. Jeff Bezos's wealth grew from $113 billion to $150 billion in that same time frame. This amounts to the largest wealth transfer in human history, accelerating existing trends of wealth concentration and inequality that existed prior to the pandemic.

If there is a silver lining to all of this it is that the public is starting to realize they have been duped on multiple levels and are starting to reassess their belief structures as it pertains to the media and government intentions. Only 28 percent of adults reported receiving the updated COVID vaccines by early 2024 and the numbers do seem to be decreasing more and more, although this is highly stratified demographically when you look at who is taking them now.

To close, I believe we must all come to terms with the past and realize there is a larger agenda at play here, designed to control our perceptions and in turn control our behavior. Trust is something that needs to be earned, not just given because people in a position of authority demand it of us.

This weaponization of mass communication created a perfect storm that has fueled not only the COVID era but has been ever present in our lives for decades. This is how we got here. Now the questions we should all be asking ourselves are, why and what do we plan on doing about it?

Sources:

https://www.amazon.com/They-Thought-Were-Free-Germans/dp/0226511928

https://www.dictionary.com/browse/propaganda

https://www.wilsoncenter.org/article/war-and-politics-libya-yemen-and-syria

https://foreignpolicy.com/2013/07/14/u-s-repeals-propaganda-ban-spreads-government-made-news-to-americans/

https://web.archive.org/web/20120725080310/http://thornberry.house.gov/News/DocumentSingle.aspx?DocumentID=296108

https://www.tabletmag.com/sections/news/articles/guide-understanding-hoax-century-thirteen-ways-looking-disinformation

https://www.cdc.gov/respiratory-viruses/data-research/dashboard/vaccination-trends-adults.html

https://usafacts.org/visualizations/covid-vaccine-tracker-states/

https://www.pewresearch.org/science/2024/03/07/how-americans-view-the-coronavirus-covid-19-vaccines-amid-declining-levels-of-concern/

https://www.pewresearch.org/short-read/2023/03/02/mental-health-and-the-pandemic-what-u-s-surveys-have-found/

https://www.statista.com/statistics/1202074/share-of-population-vaccinated-covid-19-by-county-worldwide/

https://www.kff.org/mental-health/issue-brief/the-implications-of-covid-19-for-mental-health-and-substance-use/

CHAPTER 35

The Gaslighting of the Masses

C. J. Hopkins

Playwright, Novelist and political satirist

C. J. Hopkins is an award-winning playwright, novelist, and political satirist. His plays have been produced and have toured at theatres and festivals including Riverside Studios (London), 59E59 Theaters (New York), Traverse Theatre (Edinburgh), Belvoir St. Theatre (Sydney), the Du Maurier World Stage Festival (Toronto), Needtheater (Los Angeles), 7 Stages (Atlanta), the Edinburgh Festival Fringe, Adelaide Fringe, Brighton Festival, and the Noorderzon Festival (the Netherlands), among others. His writing awards include the 2002 First of the Scotsman Fringe Firsts, Scotsman Fringe Firsts in 2002 and 2005, and the 2004 Best Play of the Adelaide Fringe. His political satire and commentary has been published by Consent Factory, OffGuardian, ZeroHedge, ColdType, Rubikon, CounterPunch, Dissident Voice, and many other publications, and has been widely translated. His dystopian science fiction novel, Zone 23, is published by Snoggsworthy, Swaine & Cormorant. (This essay provided by C.J but was originally written in late 2022)

For students of official propaganda, mind control, emotional coercion, and other insidious manipulation techniques, the rollout of the New Normal has been a bonanza. Never before have we been able to observe the application and effects of these powerful technologies in real-time on such a massive scale.

In a little over two years, our collective "reality" has been radically revised. Our societies have been radically restructured. Millions (probably billions) of people have been systematically conditioned to believe a variety of patently ridiculous assertions, assertions based on absolutely nothing, repeatedly disproved by widely available evidence, but which have nevertheless attained the status of facts. An entire fictitious history has been written based on those baseless and ridiculous assertions. It will not be unwritten easily or quickly.

I am not going to waste your time debunking those assertions. They have been repeatedly, exhaustively debunked. You know what they are and you either believe them or you don't. Either way, reviewing and debunking them again isn't going to change a thing.

Instead, I want to focus on one particularly effective mind-control technology, one that has done a lot of heavy lifting throughout the implementation of the New Normal and is doing a lot of heavy-lifting currently. I want to do that because many people mistakenly believe that mind-control is either (a) a "conspiracy theory" or (b) something that can only be achieved with drugs, microwaves, surgery, torture, or some other invasive physical means. Of course, there is a vast and well-documented history of the use of such invasive physical technologies (see, e.g., the history of the CIA's infamous MKULTRA program), but in many instances mind-control can be achieved through much less elaborate techniques.

One of the most basic and effective techniques that cults, totalitarian systems, and individuals with fascistic personalities use to disorient and control people's minds is "gaslighting." You're probably familiar with the term. If not, here are a few definitions:

"the manipulation of another person into doubting their perceptions, experiences, or understanding of events." American Psychological Association

"an insidious form of manipulation and psychological control. Victims of gaslighting are deliberately and systematically fed false information that leads them to question what they know to be true, often about themselves. They may end up doubting their memory, their perception, and even their sanity." Psychology Today

"a form of psychological manipulation in which the abuser attempts to sow self-doubt and confusion in their victim's mind. Typically, gaslighters are seeking to gain power and control over the other person, by distorting

reality and forcing them to question their own judgment and intuition."
Newport Institute

The main goal of gaslighting is to confuse, coerce, and emotionally manipulate your victim into abandoning their own perception of reality and accepting whatever new "reality" you impose on them. Ultimately, you want to completely destroy their ability to trust their own perception, emotions, reasoning, and memory of historical events, and render them utterly dependent on you to tell them what is real and what "really" happened, and so on, and how they should be feeling about it.

Anyone who has ever experienced gaslighting in the context of an abusive relationship, or a cult, or a totalitarian system, or who has worked in a battered women's shelter, can tell you how powerful and destructive it is. In the most extreme cases, the victims of gaslighting are entirely stripped of their sense of self and surrender their individual autonomy completely. Among the best-known and most dramatic examples are the Patty Hearst case, Jim Jones' People's Temple, the Manson family, and various other cults, but, the truth is, gaslighting happens every day, out of the spotlight of the media, in countless personal and professional relationships.

Since the Spring of 2020, we have been subjected to official gaslighting on an unprecedented scale. In a sense, the "Apocalyptic Pandemic" PSYOP has been one big extended gaslighting campaign (comprising countless individual instances of gaslighting) inflicted on the masses throughout the world.

Basically, what happened was, a Pfizer executive confirmed to the European Parliament last Monday that Pfizer did not know whether its COVID "vaccine" prevented transmission of the virus before it was promoted as doing exactly that and forced on the masses in December of 2020. People saw the video of the executive admitting this, or heard about it, and got upset. They tweeted and Facebooked and posted videos of Pfizer CEO Albert Bourla, Bill Gates, the Director of the CDC, official propagandists like Rachel Maddow, and various other "experts" and "authorities" blatantly lying to the public, promising people that getting "vaccinated" would "prevent transmission," "protect other people from infection," "stop the virus in its tracks," and so on, which totally baseless assertions (i.e., lies) were the justification for <u>the systematic segregation and persecution of "the Unvaccinated,"</u> and <u>the fomenting of mass fanatical hatred of anyone challenging the official "vaccine" narrative</u>, and <u>the official New Normal ideology</u>, which hatred persists to this very day.

The New Normal propaganda apparatus (i.e., the corporate media, health "experts," et al.) responded to the story predictably. They ignored it, hoping it would just go away. When it didn't, they rolled out the "fact-checkers" (i.e., gaslighters).

The <u>Associated Press</u>, <u>Reuters</u>, <u>PolitiFact</u>, and other official gaslighting outfits immediately published lengthy official "fact-checks" that would make a sophist blush. Read them and you will see what I mean. They are perfect examples of official gaslighting, crafted to distract you from the point and suck you into an argument over meaningless details and definitions. They sound exactly like Holocaust deniers pathetically asserting that there is no written proof that Hitler ordered the Final Solution ... which, there isn't, but it doesn't fucking matter. Of course Hitler ordered the Final Solution, and of course they lied about the "vaccines."

The Internet is swimming with evidence of their lies ... tweets, videos, articles, and so on.

Which is what makes gaslighting so frustrating for people who believe they are engaged in an actual good-faith argument over facts and the truth. But that's not how totalitarianism works. The New Normals, when they repeat whatever the authorities have instructed them to repeat today (e.g., "trust the Science," "safe and effective," "no one ever claimed they would prevent transmission"), could not care less whether it is actually true, or even if it makes the slightest sense.

These gaslighting "fact-checks" are not meant to convince them that anything is true or false. And they are certainly not meant to convince us. They are official scripts, talking points, and thought-terminating clichés for the New Normals to repeat, like cultists chanting mantras at you to shut off their minds and block out anything that contradicts or threatens the "reality" of the cult.

You can present them with the actual facts, and they will smile knowingly, and deny them to your face, and condescendingly mock you for not "seeing the truth."

Consent Factory
@consent_factory

···

You can show the New Normals the video, and they will watch it, and then look you right in the eye and deny it.

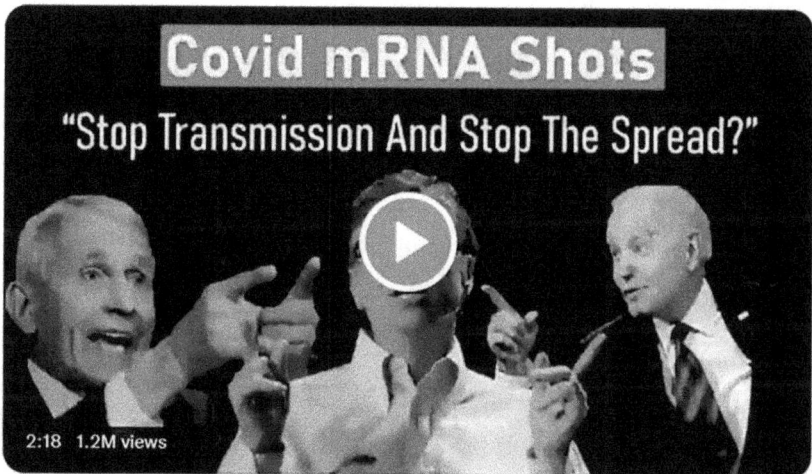

Covid mRNA Shots
"Stop Transmission And Stop The Spread?"

2:18 1.2M views

From **Mark Bayly**

Moon of Alabama @MoonofA · Oct 13
Well, it was never advertised to 'prevent transmission' because no vaccine can. It's scandalous that some are dumb enough to believe it was.
twitter.com/theblaze/statu...

But here's the tricky thing about gaslighting.

In order to effectively gaslight someone, you have to be in a position of authority or wield some other form of power over them. They have to need something vital from you (i.e., sustenance, safety, financial security, community, career advancement, or just love). You can't walk up to some random stranger on the street and start gaslighting them. They will laugh in your face.

The reason the New Normal authorities have been able to gaslight the masses so effectively is that most of the masses do need something from them ... a job, food, shelter, money, security, status, their friends, a relationship, or whatever it is they're not willing to risk by challenging those in power and their lies. Gaslighters, cultists, and power freaks, generally, know this. It is what they depend on, your unwillingness to live without whatever it is. They zero in on it and threaten you with the loss of it (sometimes consciously, sometimes just intuitively).

Gaslighting won't work if you are willing to give up whatever the gaslighter is threatening to take from you (or stop giving you, as the case may be), but you have to be willing to actually lose it, because *you will be punished for defending yourself*, for not surrendering your autonomy and integrity, and conforming to the "reality" of the cult, or the abusive relationship, or the totalitarian system.

I have described the New Normal (i.e., our new "reality") as patholo-gized-totalitarianism, and as a "a cult writ large, on a societal scale." I used the "Covidian Cult" analogy because every totalitarian system essentially operates like a cult, the main difference being that, in totalitarian systems, the balance of power between the cult and the normal (i.e., dominant) society is completely inverted. The cult becomes the dominant (i.e., "normal") society, and non-cult-members become its "deviants."

We do not want to see ourselves as "deviants" (because we haven't changed, the society has), and our instinct is to reject the label, but that is exactly what we are ... deviants. People who deviate from the norm, a new norm, which we reject, and oppose, but which, despite that, is nonetheless the norm, and thus we are going to be regarded and dealt with like deviants.

I am such a deviant. I have a feeling you are too. Under the circumstances, it's nothing to be ashamed of. On the contrary, we need to accept it, and embrace it. Above all, we need to get clear about it, about where we stand in this new "reality."

We are heading toward New Normal Winter No. 3. They are already cranking up the official propaganda, jacking up the fabricated "cases," talking about the next pandemic - fomenting mass hatred of "the Unvaccinated," and so on. People's gas bills are doubling and tripling. The global-capitalist ruling classes are openly embracing neo-Nazis. There is talk of "limited" nuclear war. Fanaticism, fear, and hatred abound. The gaslighting of the masses is not abating. It is increasing. The suppression of dissent is intensifying. The demonization of non-conformity is intensifying. Lines are being drawn in the sand. You see it and feel it just like I do.

Get clear on what's essential to you. Get clear about what you're willing to lose. Stay deviant. Stay frosty. This isn't over.

https://consentfactory.org/2021/03/29/the-unvaccinated-question/

https://consentfactory.org/2021/10/12/the-great-new-normal-purge/

https://consentfactory.org/2021/06/20/manufacturing-new-normal-reality/

https://www.politifact.com/factchecks/2022/oct/13/instagram-posts/alleged-revelation-about-pfizer-vaccine-trial-noth/

https://www.reuters.com/fact-check/preventing-transmission-never-required-covid-vaccines-initial-approval-pfizer-2024-02-12/

https://apnews.com/article/fact-check-pfizer-transmission-european-parliament-950413863226

https://consentfactory.org/2021/11/22/pathologized-totalitarianism-101/

https://consentfactory.org/2020/10/13/the-covidian-cult/

CHAPTER 36

How Science Stripped Morality From Truth

Robin Monotti

Architect, designer, cultural theorist and commentator

Robin Monotti Graziadei is a London based Italian architect, designer, architectural, urban, film & cultural theorist and commentator, published translator (Curzio Malaparte, Woman Like Me), former University lecturer (London Metropolitan University & University of Greenwich) and film producer (The Book of Vision, produced with Terrence Malick).

What's the design flaw of humanity?

I think the main design flaw is actually gullibility.

Humans are incredibly gullible. We love stories. We need stories. And when stories are told to us, we find it very difficult not to believe them.

Especially this story that's been told to us for the last few hundred years or so, maybe more, which is the story of science, and the story of medicine. We are witnessing, and we kind of all know it, that for three years there's been a fight over science, and there's been a fight over medicine. Each side is holding their banner and saying:

"This is my science. This is my medicine."

The other side saying:

"No, this is *my* science, this is *my* medicine!"

And it's like trying to shout each other out.

And it has become, using dirty tricks, one science versus another. And then you've got the people in the middle. Who in some ways have to make a choice. But the choice they will make is not really based on the numbers that are thrown at them or the diagrams, or really understanding the scientific spend.

It tends to be a basic group choice. Which group do I think will protect my interests better? Or which belief is accepted, because ultimately it's a belief, more in my group? So if I'm in a specific area of work I should believe this, otherwise I may lose my income. I may lose my friends. So, ultimately it's a group decision. It's not about what it claims to be; it claims to be about some kind of ideal form of knowledge.

And so the question is: how long can it go on? Because it can really go on forever. One person says: this is science. The other person says: it is that. And ultimately it will polarise in two different directions, with two different mythologies of what real science may be. And we, you and I, may think that one side is totally false and the other side is totally true, but that's not going to take us very far.

Another 60 or 70 percent of people are going to think that what is false is true. So this opens up a question of: what is true? And therefore, what is science? These are not the same thing. I think the first thing to try to bring back into these discussions is that science does not mean truth, just because people think it's true. It's been very effective as a tool to switch off people's brains and switch on the full gullibility mode in a lot of people; we've seen that with climate fallacies, we've seen that with COVID, with all sorts of potential epidemic diseases, bird flu and chicken flu, monkeypox, and medicine as a whole.

So the question is, why do we believe any of it? Why and how have we come to believe that there's this thing called science, which is truth by default, when actually it isn't? It's just an ideology. Like all the other ideologies that have been proven wrong when they were pushed to extremes. History has shown that these dogma have led to World Wars to defend a dominant ideology.

We're in the same position yet again. Why do I say it's ideology? Because on one side there is the myth, the narrative, which is this: there's something called the scientific method. The scientific method leads to people being objective, having total detachment from what they're looking at, and putting some input into an experiment and coming up with an answer. That answer is the truth. But that's an ideology. It doesn't happen like that. Ultimately we've got human beings involved, and when you've got humans, you've got bias. The way the experiment is laid out is full of bias. The way the results are collected is full of bias. Then, the way the results are presented is full of bias. The way the conclusions are written is to please funders.

For over a year, I was reading a lot of science. I was reading everything that I could find to try and get a feel for myself of where the truth lay. The one thing that happened again and again, was that I would read a research paper, some kind of method, some kind of discussion, and I'd be thinking: this is really saying *this*. Then I'd read the conclusion and realise that it was contradicting everything that had been said before. I saw that time and time again. People would isolate a sentence in the conclusion and say: this is what the truth is. But in reality, the study, no matter how biased it was, was really indicating the opposite.

It's not only that science is not truth: it's a highly confusing journey, Kafkaesque and labyrinthine in the way of Argentinian writer Borges, with numbers and data which contradict each other, which then are turned on their head in the conclusion. If you don't have experience in reading these scientific studies, it's hard to tell what's false. The starting point is not the one of truth. We've had John Ioannidis of Stanford who analysed the output of science. Not an experiment in itself: but analysing the output and coming to the conclusion that actually most scientific research is false.

So if I give you a piece of published science in a journal, medical journal or any scientific journal, chances are that it is false at quite a fundamental level. Although some of those experiments may be actually valid, in many cases they're not. In many cases there's data fraud and there's all sorts of other things which as lay readers we cannot pinpoint. So if we say that science is the study of evidence, and that most of that evidence is false, then we can only come to the conclusion that it's not true that science is a better way to truth than what you and I can get a feel for.

Just by listening to a gut feeling, we've probably got a bigger chance at truth. Better the gut, rather than picking up a scientific experiment and saying this is the whole truth. I think we need to rethink the relationship between what we perceive as truth and science altogether, because other-wise we are really setting ourselves up for the next one.

484 | Canary In a (Post) Covid World

We know what it's coming from: climate fear mongering. But we also know that there are repeated attempts at manufacturing so-called pandemics and diseases. We need to be ready for this, skepticism in hand, in the sense that anyone could pop up and say:"I am the chief scientist of X and Y and this is what's happening." As things stand today, the less skeptic among us will automatically believe that. I think the default position should probably be the opposite.

When considering such announcements, we should consider the person making them. To get to that position of power, what did the person do to get there? What happened to all the other people who didn't get there? Were they perhaps more truthful? Who's profiting from this person?

Let's rewind a little bit, see how we got here? It wasn't always like this. The culture that I come from is essentially a Classical culture, integrated by Christianity. That's the world I come from. I feel that truth is not in the body of scientific research: it's what needs to be said. It's what rings true to me. Some people say, "but what if what *he* says is false?" It could be so, but when people talk to each other, when people question each other, there's more chance that truth will float to the surface. We can blame French philosopher Descartes for landing us where we are now, because he postulated that the mark of truth is evidence.

The idea that in order to say something truthful, we need to present evidence, comes from Descartes. But this is only one approach and I believe one that forgets how we got to this point. As we have seen clearly over the last three years, and we're seeing now with the climate charade, I can have a whole body of "evidence" with all the top experts singing from the same song sheet, but that I can still be lying. I can have all the graphs, I can have all the people I know in movies, in politics, and layers of other "evidence" and I can still be lying. Evidence is not the mark of truth. We should be highly suspicious of evidence. Let's bring the search for truth back to other criteria, which we can talk about.

One of them is that gut feeling; intuition. Before Descartes, what did we have? We had Christianity. In Christianity, truth was understood as a belief in a certain set of moral teachings as codified in very specific books. That was the truth: it's there, it's written out, it has to do with morality. And what has that been replaced with? It has been replaced with the belief that truth is science.

Something went missing. We lost something along the way. What is it? It's morality. You see what happened? Where is the morality inherent in science? There is none, as such. So, in this passing from the belief in Christianity to the belief in science, we've done away with morality. I don't think that was accidental.

We are holding onto these beliefs of control. Eugenics for example, was born with scientific so-called progress, this belief that there are human beings who are biologically superior and therefore we can dispense with those who are inferior. The same thing with race. I know a lot of people try and argue that's not what he meant, but in the subtitle of Darwin's *The Origin of the Species*, he writes: the preservation of favoured races. He means it in a biological sense, but it's all there in a subliminal sense. It's all already there. It's setting the world up for eugenics, which is basically a form of control over other humans. That is what happens when you dispense with morality altogether.

I think we should consider that evidence was maybe the wrong place to put our hopes in truth. I produced a film called *The Book of Vision*, which is about modern medicine turning the human into an object, or a set of objects, which are the organs. It's almost as if what we did with evidence is this: we've objectified truth. So truth doesn't exist, except in an object, and the object is the evidence. That's what Descartes has done. In parallel, what we try to address in the film, *The Book of Vision*, is that *that* it is not where truth lives. It's not in objects as such, it's actually in certain practices that as humans, we do.

It becomes an active practice. It's actually something that we are doing now, by talking, or what we do when we go on some social media platform that allows it, which may be *Telegram*, maybe *twitter*, that incidentally now tends to allow quite a lot of free ranging discussion. We go there and we say something and we say it to others because that's what we are there for, and we say something, as a practice of searching for the truth. There are some technologies which allow for a form of truth searching, not necessarily truth arriving, but truth searching.

In Christianity truth searching was turned into monastic practices of stripping away superfluous things: asceticism. It's about stripping away the superfluous, looking within, and finding that moral core within a person to really tune into. Then you would become a purified being. That was very much directed toward the self because the external truth had already been decided in various books.

I'm not saying that this method of truth seeking is where we should go back to. I'm saying that this should be as important as anything that we see as science. The whole history of cultural, moral teachings as codified in religious books is just as important as anything we call science. One has not supplanted the other, one is not better than the other, as we've been told.

First, I would put them at the same level, *at least*. Let's practice these together so that we don't lapse into the same to and fro, where science became dominant because the codified books became too restrictive. Let's go even further back in philosophy and look at ancient Greece and the Socratic dialogues; the practice of speaking to each other and speaking truth. Truth-telling, or free speech, was a practice for this they had a word; *parresia*. That was quite fundamental for democracy. The person who speaks freely, they know they speak the truth. It's difficult for us to understand because we are so caught up in the Cartesian view that you need evidence, that we find it difficult to understand that at that time they had an idea of truth, and it was not linked to evidence. They would probably have laughed at you if you'd brought an object and said: "This is my evidence!"

We've turned this whole approach on its head. Back then you knew that you were speaking the truth because you really felt it, because what you spoke coincided with a moral, ethical self, within you, that wanted you to really *feel* for something so that you'd speak what you'd consider the truth. No one would doubt that that was what you thought the truth to be, and therefore, that was true. Speak your truth.

It's a bit like a poker game. You put all of your money on the table and you say, this is as much as I'm going to put in. In order to truly speak freely, you need to take a degree of risk. If there is no risk, there is no truth because then it is just common sense: no one needs to say it, right? So to define what the truth is, rather than going to a scientific article, you also need to think: what risks am I taking to say something that I feel to be true? What danger am I putting myself in? If it's none, you're probably not truth-telling. What you say may be true, but it's not truth-telling. It's not really helping anything or anyone.

In their form of democracy in Athens, there were different categories of people. Not everyone was a citizen. There were citizens, and then there were slaves. The main difference when it comes to truth-telling, and the reason why people didn't want to be exiled from Athens (one reason may be that you spoke too much truth), because if you were exiled to another city-state, you would not have the rights of citizenship, if you had them in Athens. If you had the right of citizenship in Athens, you were allowed to speak the truth. If you were a slave, you were not allowed to speak the truth. So this truth-telling was a definite sense that belonged to the democracy or proto-democracy that they had: that to be a citizen, you *had to* practice this truth-telling. If you lost citizenship, you couldn't do it anymore.

If we cast our eye over what has happened recently, you realise that everyone who is afraid of speaking the truth, is afraid because they don't want to take the risk, that risk that has been there since classical times. There are records in the classical literature of people acknowledging the risk they were taking. There are stories of Socrates being poisoned for too much truth, so we know it was real. If we the people don't do that today, we are voluntarily putting ourselves in the role of a slave in Athens, in that proto-democracy.

I know a lot of people who do that. We are in a situation in which a lot of people have become so scared of risk. So scared of danger. Where did that come from? Why are people so afraid? Money? Or is it materialism? Or being ostracised by the community? Once you strip out morality and you say that science is everything, you relinquish what people think is truth, to science. Our contemporaries say, "People like you and I should *just be quiet and stay in our lane*: let the scientists do the talking, as we have no way to know what the truth is. So we should just be quiet." But No! What I'm saying is that it's the opposite: if we want to participate in any form of democratic system, what we have to remember is that truth-telling, in classical Greece, was considered a duty. If you didn't do that, the city itself would deteriorate and become so overwhelmed with lies, it would look like the world in 2023: they knew it would lead to this.

It's clear as day in classical literature, this notion that truth-telling as an act is necessary for democracy. That risk and danger, including the risk of death, are inevitable risks. We all need to take the risk of truth-telling, for the sake of the city so that it does not rot under a veil of lies, which is where we find ourselves now in 2023.

We should seek this truth in a sense of morality, which may be aligned with certain religious books that remind us of where morality lies. We can be informed by those, but ultimately we find it also within ourselves. We have a sense of when we should speak out. Sometimes we do it knowing that we are putting ourselves at huge risk.

I remember how it felt in 2021. The pharmaceuticals were being rolled out and anyone who was suspicious was "against the science." In that climate, I remember so clearly that there was a sense that you were taking a risk in truth-telling. Then by way of confirmation, you'd get removed from social media. Next came endless negative articles, without apparent end. Back to Descartes and the evidence of truth. It's not in the scientific proof, it's in that element of risk.

A good way to sniff out the truth is to ask if the people voicing it have ever been cancelled from anywhere? If they were, there was an attempt to truth-tell. Do bots come up on their social media posts that are clearly artificial , that insult and try to steer the narrative elsewhere? Well, that means they're taking some kind of risk and that means that there is a chance they may be exercising this form of truth-telling. If we can *all* somehow get back to wanting to take risks, accepting the dangers, *not just a couple of us, but all of us,* I think the situation would improve dramatically.

If we stop saying, "where's your evidence?" and instead searched for sincerity, we might be closer to truth. I share a Telegram channel with Dr. Mike Yeadon and what interested me about him first, wasn't that I looked at his scientific resumé and thought, "Oh, he's done this drug, and therefore, of course that means that he knows what he was talking about." I just listened to him and I thought: "This guy sounds sincere to me."

I don't necessarily have to agree with him on everything, and I still don't agree with him on everything. He knows that, we both know that. But when he talks, I think this: he is being sincere. He truly believes what he says. He's speaking the truth, not because of his PhD. He's speaking the truth because he's a courageous person who is willing to say what he believes. You can hear it in the way he says it. So that for me is truth, not the scientific version of it.

We must try to counteract this belief in science as truth. I don't think science is going to die or disappear. I think as a practice we will keep on using it. But I think we just need to be a little bit less gullible about it, to understand that just because something wears the cloak of science, it doesn't mean it's true. I'm saying we should just look at science like everything else that humans do: some of it is good, some of it is bad.

On average, it's probably bad (as Ioannidis himself has proved).

Chapter 37

Blueprint for The Covid Psychological Operation

Jason Christoff

Researcher in behavior modification
& psychological manipulation

Jason Christoff is a Canadian health advocate, educator, and researcher in behavioral psychology, widely recognized for his outspoken stance on medical freedom and his insights into the psychological impact of media on public perception. With a research background in health sciences and psychology, Christoff has spent years studying how societal behaviors are influenced by media and authority, particularly during times of crisis.

During the COVID-19 pandemic, Christoff emerged as a prominent voice in global health debates, speaking at COVID hearings and conferences around the world, including influential platforms such as the Romanian Palace of Parliament. His focus on exposing the effects of media mind control and the manipulation of public behavior has resonated with those concerned about governmental overreach and the suppression of alternative perspectives on health and freedom.

Christoff's work highlights the importance of critical thinking and individual autonomy in the face of widespread propaganda. Through his speeches, writings, and public appearances, he continues to advocate for personal responsibility, informed decision-making, and a greater understanding of the psychological techniques used to influence society.

Here are several important questions; was the government's global response to COVID based on clinical virology or behavioural psychology? Does the media have the power to make our decisions for us through the use of psychological group pressure tactics? Did our fear of the crowd force us to make illogical decisions which weren't in the best interest of ourselves, our loved ones or our communities? Was the public exposed to group pressure and psychological manipulation tactics during the COVID operation?

The Asch experiment is a good way to demonstrate very clearly the power of group pressure to modify human behavior. It's one of psychology's oldest and most popular pieces of research. A volunteer is told that he's taking part in a visual perception test. What he doesn't know is that the other participants are actors, and he's the only person taking part in the real test, which is actually about group conformity. There are four lines on a white board. One, to the left, three to the right, of differing lengths. The participants are asked to choose which line on the right is the same length as the one on the left. The correct answer for the first test is two. The participant answers two, the actors all answer one. The second time around, the correct answer is two, the actors answer three, and so does the participant.

The experiment has been repeated many times and the results have been supported again and again. Mostly, we will conform to the group. We're very social creatures. We're very much aware of what the people around us think. We want to be liked. We don't want to be seen to rock the boat. So we will go along with the group. Even if we don't believe what people are saying, we'll still go along. Group dynamics are one of the most powerful forces in human psychology.

The results of the Asch conformity experiment were shocking. Over fifty percent of participants conformed to fabricated group pressure and gave the wrong answer, with the majority knowing that the answer was wrong. Secret answers given on paper to the instructor reduced group conformity to only 12 percent. So if your answer was secret, you would be less likely to conform to the group pressure. Only 25 percent of people stood up to the fabricated group pressure to give the right and truthful answer. In psychology, we call them fully functional adults. The people who conformed to group pressure and gave the wrong answer, were basically low status, high need for approval types. Most were also from cultures that honored obedience to authority. Most were people who defined their self-worth by what others thought of them. In clinical psychology, there are people who are weak, mentally known as the forever child, people who have somehow bypassed their proper rite of passage from child to adult. These people are the most conformist in a society of adults who act, talk and think like children.

There are also other factors that increase group conformity. The more psychological fear a person is in, the more they conform to group pressure. Based on fear based changes in brain function, the more chemical fear a person is in - caffeine, alcohol, junk food - the more they conform to group pressure because it's the same changes in brain function. Your body is afraid of poison, and this is why the bottle shops, the weed shops in Canada, the fast food restaurants and the corner stores were open during the health crisis. Fear shuts down critical thinking and increases conformist behavior, irrational and illogical behavior as well. And has anybody seen any members of the public exhibiting irrational and illogical behavior from 2020 forward? Obviously the answer would be yes.

Dr. Joost Meerloo, author of the books *Rape of the Mind* and *Psychology of Thought Control,* recounted that keeping a victim confused is the best way to achieve psychological control and manipulation. Dr. Meerloo also showed us that as with the training of any animal, it's best to train the human animal in isolation away from the others. It's similar to training horses, similar to training dogs; you get them away from the others. Meerloo further explained, after studying Korean War POWs, that mind controlling a person was best served with periods of intense attack and fear, broken up by periods of peace and favorable treatment, again to confuse and control the victim. Edward Bernays, author of the books *Propaganda* and *Crystalizing Public Opinion,* explained that the crowd wasn't even needed physically to build the group pressure that changed the victim's mind. Sitting in a room alone with your TV during the 14 days to "flatten the curve," only perceiving the power of an imaginary group on the TV screen, can indeed bring about conformity to that imaginary group.

Stockholm Syndrome was a phrase coined by psychiatrist Nils Bergerat after a five day bank robbery standoff in Stockholm, Sweden. Under the immense trauma, fear and stress, many bank tellers taken hostage became sympathetic to their captors and even romantically involved after the heist was over.

Demonstrations of immense public power can trigger a survival response of trauma, bonding with the abusers and endorsing the abuser for fear of reprisal. And we saw many people do that in 2020. They sided with the government not because the government was making sense, but because the government was a bully.

In the Milgram experiment, we see the power of the white coat. Just over 50 percent of research subjects would follow orders to kill or injure another human being, if the order came from someone of authority, someone with a title, and someone in a lab coat. In the case of COVID we had Dr. Anthony Fauci. He is someone of authority, someone with a title, and someone in a lab coat, and he is telling people what to be afraid of. And he was also telling people how to relieve the fear. Back to the Milgram experiments; people were manipulated to potentially hurt and kill others. In the COVID experiment, it appears people were manipulated to injure and kill themselves. This is a weaponization of psychology against the public.

Was psychology used against the public during COVID? Organizations like the UK›s SAGE, standing for the Safety Advisory Group for Emergencies and the international Behavioral Insights team, admitted openly to using nudge style psychological manipulation on the public during COVID in order to achieve their desired outcomes.

These outcomes appeared one-sided and they appeared so because they treated us like animals. We were isolated, and trained effectively in that isolation, as Dr. Joost Meerloo described. Fear was up-regulated into the stratosphere in order to lower IQ and increase conformist behaviors inside the limbic system, via the fear response. When the human animals - in other words, us - were getting trained in COVID isolation by our instructor - the TV set - the opinion of the perceived crowd was repetitively imprinted into us by the media, leading to behavior and belief altering group compliance, as Asch had documented, without the group being physically present.

As Bernays has explained, the public was kept in perpetual states of confusion with contradictory messages. Gyms had to close during the health crisis, but bottle shops were open. We were told initially that masks weren't necessary. Then one was necessary, then two, then no masks, then masks back on for everybody. Then suddenly, magically, masks did not matter. The virus attacked at 10:01 pm, but not at 9:59pm in places where there was curfew, because we know the virus carried a stopwatch everywhere it went. The virus also attacked when you were standing at a restaurant, but not when you were sitting, because the virus also carried a tape measure. Confusion is the foundation of all mind control, according to Dr. Meerloo.

Then came the public exposure of people's vaccine status, with the work mandates triggering Asch's 50 percent or more compliance to group pressure compared to the 12 percent compliance level if our decisions are kept private. They outed our vaccine status to get four to five times more vaccine uptake. This, again, is a weaponization of the known psychological research. The cycling of terror, followed by more normal periods of peace and favorable treatment, were relentless, which kept the human psyche in a permanent state of instability, optimal for controlling the masses. Businesses were open, businesses were closed; you had to wear a mask, you could take off your mask. It was all very confusing, and it worked exactly as designed.

Were the police told by governments to be as heavy handed as possible in order to induce Stockholm Syndrome trauma bonding with authority? Were they told to do this to instill fear around a COVID narrative so obviously made of pure wind? The question remains, was the government's response to COVID based on clinical virology or behavioural psychology?

The public is generally aware that crimes have been committed. Morality, ethics and justice must be reinvigorated in all levels of our society from the ground up. Charges must be laid, criminal investigations initiated and criminal conspirators punished to the highest order. Never again shall such blatant psychological manipulation be used by governments against their own citizens.

God and good always win.

Help Us Spread the Word

If this book has resonated with you, we encourage you to share your thoughts by leaving a review on Amazon. Your feedback not only supports our work but also helps others find the book. Every review matters, and it plays a key role in reaching a wider audience. Thank you for being part of this journey!

www.ingramcontent.com/pod-product-compliance
Lightning Source LLC
Chambersburg PA
CBHW061230220326
41599CB00028B/5382